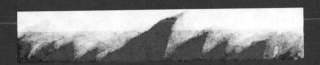

Praise for
The owner's manual for the brain

"In business today, we either change or die. To cope with change, we need a mind open to new ideas. *The Owner's Manual for the Brain* is for people who understand this: people who never stop learning, who want to improve themselves, who need to understand what motivates others."

Ed Crutchfield
Chairman and CEO
First Union Corporation

"It helps introduce us to ourselves. Drawing upon the latest research on our own mental processes, Dr. Howard presents practical applications to help us to develop our own potential as well as the potential of those with whom we live and work."

Stephen M. Stevick
Executive Director
The Sierra Club Foundation

"A *Poor Richard's Almanac* of mind-brain research. Will be valuable for anyone with intellectual curiosity."

John Kello, Ph.D.
Professor of Psychology
Davidson College

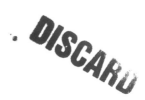

"An outstanding and very user-friendly resource packed with up-to-the-minute information. Whether you're a professional who needs easily accessible, current research on how we use our brains or an intellectually curious person who wants to browse, there's something here for everyone."

Janice M. Gamache, Ed.D.
Consulting Partner
Drake Beam Morin

"A wonderful job of taking an opaque, arcane, and obscure literature and translating it into understandable, tantalizing, highly usable, helpful information."

Ron Zemke
Coauthor of the *Knock Your Socks Off Service* books

"Full of knowledge that is useful to me as an educator and as a businessman."

Dick Richardson
Training Manager
IBM Information Products Division

"Makes the hard-to-understand brain research accessible—with appropriate humor—for the average person."

Jill S. Flynn
Senior Vice President
First Union National Bank

"To upgrade your old, slow, low-capacity computer with bigabytes of memory and a more agile and reliable processor, with room for all the latest software programs and utilities, just read *The Owner's Manual for the Brain* and practice its recommended applications."

James G. Martin, Ph.D.
Former Governor of North Carolina

"The successor to Maxwell Maltz! *The Owner's Manual for the Brain* can be a key to unlocking the rich and exciting potential of your mind."

Ty Boyd
Motivational Speaker

"Finally, a book about brain research that human resource professionals can understand and use!"

Sara Cohen
Human Resources Representative
Glaxo, Inc.

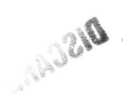

"A painless and fascinating way for everyone to understand the latest in brain research. But more important, *The Owner's Manual for the Brain* is a valuable resource for all of us who, as organizational change professionals, create change through people."

Joanne C. Preston, Ph.D.
Professor of Organization Development
Pepperdine University
Editor of the *Organization Development Journal*

"A quick and easy way for busy professionals to get caught up on the many fronts of brain research."

Richard M. Furr, Ph.D.
Licensed Industrial/Organizational Psychologist

"Combines and interprets research on the brain and its functioning in a very understandable fashion even for the lay reader—a very difficult task pulled off amazingly well. It will be a useful tool for people in many professions and frames of reference."

"A must-read for every manager, trainer, and person curious about the final frontier! An invaluable tool—full of practical features, insightful uses, and surprising benefits."

"Really enjoyed it! Makes the current research findings easy to understand and apply."

"Highly recommended for those who want to keep abreast of a significant learning curve. It puts the reader in touch with the flood of research on the brain and helps to distinguish promise from delivery in the cognitive sciences."

"A scientifically sound, well-written, and entertaining review of the many central nervous system influences that affect the way we feel and function. As a practicing physician, I believe that this book will provide my patients with extremely useful information that will help them lead happier and more productive lives."

The owner's manual for the brain:

Everyday applications from mind-brain research

Pierce J. Howard, Ph.D.

Leornian Press

A BARD PRODUCTIONS BOOK

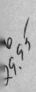

ISBN 0-9636389-0-4 *paperback*
ISBN 0-9636389-1-2 *hardcover*

The author may be contacted through:
    CentACS *Center for Applied Cognitive Studies*
    719 Romany Road
    Charlotte, North Carolina 28203
    704-331-0926 *(phone)*   704-331-9408 *(fax)*   centacs@fx.net *(E-mail)*

A BARD PRODUCTIONS BOOK
    Austin, Texas
Copyediting and proofreading: Helen Hyams
Index: Linda Webster
Illustrations: Kim Allman

Table of contents

Part five: **Creating new mental paths:**
Memory, creativity, and problem solving

Quick content guide

While everyone will find each chapter in this book relevant to his or her life in some way, those who fill special roles may find certain chapters of particular interest. The first eight chapters deal with subjects like sleep and diet that affect everybody every day; therefore, we suggest that all readers, regardless of their roles, would benefit from the materials in these chapters.

Below are listed several role categories and the additional chapters that may be of special interest to them.

Role:	Chapters:
Teachers, trainers, and coaches	9–10, 12–15, 18–26
Managers	9–10, 12–17, 19, 21–26
Students	12–23
Mental health professionals	All
Salespeople	9–10, 13–15, 19, 23
Doctors, lawyers, and others in professional practice	9, 16–17, 19, 23–26
Human resource professionals	All
Parents	All
Religious professionals	9–15, 18–20, 24–26
Negotiators	10–12, 23, 24–26
Research and development professionals	12–17, 21–23

Preface

Why this book? Tomes about the mind and brain pepper the shelves of airport kiosks and bookstores from Phoenix to Philly. This is the fourth year of the Decade of the Brain, but that is insufficient reason for yet another book, just as, for example, World Series time alone is not sufficient reason for another book on baseball.

The available books about the brain can be divided into two categories: research reports and practical applications. Neurobiology texts belong in the first category, and how-to books (*How to Increase Your Memory, How to Be More Creative*) belong in the second. This book serves to create an explicit overlap between these two categories. Research books generally decline to identify the everyday applicability of their findings—indeed, that is not their purpose. Practical books generally omit making the explicit connection between a piece of advice and its basis in research. The intention of this book is to yoke the two together as a team, by saying, "Here's what we know about memory storage in the brain, and here's how that knowledge can help us improve our recall of information."

Why me? I'm not an academic who must publish or perish, and I'm not a natural writer possessed with an irresistible urge to put pen to paper (or, more aptly, fingertips to keyboard). In fact, I'm a very extraverted guy for whom writing is the ultimate act of self-discipline—it doesn't come easy. Reading has traditionally been my introverted activity of choice. So why did I write this book? A story will explain.

All my life I had viewed myself as a dilettante. That changed in the spring of 1988, when I read Morton Hunt's *The Universe Within*. Hunt, a science popularizer, introduced the English-reading world to cognitive science—the interdisciplinary approach to understanding the workings of the mind-brain. Each chapter of his book summarized research in an area that had been of interest to me: problem solving, creativity, learning theory, and so on. Voilà! I was no longer a dilettante; I had a focus. I began to read everything I could find dealing with this new field (which is described in Chapter One), and I found that the extensive scientific literature on brain research provided me with a basis for my applied interests.

In December 1988, I began serving a term on the program committee of the local chapter of the American Society for Training and Development (ASTD). The committee asked for program suggestions for monthly meetings in 1989, so I suggested that we bring in a speaker on the subject of cognitive science. After hearing my justification, they agreed that the chapter would benefit from such a program and asked me to find a speaker. I was able to find speakers who were expensive and practical in their approach, or speakers who were inexpensive and theoretical in their approach, but I had to report that I was unable to find anyone we could afford who was willing to present an application-oriented program to our group. I argued, and they agreed, that the more theoretical speakers would

> "There are two ways of spreading light: to be
> The candle or the mirror that reflects it."
>
> **Edith Wharton**

be hooted out of the hall. As a result, they asked, "Pierce, why don't you do a program?" I agreed.

I presented the program—"Brain Update"—in August 1989. After an encouraging reception, I presented the program in two other cities and then at the regional meeting in Gatlinburg, Tennessee, in the fall of 1990. After each of the four presentations, people came up to me and asked, "What have you written? Your content is fascinating, but we'd like something written to consider in more depth." Responding to this encouragement as evidence of a genuine need, my wife and partner, Jane, and I decided that I should cut back on my consulting duties and write a book. That was in August 1991. For the next year I wrote and read to fill in the gaps. As I write this preface, I find myself closing in on fulfilling my commitment to provide you with written documentation of what I enjoy doing so well from the front of the classroom.

How is this book unique? First, it stands with one foot in the research camp and the other in practice. Second, it reflects my twenty-plus years' experience as a management consultant. (I cannot apologize for the fact that this book is limited to the part of the world with which I am familiar.) Third, I have included only brain research findings that have widespread practical applications. Findings that are interesting but not generally useful have not been included. Fourth, for the most part, the structure is aimed at those using the research, not the researchers themselves.

The basic structure of the book employs what I like to refer to as the "So what?" format. The typical response to reported research findings is "So what?" For example, research shows that the level of the hormone melatonin is directly related to the quality of our sleep. You may say, "So what?" Well, this book is designed with that question in mind. Every piece of research reported is followed by one or more specific suggestions for its application. Here is an example of what you will find.

Topic 7.4 Melatonin and sleep

Research findings indicate that levels of the hormone melatonin in the body are directly related to the quality of our sleep. The higher our melatonin level, the better we sleep. The production of melatonin is triggered by consuming dairy products and is suppressed upon exposure to light.

Applications

1   Have milk, cheese and crackers, ice cream, or yogurt before sleeping. Better yet, have warm milk—it metabolizes more quickly.

2   Make sure your sleeping area is completely dark—for example, use a mask or install opaque, overwide shades.

The book is organized around these Topics (except for Chapters One, Two, and Twenty-Seven). The numerical identifier refers to the chapter number and the sequence within that chapter. While most of the application ideas are mine, several of my readers have suggested additional ideas. I have indicated their authorship following the suggestion. I look forward to including suggestions from other readers in subsequent editions of this book.

In its most general sense, this book is for people who want to use their heads. More specifically, it is for lifelong learners, professionals who value keeping up and/or ahead of the game, people developers, human resource professionals, leaders, consultants (internal and external), supervisors of teachers, training managers, teacher educators, adult education professionals, train-the-trainer professionals, curriculum writers, curriculum designers, industrial and organizational psychologists, writers, and research-and-development professionals. I could summarize this list by reducing it to five types of readers: lifelong learners, educators, consultants, managers, and psychologists. Readers will gain insights into improving their personal effectiveness without having to wade through the tedium of academic detail (I've done that for them) or the fluff of wordy popularizers (I've cut away the padding).

This book is not:

- A biology or medical text
- A psychology text
- An in-depth treatment of specific research findings
- A collection of esoteric findings that are interesting but not useful
- An in-depth treatment of general subjects (I only report the brain research findings that are relevant to the subject)
- A reference work for research scientists

This book is:

- Application-oriented
- A reflection of my experiences as a management consultant
- Composed of findings that have practical applications
- A reference work for consumers
- Centered on the *what* and the *why*—what brain research suggests we could do for personal improvement and why we should do it

This book is designed to be something of an encyclopedia or resource book of application ideas. I suspect that a few people will read it from cover to cover, with most preferring to browse according to which sections are of the most current interest to them. Where the understanding of a chapter or Topic is particularly dependent on material covered elsewhere in the book, I have attempted to indicate that fact. In order to group the chapters for the convenience of most readers, I have divided the book into six parts.

Part One serves as an introduction to the field of cognitive science; Chapter One provides an overview both of the field of cognitive science and of the book itself and Chapter Two reviews some of the basics of brain functions. If you have a strong or recent background in cognitive science, you may choose to skim or skip these first two chapters. Part Two will prove to be of the greatest interest for most people, covering findings related to gender, aging, diet, drugs, sleep, handedness, exercise, and disease. Part Three focuses on aspects of personality—traits, emotions, and intelligence—and how they should be viewed in light of current research on the nature-nurture controversy. This section will be of particular interest if you are interested in personnel selection, parenting, or similarities and differences in personal styles at work and at home. Part Four deals with motivation and workplace design and should be of particular interest if you are a people manager. Part Five is designed for the teacher in us all; it discusses how we learn and remember, facilitate learning, and maximize our creativity and problem-solving ability. The topic of Part Six—epistemology—may at first glance seem somewhat esoteric. However, epistemology is the ultimate domain of brain science. It is through appreciating the structure of knowledge that we develop peace in relationships, both in our homes and among nations. This final section should be of particular interest to those in peacemaking roles, such as ministers, diplomats, and negotiators.

I've chosen to exclude several subjects that could have been covered: artificial intelligence (because it seems to be confined to a more specialized audience than this book is intended for), chaos theory (because I'm not sure yet how to treat its general applicability), and hypnotism (because the research ranges from rejecting it altogether as a legitimate state of consciousness to at best acknowledging it as an alternative relaxation technique). Perhaps there will be more extensive treatment of these subjects in subsequent editions.

My main purpose in writing this book is to help you discover ways to improve. By giving specific suggestions along with their research justifications, I hope to tweak your interest in opportunities for personal improvement. Because the scope is so inclusive, some of you may be frustrated by finding insufficient information on these pages to enable you to immediately implement an idea. To solve this problem, I would like to suggest several possible resources that could be helpful in leading you to further information or skill mastery:

- Talk with your public library's reference staff.
- Consult the continuing education department of a school of higher education near you.
- Consult officers in your local chapters of the ASTD or the National Society for Performance and Instruction (directories are available in your library).
- Write the authors of books mentioned in a specific Topic.
- Read the materials listed at the end of each chapter and in the Bibliography that relate to ideas in which you are interested.

If, in your search to improve your skills, you seek out workshops on a particular subject mentioned in this book, be sure to evaluate the content of the workshop before attending. For example, don't just go to a "motivation" workshop. Find out whose theories or work the session is based on. Many workshops today use outmoded information. But that's the subject for another book.

I acknowledge debts to many in writing this book. To my readers, who've provided helpful suggestions and criticism: Rick Bradley, Sara Cohen, Lynne Ford, Dr. Richard Furr, Dr. Janice Gamache, Dr. John Kello, Dr. Greg Lanier, Laura Lenhardt, Dillon Robertson, and Jack Wilson. To the readers whom my publisher recruited: Montgomery Scott Bard, Sandra Hirsh, Dr. Gary John, Dr. Ann McGee-Cooper, Dr. Luis Picard-Ami, John Shamley, and Dr. Claire Ellen Weinstein. To members of the University of North Carolina at Charlotte Cognitive Science Academy: Dr. Paul Foos, Dr. Paula Goolkasian, Dr. Mirsad Hadzikadic, Dr. Haas Raval, Dr. Larry Upton, and Dr. Laurie van Wallendael. To Dr. Chip Bell, who has encouraged me to write and who introduced me to Ray Bard. To Kim Allman, my illustrator, for his wide-eyed enthusiasm. To Ray Bard, my publisher, for his wise counsel and constant support. To Helen Hyams, my editor, for her insight and unflagging attention to detail. To my daughters, Allegra and Hilary, whose excitement in the process fueled me to return to the keyboard. And to Jane, my wife and partner, for bearing the brunt of the financial and emotional cost associated with writing a first book—to her I dedicate this work.

The author

Pierce J. Howard is director of the Center for Applied Cognitive Studies (CentACS), a consulting firm headquartered in Charlotte, North Carolina. His wife, Jane, is director of programs at CentACS. Together, they develop both public and organizational programs based on the most current research in cognitive science. These programs include workshops, breakfast seminars, speeches, retreats, custom-designed programs, and a quarterly newsletter, *Brain Update*.

In addition, for the last twenty years, Dr. Howard has been an organization development consultant. His motivation and, hence, his own professional development stem from a deep-seated desire to help others learn how to overcome their obstacles. He has attended numerous workshops and professional meetings, read extensively in the field, conducted computer data base searches, and created hundreds of workshop designs in an unrelenting effort to find the best ways to help people to solve problems, make decisions, create new approaches, and understand themselves and others—in effect, to take responsibility for their own growth and development both as individuals and as members of teams and organizations. Dr. Howard's skill and interest in debunking myths and in finding the most effective ways to help others learn has served him well in the business community.

Dr. Howard grew up in Kinston, North Carolina. He received his B.A. degree in 1963 from Davidson College and his M.A. degree in 1967 from East Carolina

University, both in English. In 1972, he received his Ph.D. degree in education with a special interest in curriculum and research from the University of North Carolina at Chapel Hill. His college years were interrupted by a three-year tour with the U.S. Army in Germany, where he served as an intelligence specialist.

His professional affiliations include the Cognitive Science Society, the American Psychological Association, the North Carolina Psychological Association, the Mecklenburg Psychological Association, the American Society for Training and Development, and the Southeast Organization Development Interest Group. He has written and published numerous workbooks, tests, and other materials for clients. For relaxation, he and Jane enjoy walking, cooking, chamber music, choral singing, reading, and camping.

The author

Part one

Catching up on how the brain works:

The latest news
from cognitive science

Catching up on how the brain works:

The latest news from cognitive science

1

Getting started: A framework for

World War II started something. The pain and tragedy of head injuries catapulted brain research into the foreground of scientific and pseudoscientific investigation. From the popular claims of split-brain research to the profound findings of neurotransmitter studies, discoveries by increasing numbers of researchers and readers have focused on learning how the brain works.

This explosion of research has given birth to a new field of knowledge: cognitive science, also known as brain science. One feature that makes this field unique is that it is interdisciplinary—it is made up of more than one traditional field of study. The research has been conducted by investigators from six broad fields, although some subdivisions of these fields are more germane to cognitive science than others; for example, psychopharmacology is more germane than social psychology. The fields are:

1 Neurobiology   4 Philosophy
2 Psychology   5 Anthropology
3 Information science   6 Linguistics

Prior to World War II, communication among scholars in these fields was minimal. But the momentum increased noticeably soon after the war ended. Most people seem to date the beginning of cognitive science as a formal interdisciplinary field of study from September 1948 (Gardner, 1985), when scientists

exploring mind-brain concepts

assembled at the Hixon Symposium at the California Institute of Technology, which was titled "Cerebral Mechanisms of Behavior." Presenters included John von Neumann and Karl Lashley, representing mathematics and psychology. Many regard this meeting as the sounding of the death knell for the behaviorism of B. F. Skinner, Ivan Petrovich Pavlov, Edward Lee Thorndike, and John B. Watson, which had held sway until then. No more would strict stimulus-response explanations of human behavior be ascendant. With the rise of cognitive science came the doctrine that human behavior was more than conditioned responses, that the human mind was indeed able to create, to choose, to reflect—in short, to explore the universe between stimulus and response. Stephen Covey (1990, p. 69) suggests that between stimulus and response, man has the freedom to choose. Or, as Richard Restak (1991, p. 50) observes, we are moving from Socrates' "know thyself" to Kierkegaard's "choose thyself."

Emerging from over thirty years in the relative obscurity of academia, cognitive science had its coming-out with the publication in 1982 of Morton Hunt's *The Universe Within: A New Science Explores the Human Mind.* His highly readable volume introduced many to this new field. Drawing from examples in areas such as problem solving, creativity, decision science, epistemology, moral development, personality theory, artificial intelligence, logic, linguistics, learning theory, and memory, he showed how cognitive science has brought together previously

> "Few minds wear out;
> more rust out."
>
> **Christian Nestell Bovee**

isolated fields into one common alliance committed to describing how the mind works. He related how this alliance of scholars is collaborating to describe the mind's functioning from both the detailed, microscopic, bottom-up perspective, as in cellular neurobiology, and the big-picture, global, top-down perspective, as in discussions of primary personality traits. The excitement of this multipronged scientific movement lies in the moment when the bottom-up, or *molecular,* studies become recognized as equivalent to the top-down, or *molar,* studies.

An example of such a "meeting at the middle" can be found in Hans Eysenck's *The Biological Basis of Personality* (1967), in which he begins to establish the relationship between the reticular activating system (RAS) in the brain (a molecular structure) and the personality traits of extroversion and neuroticism (molar behaviors). Paul MacLean (1990) describes the bottom-up perspective as "objective" and the top-down approach as "subjective." The point where they meet defines the discipline of *epistemology* (see Part Six). For an excellent and timely discussion of this molecular-molar relationship, see Cacioppo and Berntson (1992).

The mind-brain dichotomy

As we slip into the content proper of this book, you will notice that the terms *brain* and *mind* are used interchangeably. IBMer E. Baird Smith has a comedy routine in which he asks, "Is your mind a part of your brain, or is your brain all in your mind?" In the nineteenth century, English scholar Thomas Hewitt Key played with this semantic difficulty by asking, "What is mind? No matter. What is matter? Never mind." This semantic puzzle needs attention! Dealing with the historical debate between mind and brain is beyond the purpose of this book. Understandable treatments are available in Gardner (1985) and Hunt (1982). In the seventeenth century, René Descartes argued for *dualism,* with "mind" a kind of software and "brain" a kind of hardware; he apparently developed this idea as a result of a rift with the church authorities, who allowed him to continue his work as long as he stuck to the body and let the church take care of the mind and spirit. Later, behaviorists like Skinner argued for *monism* (nothing exists other than cells), whereas current thinking argues for an interactionist approach. This approach describes the intimate, sensitive way in which mind (ideas and images) and body (cells, chemicals, and electricity) directly and immediately influence each other. As a simple example, we know that a joyful disposition (mind and spirit) can increase the number of "helper cells" in the immune system (brain and body), and that, conversely, a reduction in the number of helper cells can dampen a joyful disposition. We also know that using our memory and skills tends to preserve nerve cells ("use it or lose it") and that, conversely, losing nerve cells over time interferes with memory and skills.

Catching up on how the brain works

To say "use your mind" or "use your brain" is to say the same thing. It is like saying "use your computer" versus "use your word-processing program." The features of one influence the features of the other. Ira Black (1991, p. 8) argues that our mental software and hardware are one and the same when he speaks of "the essential unity of structure and function." When the computer is turned off, the word-processing program cannot function. Yet just because the computer is turned on, that doesn't mean the program is being used, or being used to capacity. When the brain is dead, the mind cannot function. Yet just because the brain is alive, that doesn't mean the mind is being used, or being used to capacity. In a sense, then, the best definition of mind is that it is the state that occurs when the brain is alive and at work. Richard M. Restak, who wrote the books and television series *The Mind* (1988) and *The Brain* (1984), despaired of a crisp, clear definition that could distinguish between the two, concluding, "Mind is the astounding interplay of one hundred billion neurons. And more" (1988, p. 31). J. A. Hobson (1988, p. 230), in *The Dreaming Brain,* writes, "I believe that when we have truly adequate descriptions of brain and mind, dualism and all of its dilemmas will disappear. We will speak of the brain-mind as a unity, or invent some new word to describe it." To talk of the brain is to refer to the more molecular aspects of a phenomenon, while to talk of the mind is to refer to the more molar aspects. *Cognitive* and *cognition* are our only words that refer to both brain and mind, and the public finds them smacking of the ivory tower. We do need a new word that the public will accept—perhaps something like *processor* or *reactor, main* or *brind*. Send me your suggestions, and I will publish them in my newsletter, *Brain Update*. (Information on ordering the newsletter is given in the back of the book.)

> "I believe that when we have truly adequate descriptions of brain and mind, dualism and all of its dilemmas will disappear."
> **J.A. Hobson**

Human or animal—what's the difference?

Humorists, philosophers, scientists, theologians—all have made stabs at defining the difference between humans and animals. Consider:

> "No animal admires another animal." **Blaise Pascal**

> "Man is the only animal that blushes. Or needs to." **Mark Twain**

> "The desire to take medicine is perhaps the greatest feature which distinguishes man from animals." **Sir William Osler**

The parade of quotes could quickly become tiring. I will, however, summarize both the popular and scientific efforts to describe this difference by one top-down and one bottom-up observation. The top-down observation: that

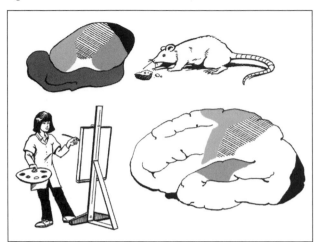

Cortical commitment.

A comparison of committed (shaded) and uncommitted (unshaded) regions of the cerebral cortex in (top) rat and (bottom) human.

Figure 1.1

humans can introvert, while animals can't. The bottom-up observation: that humans have a proportionately greater area of uncommitted cerebral cortex, or cortex in which unused synapses are available to be committed to new learning (see Figure 1.1). The cerebral cortex (see Chapter Two for further discussion) is the part of the brain that houses the rational functions—for example, problem solving, planning, and creativity. The comparison between a rat's brain and a human brain is dramatic. All but a sliver of the rat's brain is "committed" to motor, auditory, somatosensory, olfactory, and visual functions—that is, survival activities. These committed, or dedicated, areas can't be used for any other function, such as memory or problem solving, in much the same way that a word-processing machine can't be used for other computing functions. In contrast, well over half of the human brain is uncommitted and thus available for forming new synapses in the service of creativity, problem solving, analysis, memory—in short, of civilization itself. In other words, we have a greater capacity for learning. (See the discussion of synapses in Chapter Two.)

What is the mind-brain?

Metaphors abound to explain the physical process that governs our behavior. Some explain it as a power plant, emphasizing the electrochemical ionic transfers that culminate in the nervous system's capacity to supply enough power to illuminate a twenty-five-watt light bulb. Others explain it as a computer, using the analogy of RAM and ROM and bits and bytes and memory and storage to describe the brain's capacity to store 2.8×10^{20} bits of information. Still others see the brain as a library that can store ten million 1,000-page books. And some see the brain as a minigovernment that administers a vast array of bodily functions, from breathing and blood flow to meditation and stock market analysis.

May I have the envelope, please? The winner is—all of these and more. The closer we get to understanding the structure and function of the mind-brain, the more anomalies slip through the cracks of our descriptions. Should our goal be to have complete understanding? Probably. Settling for a lesser goal may blind us to new insights: if we do not expect large gains in scientific progress, we are less likely to experience them. However, to the degree that we can humbly marvel in wonderment at the vast unexplained mystery of mind, brain, and behavior, we are more likely to live in peace with ourselves and our neighbors. With admitted imperfection of the self comes the humility necessary for developing satisfying relationships.

The core principles of cognitive science

In reflecting over the vast mind-brain literature, we see several patterns emerge. These patterns may best be described as the core principles of cognitive science—the concepts essential to making sense out of the thousands of pieces of research available to us. As an aid to browsing through this book, I will state here what I see as the core principles. We will revisit them in the final chapter, after having had a chance to see them at play in Chapters Two through Twenty-Six.

Nativism. The principle of nativism holds that we inherit our behavior, and that our environment can either nurture it to develop naturally or distort it by withholding nurturance (food, shelter, warmth, touch, affection, attention, etc.).

Unity. The principle of unity holds that the body and the mind are one and the same, and that a change in one results in a change in the other.

Connectivity. The principle of connectivity holds that the establishment of new connections between prior learnings is the essence of growth and development, and that the condition of the connection points, like the condition of the gap in a spark plug, determines how well we function.

Interconnectivity. The principle of interconnectivity holds that each identifiable element in our vast storehouse of experiences and learnings is connected to each of the other elements, some more strongly or closely and others more loosely or distantly (thus, to remember a name, we silently say the alphabet until the name pops out).

Control. The principle of control holds that the health of the human (and animal) organism is a function of the degree to which the individual feels in control of his or her situation, with less perceived control resulting in poorer health and performance and greater perceived control resulting in better health and performance.

The scientific method—a warning

Many of us tend to react to the reported results of scientific research as isolated fragments of absolute truth that identify predictable cause-and-effect relationships. The misery that can accompany such gullibility comes chiefly from two kinds of scientific report formats: the *correlation* and the *comparison of means.*

Correlation

Correlations are reported in statements such as "The more melatonin, the better you sleep" or "Melatonin is positively correlated with sleep" or "Melatonin and sleep are positively related" or "Melatonin and wakefulness are negatively related." We misunderstand these statements because they don't say that melatonin *causes* good sleep, just that good sleep is more common among persons who have more melatonin. The correlation doesn't say, and probably doesn't take into account, other influences that might disrupt this relationship—daylight; other hormones; body weight; recency of eating a big meal, drinking alcoholic or caffeinated beverages, or consuming artificial sweeteners; high stress levels; the subject's age; the source of the melatonin; the environment (lab, airplane, bedroom, hotel) where the sleep was measured; and so on. It also doesn't specify whether the quality of the sleep was self-reported or was measured by an objective observer. All we know is that, for some people, more melatonin means better sleep, but it may not be true for me or for you.

Recommendation. You must approach such conclusions with a cautious, experimental spirit. For example, try a warm cup of milk, which triggers melatonin production, before bedtime to see if you sleep better. If you don't, look for a possible influence that prevents the melatonin from "working," assuming that it really works. For example, don't drink alcohol close to bedtime.

Comparison of means

Comparisons of means are reported in statements such as "Males score higher on mathematics achievement tests, while females score higher on language achievement tests." We misunderstand this type of statement because it doesn't say how much higher each sex scores. The gender difference in math achievement scores is extremely small and is of little or no practical significance. The comparison also doesn't say which subtests are involved and whether the differences are true for all subtests. It doesn't say what time of day the tests were administered—some evidence suggests that males' lower testosterone levels in the afternoon influence their achievement and females' lower estrogen-progesterone levels during the seven to fourteen days following ovulation influence theirs. In fact, if half the females in the sample took the tests during the two weeks following ovulation, which is a reasonable assumption, this could more than account for their lowered scores. In addition, we do not know whether the differences hold for all possible cultural groups—socioeconomic, ethnic, educational, and international. And the comparison doesn't say whether the range of scores of one group was similar to that of the other group. One group might score somewhat higher but with a very narrow range of scores, while the second group might

Catching up on how the brain works

Why statistics may be misleading

A statement relating to the three boxes below might claim that one group scores higher than another. However, this statement does not, by itself, give you much information.

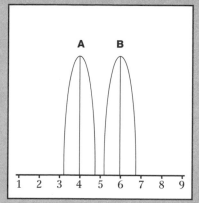 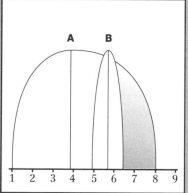 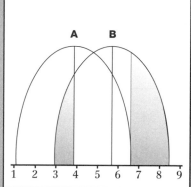

Why is this information incomplete?

- In all three examples, Group A scored an average of 4, while Group B scored an average of 6.
- In the left-hand box, however, *everyone* in Group B scored higher than anyone in Group A (this is very unusual).
- In the middle box, everyone in Group B outscored the average of Group A, but a substantial number in Group A outscored Group B altogether (shaded area).
- In the right-hand box, most of those in Group B outscored the average of Group A, but only a few outscored the highest scorers in Group A (right shaded area), and some scored below the average of Group A (left shaded area). Beware!

Why might a research finding not apply to you?

- Experiments conducted in clinics don't always apply to the everyday world.
- You may exhibit a particular feature that the research didn't account for, such as living in an unusual climate, having unusual dietary or exercise patterns, or being subject to environmental influences of which you may or may not be aware, such as gases or X rays.
- Your genetic code may render you resistant to the finding.
- You may be affected by medication you are taking, an illness you have or have had, or stress.
- Cultural differences may affect the findings.
- The statistics may be incompletely or misleadingly represented.
- The researchers may have made one of two basic errors:
  1. Saying that relationships or differences are present when in fact they are not.
  2. Saying that relationships or differences are absent when in fact they are present.

Figure 1.2

score somewhat lower but with a wide range of scores. In forming two basketball teams, for example, you would be more likely to pick a winning team from the latter group (lower average points scored but a wide range of scores) than from the former (higher average points scored but a narrow range of scores).

Recommendation. Realize that differences in average scores are differences in groups, not differences between individuals. Any individual may outscore or underscore members of another group, except in the rare circumstance in which the ranges of scores do not overlap. The value of knowing about group differences is that it explains variations on some basis other than personal deficiency. For example, males tend to have better day vision, females better night vision, and this difference, where it is true, tends to increase with age. Here's how it applies to me: I typically do the laundry chores in our home, but if I do laundry in the evening, Jane sorts the socks. Acknowledging that this difference applies to us keeps her from accusing me of shirking!

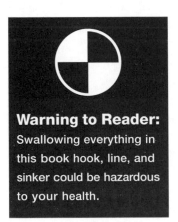

Warning to Reader: Swallowing everything in this book hook, line, and sinker could be hazardous to your health.

The Caveat Box

As a way of reminding you of the pitfalls of inappropriate reactions to scientific research results throughout this book, I have come up with the Caveat Box.

This message will appear throughout as a reminder to take statements with a grain of salt. I hope you will view it both as a personal disclaimer—hey, I'm just passing on research reports—and as a consumer warning: life is not drawn in black and white, nor should our judgments be. A demonstration of the problems involved in accepting statistics without question is given in Figure 1.2. Helpful hints for detecting misleading presentations in statistical graphs and charts are also found in Darrell Huff, *How to Lie with Statistics* (1954)—a classic still available in paperback.

Suggested readings on cognitive science
Gardner, H. (1985). *The Mind's New Science: A History of the Cognitive Revolution.* New York: Basic Books.
Huff, D. (1954). *How to Lie with Statistics.* New York: W. W. Norton.
Hunt, M. (1982). *The Universe Within: A New Science Explores the Human Mind.* New York: Simon & Schuster.
Restak, R. M. (1984). *The Brain.* New York: Bantam.
Restak, R. M. (1988). *The Mind.* New York: Bantam.
Restak, R. M. (1991). *The Brain Has a Mind of Its Own.* New York: Harmony.

Catching up on how the brain works

2

Brain basics: A refresher course

Once upon a time there were only lizards and other such reptilian creatures. The *lizard brain* was simple, geared only to the maintenance of survival functions: respiration, digestion, circulation, and reproduction. Over evolutionary time, the leopard and other such mammalian creatures emerged. Extending out from the lizard brain stem, the *leopard brain* (now called the limbic system) added to animals' behavioral repertoire the capacity for emotion and coordination of movement. This second phase of brain evolution yielded the well-known general adaptation syndrome (GAS), or fight-or-flight

Figure 2.1

Two views of the evolution of the brain.

A. The dark area represents the earliest appearance of the brain— the lizard or reptilian brain; the shaded area, the leopard or early mammalian brain; the light area, the learning or late mammalian brain. **B.** Alternate illustration of these levels of brain development.

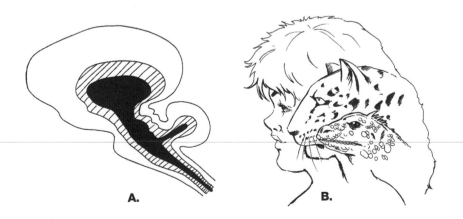

A.   B.

in hardware and hormones

response (Selye, 1952). The evolutionary advantages of this syndrome are attested to by the disappearance of many reptilian species. The third phase of evolution was the *learning brain*—the cerebral cortex. It is this third and most recent phase of brain evolution that provided the ability to solve problems, use language and numbers, develop memory, and be creative. MacLean (1990) refers to the three stages of brain evolution as protoreptilian, paleomammalian (early mammal), and neomammalian (late mammal). Figure 2.1 contrasts the three brain stages.

The millions of years of brain development from lizard to leopard to learner are repeated in each human embryo during the nine months in the womb. Thus, the development of an individual embryo (ontogeny) retraces (recapitulates) the evolutionary path of its ancestors (phylogeny). Scientists summarize this complex concept with those three words: ontogeny recapitulates phylogeny. The consequences of poisoning the brain with drugs or alcohol during pregnancy can be seen in infants whose development was arrested or thwarted at the lizard or leopard level. More complete yet highly readable treatments of brain development and function are available in Hunt (1982) and Restak (1984, 1988); a detailed encyclopedia of information is available in Gregory (1987).

Because this book is concerned with the day-to-day applications of brain science, I will not attempt to provide a complete physical description of the brain

> "We need education in the obvious more than investigation of the obscure."
>
> Attributed to
> **Oliver Wendell Holmes, Jr.**

and all of its functions. It is not really important for you to know, for example, what the hypothalamus is or even what it does. I will dwell only on the physical aspects that you should understand in order to apply the ideas presented here to everyday life. Two such physical aspects are the reticular activating system and the synaptic gap.

Two key features of the brain: RAS and the gap

A kind of "toggle switch" controls whether the leopard brain or the learning brain is currently in charge. This toggle, the *reticular activating system* (RAS), is located in an area beginning in the upper brain stem and continuing into the lower reaches of the cerebral cortex (see Figure 2.2). RAS switching appears to occur at one of two times: when we become emotionally charged up or when we relax. When we become emotionally charged, as in the fight-or-flight response, the RAS shuts down the cerebral cortex, or learning brain. For all practical purposes, when the cortex is shut down, we proceed on "automatic pilot," where instinct and training take over. When the limbic system, or leopard brain, is shut down as a result of general bodily relaxation and removal of threat, the RAS switches the cortex back on and allows creativity and logic to return to center stage. The RAS is a large, diffuse neural process, and its effective functioning is important to both our personal survival and our ability to enjoy life.

Another key feature of the brain is the *synapse*. The synapse is the point at which neurons, or nerve cells, connect with one another; its effective functioning is vital to our quality of life. A typical nerve cell is composed of a main cell body (with nucleus) and two branches, one outgoing and the other incoming, that serve as communication links with other nerve cells. The outgoing branch is called the axon, while the incoming branch is called the dendrite. The axon and the dendrite both have many connector points, so that a neuron can receive many messages through its dendritic terminals and send many different messages through its axonic terminals. The space where the axon of one neuron establishes a connection with the dendrite of another neuron is the synapse, or synaptic gap (see Figure 2.3).

Just as the condition of the gap in an automotive spark plug is important to effective operation of a car, the synapse must be clean and in good condition

Figure 2.2

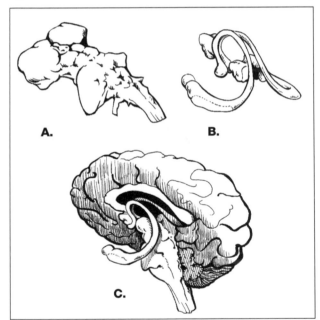

A.   **B.**

C.

Control elements in the brain.
A. The reticular activating system (RAS), which serves as a kind of toggle switch to allow either **B.** the limbic system or **C.** the cerbral cortex (shown with the RAS and limbic systems) to be in control of the brain at any one time.

Catching up on how the brain works

for our nerves to work properly. You can clean the gap of a spark plug with a wire brush, and you can also clean the synaptic gap. Normal maintenance of the synapse is accomplished by the presence of calpain, a compound derived from calcium. Calpain acts as a kind of cleanser, dissolving protein buildup at the synaptic gap like a miniature PacPerson (remember the PacMan video game of the early 1980s in which a moving circular head gobbled a diet of dots?). The dietary source of the cleanser calpain is dairy products and leafy green vegetables. Too little calcium in the diet results in protein buildup at the synapse, with resulting loss of mental performance (e.g., memory), as the buildup interferes with the ability of neural messengers to "jump" the synapse. On the other hand, if there is too much calcium in the diet, the excess calpain itself begins to interfere with neural transmissions. One drastic solution to remove protein from the synaptic gap is electric shock. Studies have shown that for aged patients with severe memory loss, improvements in memory lasted up to six months following shock treatment.

In a sense, RAS switching is the major determinant of our primary *strategies* from situation to situation (proactive-cortical vs. reactive-limbic), whereas the condition of the synaptic gap determines the effectiveness of the *tactics* we employ (memory, logic, creativity, movement, coordination, perception, etc.). The consequences of ineffective RAS switching are devastating. Recent studies have revealed tumors in the brains of some criminals. These tumors are hypothesized to have prevented RAS switching from the limbic system to the cortex, thus maintaining a level of rage behavior. In 1980 in Sacramento, California, a man turned himself in to authorities after repeated violent outbursts. His physician discovered that a tumor was causing pressure in a way that sustained limbic arousal. After surgical removal of the tumor, the pattern of rage disappeared. Apparently, the tumor had caused this man's RAS to lock up. Experimental efforts (Restak, 1984) to create the same type of uncontrollable rage have been carried out by implanting electrodes into the brains of bulls and cats. Activation of an electrode is the equivalent of constant pressure from a tumor. By simply turning a switch on or off, experimenters could turn rage and aggression on and off. An implanted cat in the middle of attacking a mouse would instantly turn friendly when the experimenter turned off the switch.

Figure 2.3

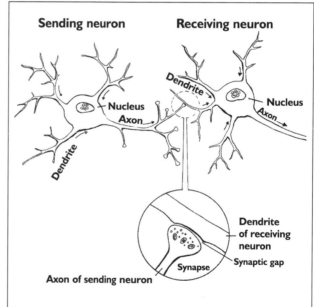

Basic neuronal structure.
The lower enlarged area shows the synapse in some detail, while the upper area shows how it fits into the overall neuronal structure.

Neurotransmitters: The alphabet of personality

We are born with 100 billion brain cells, or *neurons*. We then proceed to lose about 100,000 neurons each day for the rest of our lives, a rate that increases when our brain is subjected to toxins such as alcohol, drugs, chronic illness, long-term medication, and sustained stress. That adds up to 36.5 million neurons a year, or 3.65 billion over 100 years. However, we still have about 96.35 billion neurons left at age 100! It is not the number of neurons itself that determines our mental characteristics—it is how they are connected. Each cell reaches out to other cells through its axon (it "acts-on" other cells), with end points of the axon pairing up with receiving points on the dendrites ("end-right") of neighboring cells. Each neuron is connected to hundreds of other neurons by anywhere from one thousand to ten thousand synapses. Edelman (1992) estimates that it would take some 32 million years to count synapses in the cerebral cortex alone.

Learning is defined as the establishment of new synapses. Gary Lynch of the University of California, Irvine, is one researcher who has confirmed that new synapses appear after learning. It is the *density* of the brain, as measured by the number of synapses, that distinguishes greater from lesser mental capacity. Ira Black (1991) defines knowledge as the "pattern of connectivity" among neurons, and learning as modifications to this pattern of connectivity. The number of synapses and their condition form the stage upon which our electrochemical language plays out its drama. The alphabet of this physiological language is composed of over forty *neurotransmitters*.

Neurotransmitters are chemicals secreted at the synapse that affect the formation, maintenance, activity, and longevity of synapses and neurons. They are like the letters of the alphabet, with their "words" corresponding to behaviors. As words are composed of letters, with individual letters having predictable phonetic effects and groups of letters having predictable semantic effects, so behaviors are composed of neurotransmitter activity, with individual neurotransmitters having predictable physiological effects and groups of neurotransmitters having predictable behavioral effects.

Neurotransmitters create two broad categories of effect: *excitation* (or *activation*) and *inhibition*. For example, one neurotransmitter will activate sleep and another will inhibit it. Drinking milk will trigger the release of melatonin, the neurotransmitter that activates sleep (and, along with the neurotransmitter serotonin, depression), but eating chocolate, which contains caffeine, will interfere with sleep. Still other chemicals serve as neuromodulators, affecting the intensity of excitation or inhibition. Intensity of transmission is measured by the *action potential,* an electrical charge with wave properties (see Figure 2.4).

The nature of the action potential is a key to understanding individual differences. Neurons don't even fire (react to a stimulus), for example, if the stimulus is too weak to cross the response threshold. The threshold for activation of a particular neuron is determined by a complex interplay of one's genetic code, physical condition (tired, pained, alert), and environment (noisy, light, cold, stimulating). Thus, while neurotransmitters constitute a kind of alphabet, other factors affect the nature of neural communication, in much the same way that volume, pitch, and speed affect how our spoken words are understood. For example, I once counseled a young female manager who felt that she was being passed over unjustly for promotion to a field management position. Her manager declined her requests, saying that she was too valuable to be promoted. Her manner was so contrite that I speculated to her that her manager had most likely not heard her pleas for promotion; her voice and emotional level had not crossed his "threshold" for acknowledgment. She practiced a more forceful presentation, delivered it to her manager, and was promoted within days!

Neurons average about three neurotransmitters apiece: some may contain channels for only two neurotransmitters, while others may have channels for five. Each neurotransmitter can exist in a continuum of states— weak, medium, and strong—so that the types of information transmitted in one synapse can range from a dozen to a thousand. I have often thought of the human personality not as a computer but rather as something of a giant equalizer (see Chapter Nine), the contraption stereo buffs use to modulate and transmit sound from their records, tapes, and CDs. Surely you've seen those electrical units with their levers and gauges hooked up to a stereo system. Well, the levers of the equalizer are analogous to the neurotransmitters and neuromodulators—where one affects the quality of sound, the other affects the quality of behavior. A little less serotonin and more testosterone, a little less of the endorphins, the body's own tranquilizer— now we've got a real Bengal tiger on our hands! Add more serotonin—ah, now we're purring.

Figure 2.4

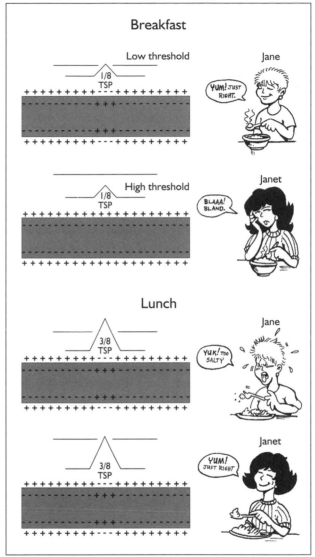

The action potential.

Jane has a lower threshold for tasting salt (i.e., she doesn't need as much for the same effect) compared to Janet.

But this process is complex. Don't let my effort to simplify obscure the vast interconnectedness of cells, chemicals, and systems. Black (1991, p. 37) writes: "Consideration of synaptic transmission has illustrated that the synapse is hardly a simple digital switch, enslaved to a few, simple physiological variables. Quite the opposite occurs. Synaptic communication is a remarkably flexible and changing process, subject to modification by intraneuronal, extraneuronal, local microenvironmental and even distant regulatory mechanisms."

Black goes on to describe the range of complexity of a single neuron. My summary of his description follows:

- Circuits of neurons are electrochemically coded.
- The circuits of a single neuron may use from two to five transmitters, or coded signal types.
- One transmitter may respond to stimuli independent of other transmitters.
- Each transmitter has multiple states (from two or three discrete states to a continuous state).
- So, for example, four transmitter types with three states each (weak, medium, and strong) would possess the potential for eighty-one distinct neuronal states.
- The number of neuronal states for a typical neuron may range from just under 100 to the thousands.
- Multiplying these numbers by 10^{11} neurons gives you some idea of the complexity of the system.

Some of the neurotransmitters that appear frequently in the literature are:

Norepinephrine (also called noradrenaline): Serves as a kind of "printer" that fixes information into long-term memory and helps establish new synapses associated with memory. Rats deprived of norepinephrine can still learn but can't remember. The norepinephrine released as a result of sympathetic arousal in the fight-or-flight syndrome explains why we so vividly remember information related to moments of shock, fright, or anger.

Calpain: Serves as a cleanser when it is released by calcium into the synaptic gap.

Endorphins: Literally, the "morphine within" the brain, serving as a tranquilizer and analgesic. They are released in the presence of pain, relaxation exercises, vigorous exercise, and hot chili peppers. Frank Etscorn, of the

New Mexico Institute of Mining and Technology, injected endorphin blockers into the bloodstream of jalapeño-pepper eaters. The result was sheer agony. Hot chili peppers are not enjoyable without endorphin release.

Serotonin: High levels are associated with aggression and appear to inhibit REM sleep (see Topic 7.1), moderate levels are associated with relaxation and sleep, and low levels are associated with depression. Serotonin is an amine that is metabolized from the amino acid tryptophan, which is produced in the pancreas by the hydrolyzing action of the enzyme trypsin on proteins. Serotonin constricts blood vessels and contracts smooth muscles; it and norepinephrine are both associated with the RAS switching mechanism: extreme levels prevent flexible switching. Serotonin is being closely observed in research on depression. While serotonin levels appear to be consistently related to depression, it cannot act alone in influencing depression. (In a 1983 UCLA study, a higher-than-average level of serotonin was found in dominant male vervet monkeys and in officers of college fraternities!)

> Serotonin is being closely observed in research on depression.

Acetylcholine: A neurotransmitter metabolized from dietary fat (fat ⟶ lecithin ⟶ choline + cholinacetyltransferase ⟶ acetylcholine). Acetylcholine is absolutely essential to the health of the neuronal membrane: the cell wall becomes brittle without it. It is also necessary for activating REM sleep. That is why a minimum level of fat is necessary in our diet (see Chapter Five).

Suggested readings on brain mechanics

Black, I. B. (1991). *Information in the Brain: A Molecular Perspective.* Cambridge, MA: MIT Press.

Cacioppo, J. T., & Tassinary, L. G. (Eds.). (1990). *Principles of Psychophysiology: Physical, Social, and Inferential Elements.* Cambridge, England: Cambridge University Press.

Gregory, R. L. (Ed.). (1987). *The Oxford Companion to the Mind.* New York: Oxford University Press.

Hooper, J., & Teresi, D. (1986). *The Three-Pound Universe.* New York: Macmillan.

MacLean, P. D. (1990). *The Triune Brain in Evolution.* New York: Plenum.

Toates, F. (1986). *The Biological Foundations of Behavior.* Philadelphia: Open University Press.

Part two

Your personal almanac:

The power of the mind-body relationship

Your personal almanac:

The power of the mind-body relationship

3

Getting along with the opposite sex:

Perhaps the facet of brain research of most general interest is the area related to gender differences in brain structure and functioning. After all, everyone can identify with some aspect of gender. There are not only males and females, but also males with female-differentiated brains and females with male-differentiated brains, as well as persons whose brain-body differentiation is somewhat ambiguous.

This chapter summarizes the findings from cognitive science research on gender differences that have some practical applications. See Appendix A for a complete listing of these differences.

A word of warning: Whenever I refer to differences between sexes, keep in mind that these differences are *averages* unless otherwise specified. This means, for example, that although males have a higher average score on math tests, some males score lower than females and some females score higher than males. In addition, only time will tell which of these reported differences are free of cultural influence. To avoid having to constantly repeat the mouthfuls *male-differentiated brain* and *female-differentiated brain,* I will use the terms *male, male brain, female,* and *female brain;* they all are intended to refer to the fuller term. I will also occasionally use the full term as a reminder. When I intend to refer to men and women and not just their brains, I will use the terms *men* and *women.*

The wiring is not the same

Topic 3.1 In the womb

It appears that, in addition to our genetic endowment, our mothers' hormone levels during pregnancy are the primary determinant of the degree to which we will have a male- or female-differentiated brain. The male-differentiated brain has a thicker right cerebral cortex, a corpus callosum (which connects the hemispheres) that is thinner relative to brain weight, denser neurons, nuclei up to eight times larger than those of the female brain, and a hypothalamus that works on the principle of negative feedback to maintain constancy. The female-differentiated brain has a thicker left cerebral cortex, a corpus callosum that is thicker relative to brain weight, neurons that are less dense, smaller nuclei, and a hypothalamus that works on the principle of positive feedback to increase fluctuation in the system—that is, highs get higher and lows get lower, resulting in more emotionality.

The result is that the two brains are hard-wired differently: the male for doing and the female for talking. The male Doer tends to become more proficient in math, spatial reasoning, and what Moir and Jessel (1991) call the five characteristics of the male-differentiated brain: aggression, competition, self-assertion, self-confidence, and self-reliance. All of these characteristics are highly correlated with testosterone level, whether in males or females. The very highest levels of testosterone, however, do not produce the highest math scores; slightly

> "There is one phase
> of life that I have
> never heard
> discussed in any
> seminar
> And that is that all
> women think men
> are funny and all
> men think that
> weminar."
>
> **Ogden Nash**

lower levels do. Females who excel in math usually also exhibit the five male traits, and females who exhibit the five male traits tend to score higher in math and visual-spatial skills. The female Talker tends to become more proficient in language, sensory awareness, memory, social awareness, and relationships. Much of this is apparently due to the relatively thicker corpus callosum in the female-differentiated brain, which allows freer communication between the two hemispheres. In an effort to describe how this differentiation looks as pictured by various measures of brain activity, Moir and Jessel (1991) provide a summary, shown in Table 3.1.

Table 3.1 Location of brain function by gender

Function	Location
Language mechanics	**Men:** Left hemisphere front and back
	Women: Left hemisphere front[a]
Vocabulary	**Men:** Left hemisphere front and back[a]
	Women: Left and right hemispheres front and back
Visual-spatial perception	**Men:** Right hemisphere[a]
	Women: Right and left hemispheres
Emotion	**Men:** Right hemisphere
	Women: Right and left hemispheres

[a]Denser, more specific, and highly localized concentrations of neural activity, which are associated with superior performance.

Note: From *Brain Sex: The Real Difference Between Men and Women* by Anne Moir and David Jessel, 1991, New York: Carol Publishing Group/Lyle Stuart. © 1989, 1991 by Anne Moir and David Jessel. Reprinted by permission of Carol Publishing Group.

The more concentrated activity for language production in females that is shown in the table may account for their verbal superiority as measured by various tests, and the more concentrated activity for visual-spatial perception in males may account for their visual-spatial superiority. The advantage of the denser concentration is apparently that fewer possibilities exist for interruption or interference of neural activity. Male-differentiated brains, in fact, find it easier to handle multitasking, such as talking while building something. Talking, which uses the left hemisphere, doesn't interfere in a major way with building, which is visual-spatial and uses the right hemisphere. Because the female-differentiated brain handles visual-spatial tasks in both hemispheres, building and talking, which both use the left hemisphere, interfere with each other.

One major structure that affects this pattern of specialization is the corpus callosum, which connects the two hemispheres. It is up to 23 percent thicker in the female-differentiated brain relative to brain size, providing the female brain with appreciably more connections, or synapses, between the two hemispheres. This degree of connection between the two hemispheres has been shown to be related to articulateness and fluency in language. The male's separation of language specialization in the left hemisphere and emotional specialization in the right helps to explain his traditional ineptitude at talking about feelings; the neural basis of his feelings has far fewer connections with his language production via his thinner corpus callosum. The female, with emotions seated in both hemispheres and with a thicker corpus callosum, has greater access to both her own feelings and the feelings of others as she produces her language. The male, with vocabulary-making powers seated in the left hemisphere only, is more proficient at developing vocabulary (hence the incredible mountains of male-created jargon and technical vocabulary), yet the female is more proficient at using what vocabulary she has.

Apparently the key to differentiation is in hormonal levels during pregnancy. The effects are easier to experiment with in animals. If a pregnant rhesus monkey is injected with testosterone, a female offspring will exhibit one or more male traits, such as aggressive play or mounting. The female chaffinch can't sing; it doesn't have the synapses for singing that are present in the male. If male hormones are injected into the female chaffinch, the appropriate synapses develop along with the accompanying ability to sing. When the ovaries of newborn female rats are removed, a check after they've reached adulthood reveals thicker right hemispheres with an accompanying increase in spatial ability—a male trait. And when the testes of newborn male rats are removed, a similar check reveals thicker left hemispheres—a female trait.

Studies are demonstrating that men who behave as if they had female-differentiated brains in fact possess lower levels of testosterone. And, in parallel, women who behave as if they had male-differentiated brains possess higher levels of testosterone. Variations in androgens (male sex hormones) and estrogens (female sex hormones) can affect the degree and direction of gender differentiation in the brain:

Excess androgen in female embryo	Male-differentiated brain with male appearance and behavior
Excess estrogen (no androgen) in female embryo	Excessively female appearance and behavior (Turner's syndrome)
Excess androgen in male embryo	"Super" male (aggressive, hairy, etc.)
Excess estrogen in male embryo	Female-differentiated brain with female appearance and behavior

Events during pregnancy that can affect the hormonal level of the unborn child include:

- Mutations within the chromosomal matter
- Major or sustained stress, such as war, rape, or bereavement; testosterone is suppressed
- Renal dysfunction, such as congenital adrenal hyperplasia; this produces too much testosterone
- Injections, as when mothers take estrogen for diabetes
- Barbiturates (taken by 25 percent of pregnant women from the 1950s through the 1980s)
- An extra chromosome (XXY in a boy yields low testosterone)
- Vigorous exercise (spurt exercise, such as tennis, increases testosterone; sustained exercise, such as a long run, lowers testosterone)

Although the brain is wired in the womb, the differences are most noticeable after puberty, when the brain becomes fully activated as a result of being bathed in hormones.

Applications

1 Do not take any medication during pregnancy until you've carefully weighed the possible consequences. If you are in doubt, consult a neuro-pharmacologist (a specialist in pharmaceuticals for the nervous system). Be especially cautious during the first four months, when neurons are migrating.

2 Be accepting of your level of performance in various areas. Work to improve, always, but accentuate your strengths. If you sense that you are stronger at spatial skills than verbal skills, don't blame fate or your parents or your boss for not having done more to develop your verbal skills. The chances are that the discrepancy in skill level is hard-wired and permanent. Work to improve a skill to its next level, but don't begrudge how far you have to go to be perfect. Have a sense of humor about your natural gifts. There is so much to learn and so little time to learn it—don't moan about what seems impossible to learn. Instead, be attracted to what seems natural. As the Delphic Oracle said, "Know thyself."

3 Value typical females for cooperation and relation building, among much else. Value typical males for competition and achievement, among much else. Know that achievement and relation building are both important for success in today's business environment. Look at them as complementary assets in terms of meeting customers' needs and competing in a Total Quality Management business environment.

Topic 3.2 The math-verbal controversy

Figure 3.1

In addition to documenting the hard-wiring differences in brain structure and their possible impact on math and verbal performance, research continues to explore a very close relationship between hormonal levels and individual performance. A higher testosterone level results in more sexual activity, more aggression, and higher math and spatial performance (and maze performance in rats). In females, performance is related to the menstrual cycle. From day 1 (the first day of menstruation) through ovulation, estrogen starts low and rises. From ovulation through the end of the cycle, progesterone is high and, for the most part, estrogen is high. This relationship is portrayed in Figure 3.1.

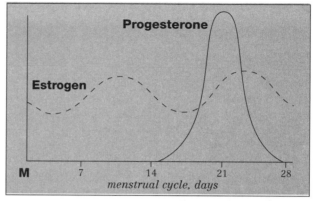

Female hormone levels throughout the monthly cycle.

M = Menstruation.

From *Brain Sex: The Real Difference Between Men and Women* by Anne Moir and David Jessel, 1991, New York: Carol Publishing Group/Lyle Stuart. © 1989, 1991 by Anne Moir and David Jessel. Reprinted by permission of Carol Publishing Group.

Regardless of hormonal levels, females perform on the average higher on verbal than on fine-motor coordination, and higher on fine-motor coordination than on math and spatial skills. But when female hormonal levels are higher, females have higher average scores on verbal skills and fine-motor coordination, yet even lower scores on math and spatial skills. In fact, during menstruation (when estrogen and progesterone are at their lowest), women score 50 to 100 percent higher on mental rotation tests. Regardless of hormonal levels, females perform on average higher on verbal skills and fine-motor coordination than males, and lower on math and spatial skills than the male average (Kimura & Hampson, 1990). Figure 3.2 illustrates this pattern.

If this same relationship of hormones to performance holds true for males, then males should do their best on math and spatial skills in the morning (testosterone levels are highest around 8:00 A.M.) and their best on verbal and fine-motor skills (although not as high as the average female) from midafternoon through early evening (testosterone levels are lowest around 8:00 P.M.). This is purely my hypothesis—as far as I know, no research exists to support or reject it. Kimura and Hampson (1990) have found that males score higher on mental rotation tests in the spring (when testosterone is lowest) than in the fall (when testosterone is highest); apparently the relationship is curvilinear—too much testosterone interferes with spatial performance.

Figure 3.2

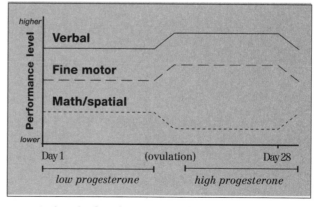

Female hormone levels and their relation to performance.

Another interesting finding relative to math performance is that the female-differentiated brain tends to solve math problems by talking them through (hence, the female Talker), while the male-differentiated brain solves math problems non-verbally. Females manipulate math concepts with verbal labels, while males manipulate the concepts in abstract mental space without conscious use of language. (My wife cannot talk while studying a map in the car; I can.) One consequence of this difference is that the female-differentiated brain takes longer to solve a problem.

Recent studies show that the gap in spatial ability between the sexes remains constant but the math gap was cut in half between 1982 and 1989. The argument rages on. In *Gender and Thought* (Benbow & Linn, 1989), Camilla Benbow says that cultural differences can't explain all the data, while her coauthor, Marcia Linn, sees the differences as continuing to narrow and as being caused by differences in sex roles. I have not seen math scores broken down by subtests—perhaps the differences are related to differences between computational skills, which would appear to be more left-brain-oriented and basically syntactical, and word-problem skills, which appear to be right-brain-oriented, since they are three-dimensional and spatial, with the computational ability more similar between the sexes and the word-problem ability more discrepant.

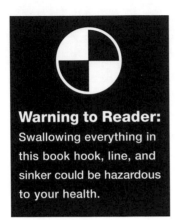

Warning to Reader:
Swallowing everything in this book hook, line, and sinker could be hazardous to your health.

Applications

1   If you are a female and you must take a math test, like an actuarial exam or a financial audit, attempt to schedule it during the first two weeks of the menstrual cycle, between the first day of your period and ovulation. It is likely that your scores will be higher during this time. If you must take a verbal test, like a graduate oral or written exam, or make a major sales presentation, attempt to schedule it during the second two weeks of the menstrual cycle, between ovulation and the beginning of your period. If you must take a test that has both verbal and math components, like the SAT, GRE, GMAT, or LSAT, schedule it according to which part of the test is your greater priority, math (first half of the cycle) or verbal (second half of the cycle).

2   If you administer tests—for example, as a human resources selection specialist or a teacher—then be flexible in scheduling tests, whether with males or females. When possible, permit people to select the time of day and day of the week that best suits them.

3   The typical school curriculum (kindergarten through adult education) is biased toward the female learner, with a predominance of oral and verbal methods and a minimum of visual and hands-on methods. In this environment, the female Talker finds it easier to excel over the male Doer. If you are a teacher or a student, examine your curriculum for its sexual fairness and recommend changes.

4 Do not administer a timed math test to women (or, actually, to anyone) unless speed at computation is a bona fide occupational qualification. See Sternberg's definition of intelligence in Topic 12.1. He makes a strong case against timed intelligence tests in *The Triarchic Mind* (1988).

5 A case could be made for females putting off written reports until the second half of their menstrual cycle, when verbal ability is higher. (contributed by Jane Howard)

6 Schedule meetings with men early in the morning when you want challenging alertness and problem-solving ability, and late in the afternoon when you want their agreement (males are less aggressive then). (contributed by Jane Howard)

7 Males should schedule math and spatial tasks early in the day, verbal tasks such as writing and conversation later in the day. (contributed by Jane Howard)

Topic 3.3 Vision

Research has shown that male-differentiated brains have better visual discrimination in the blue end of the spectrum, and female-differentiated brains have better visual discrimination in the red end. Males have better visual discrimination in bright light (day vision), while females have better discrimination in subdued light (night vision).

Applications

1 Where extremely fine color discrimination is necessary, allow for the fatigue, error, and slowdown that might accompany an attempt to concentrate on an end of the spectrum that is not your "natural" end.

2 In testing employees for color discrimination, be aware that you will rarely find employees who are equally strong at both ends of the spectrum.

3 Females may be safer drivers at night, although I have not seen any hard data to support this.

4 Be aware in work-space design that brightly lit areas are more fatiguing for females and dimly lit areas are more fatiguing for males. Allow variations in brightness throughout the facility as much as possible. Vary lighting in break areas to give individuals a choice.

5   In a romantic setting, don't assume that the male is unromantic because he wants more light, or that the female is romantic because she is comfortable with less light. Females can see better with less light, while males can't see as well.

Topic 3.4   Differences in visual and auditory perception

Research has shown that males, with their larger right hemisphere, tend to demonstrate better visual perception and discrimination, which is centered in the right hemisphere. Females, on the other hand, tend to demonstrate greater auditory perception, which is centered in the left hemisphere.

Applications

1   In setting up work assignments, remember that females tend to make fewer errors in auditory tasks, such as talking on the telephone, taking dictation, interviewing others, or listening for malfunction indicators in machinery. Males tend to make fewer errors in visual tasks, such as proofreading, visual scanning, or looking for malfunction indicators in machinery.

2   Also remember that, because they are more sensitive to auditory stimuli, females become fatigued more readily in a noisy environment. Males do not, but they do become fatigued more readily in a visually chaotic environment.

Topic 3.5   Space

Research has shown that females are more comfortable being in close physical proximity to other females than males are being close to other males. As a general rule, males require more work space than females. However, this should not be a reason to discriminate with space. Understand that accepting a smaller space is not necessarily to be taken as a sign of low ambition—some people, especially those with female-differentiated brains, are very comfortable with less space. Conversely, wanting a larger space is not necessarily to be taken as a power play—some people, especially those with male-differentiated brains, become uncomfortable, or even stressed, in a smaller space. It is possible that this difference was genetically favored back during the times when women were primarily cave dwellers during the day and men roamed the fields as hunters.

Applications

1   Allow males to create a sufficiently comfortable space between themselves and other males.

2   Trust people to tell you how much space they need in order to be comfortable.

3   When overnight accommodations are necessary, if possible, let people choose single or double rooms. Females will generally feel more comfortable sharing a room than males. (contributed by Jane Howard)

Topic 3.6 Mood

During the several days preceding the onset of the monthly menstrual period, the woman's body experiences a dramatic drop in progesterone and estrogen production. This is an example of positive feedback, in which changes tend to increase in their initial direction of change, as opposed to negative feedback, in which changes tend to return to the original state. The result of this positive-feedback phenomenon is an emotional volatility. Fifty percent of females' psychiatric and medical emergency hospital admissions occur at this time and 50 percent of females' criminal acts occur here; most female solitary confinement prison admissions take place during the premenstrual period. In September 1991, the U.S. Department of Agriculture reported that elevated (1,300-milligram) daily doses of calcium relieve some of these symptoms; American women average about 600 milligrams of calcium per day. It is not clear how the calcium works— an elevated level may result in optimum calpain production for cleaning out synapses so that the body's endorphins can work more effectively, or it may result in clogged synapses that dull a pain message. I suspect the former.

Males experience six or seven testosterone-level peaks each day.

The equivalent of a woman's hormone depletion in a man is an excess of testosterone. The normal peaks in male testosterone levels are: early in the morning (they are 25 percent lower in evening hours), during rapid-eye-movement (REM, or dream) sleep, and in early autumn (they are lowest in spring). Males experience six or seven testosterone-level peaks each day, with accompanying variations in the five male characteristics of behavior (competition, aggression, self-reliance, self-assertion, and self-confidence; see Topic 3.1). Excessively high testosterone takes these characteristics to a grotesque extreme: the *cocksure* (extreme self-confidence) *loner* (extreme self-reliance) *driven* (extreme self-assertion) *to dominate* (extreme aggression) *whatever the cost* (extreme competitiveness). Testosterone production soars in the teenage years; as a result, the highest crime rates are in the age bracket of thirteen to seventeen. Moir and Jessel (1991) talk of the two equivalent mood disorders as PMT (premenstrual tension) and VMT (violent male testosterone).

Pioneering work by British researcher Katharina Dalton (1987) has yielded two significant findings relative to PMT: first, that administration of progesterone calms the rage center of the brain, and second, that a drop in blood sugar results in a rise in adrenaline and a drop in progesterone. Holly Anderson has opened a PMT clinic based on this research—the PMS Treatment Center in Arcadia, California.

Applications

1   A simple, self-administered remedy for women with troublesome mood swings is to try snacking every two to three hours in order to sustain blood sugar levels throughout the day. Women with a tendency toward violent moods that won't go away should consult an endocrinologist for both pharmaceutical and nonpharmaceutical treatment.

2   Women need to understand if they have a tendency toward violent mood swings. They also should inform others about their mood swings and deal with them with appropriate humor after the fact. Men (and other women) need to avoid taking a woman's premenstrual mood swings personally; it helps if they can find appropriate ways to respond (such as "Wow! You're furious!" or "You have a right to be mad" or "You're right—good point") and then get on with things.

3   Men need to understand their tendency to "take no prisoners." They should follow up such episodes with humorous or self-deprecating comments, such as "Boy! I just couldn't let go of my position, could I? I was a real bastard." When an important, high-risk situation is coming up, to minimize the possibility of killer behavior, they should try preceding the situation with long, strenuous exercise (e.g., a thirty-minute run, lap-swim, or brisk walk).

Men need to understand their tendency to "take no prisoners."

4   It is important for both males and females to pick up the pieces after their hormone-driven outbursts. At a minimum, they should say, "I'm sorry" or its equivalent (such as giving flowers or some other token). At another level, decisions made during outbursts should be reconsidered.

5   Women might try consuming more calcium products, such as milk or yogurt, before their periods.

Topic 3.7 Automization

Males and females who are injected with extra testosterone show an ability to persevere at automized behaviors. These are behaviors that, once learned, do not demand excessive mental or physical exertion, but that are subject to fatigue effects over time (Moir & Jessel, 1991). Examples include solving basic arithmetic problems, walking, talking, keeping balance (e.g., standing guard), maintaining observation (e.g., as a military sniper or quality inspector), and writing. Injected groups show a lower decline in skills as the day wears on. Those who are not injected get tired and make more mistakes. The "automizers," with extra testosterone, tend to be more focused and single-minded and are more often associated with success and upward mobility. Estrogen is known to suppress automized behavior, especially just after puberty, when girls' academic performance tends to decline. Boys begin to exhibit automized behaviors during puberty, when their system ratchets to a new level of testosterone.

Applications

1 Females engaging in automized behaviors will require more frequent breaks to maintain a skill level.

2 Females can be more consistently productive in nonautomized areas—for example, sales, research and development, supervision, training and development, planning, analysis, and creative activities.

3 Promotional policies should not be based exclusively on performance at automized skills. Management itself does not consist of automized behavior, so to promote those who are good at it incurs the risk of creating managers who convert their success at these behaviors into inappropriate management behavior, such as supervising too closely and pushing, pulling, or riding employees without letup. Nonautomizers are more likely to develop effective coaching, counseling, and listening skills.

Topic 3.8 Relationships

Males are wired to do, and females are wired to talk (Moir & Jessel, 1991). Expecting a male to talk and only talk can be highly uncomfortable for the male and rather unproductive as well. Expecting a female to engage in an activity without talking can be equally uncomfortable and unproductive for the female.

Applications

1 In most male-female relationships, conflict arises when the female wants to talk and the male wants to act; the classic example is the female preference in lovemaking for greater foreplay and the male preference for immediate release. The solution to this type of conflict is to allow the other person's style to be expressed: the male agrees to talk if he is allowed to continue what he is doing, and the female agrees to work in the yard with him if he will talk with her. Males need to be willing to listen and respond while doing, and females need to be willing to "do" as a stage for talking. For example, a male and female who go to a ball game or museum may discuss family matters during appropriate lulls. Or they may just go for a drive together, with the male driving (doing) while they are talking. An alternative is to set aside exclusive times to talk without doing and vice versa.

2   Any negotiating team should include females; they provide a willingness to talk and work on relationships that balances the males' desire for a quick fix.

3   Human resource functions in organizations should have females in decision-making or advisory roles.

4   One way to get males to talk more is to make something of a game or contest out of it. A traditional male is more likely to engage in talk the more he can see communication skills as a set of tools to master. That way, he is not just "talking"; he is practicing a skill set. See the list of interpersonal communication skills in Topic 26.1.

Topic 3.9 Sexual orientation

The emerging evidence points strongly in the direction of a genetic basis for homosexuality. Richard Pillard of Boston University School of Medicine summarizes the research evidence in the June 1992 *Harvard Health Letter:*

- Homosexuality runs in families.
- Homosexuality appears randomly in birth order.
- Homosexuals exhibit early childhood gender nonconformity.
- Monozygotic twins have the highest concordance rate; if one is homosexual, there is a 50 percent probability that the other will be too.
- A recent finding suggests a major biological difference—the third interstitial nucleus of the anterior hypothalamus is of equal size among women and homosexual men but is twice as large in heterosexual men. The meaning of this discovery is unclear; it is hoped that further research will clarify it.

Apparently sex hormones are not an important determining factor. While there is a small difference in testosterone levels between heterosexual and homosexual groups, a greater difference exists within groups. In one comparative study, the highest testosterone level belonged to a homosexual subject.

Application

Homosexuality appears to be a genetically determined difference. It is not a choice and therefore it is not a moral issue. Apparently, homosexuality and heterosexuality are as natural as blond or brown hair. Accept homosexuals and heterosexuals as equals, and don't try to change a person's preference or make fun of something that cannot be changed.

Suggested readings on gender differences

Kimura, D., & Hampson, E. (1990, April). "Neural and Hormonal Mechanisms Mediating Sex Differences in Cognition." *Research Bulletin No. 689*. London, Ontario: Department of Psychology, University of Western Ontario.

Moir, A., & Jessel, D. (1991). *Brain Sex: The Real Difference Between Men and Women*. New York: Carol Publishing/Lyle Stuart.

4

Growing old: Use it or lose it!

While not all of us will be blessed with the opportunity of knowing the perspective of old age, certainly all of us have an interest in knowing what research in cognitive science has discovered about the effect of aging on mental structure and ability. This chapter focuses on findings that can help us age with maximum effectiveness and better understand those who are preceding us into the Golden Age.

Topic 4.1 General effects of aging

We are born with roughly 100 billion neurons. By establishing connections between neurons, or making new synapses, the brain increases its mass threefold until the early twenties. From that time on, the brain decreases in weight by one gram each year. This drop is the result of losing, naturally and inevitably, 100,000 neurons each day of our lives. No more than 50,000 per day are lost in the cerebral cortex. Proportionately more are lost in the frontal and temporal cortex, especially the motor cortex, which contains the long axons from the spine necessary for balance. Alcohol consumption increases the daily destruction proportional to the quantity consumed (around 60,000 neurons per day for a heavy drinker or alcoholic). Sickness, medication, and untold other assailants can also increase the rate of neuron loss. The average person loses about 10 percent of his or her brain weight in a lifetime. Men lose more than women, and men lose more in the left hemisphere, which controls language, than in the right, which controls visual-spatial skills. Females experience about a two-ounce drop in brain mass around menopause, while males experience their accelerated loss beginning somewhere around age sixty.

As a general rule, aging itself does not have a large impact on deterioration of brain function. While a debate continues to rage on this issue, it is clear that the primary assailants on neurons are:

- Medication
- Disease (especially heart disease)
- Extended grief over personal losses
- Alcohol
- A sedentary life-style
- Lack of stimulation
- A low educational level *and* absence of curiosity
  or a desire to learn
- Malnutrition
- Depression

The lesson of all this is: *Use it or lose it!* As neurologist David Krech says, "They who live *by* their wit die *with* their wit." Thomas Edison, Johann Wolfgang

> "Do not go gentle into that good night."
>
> **Dylan Thomas**

von Goethe, Victor Hugo, Margaret Mead, Claude Monet, and Titian did some of their best work in their seventies and eighties. George Bernard Shaw, Pablo Picasso, Arthur Rubinstein, Albert Schweitzer, and Pablo Casals were still active in their nineties. Also:

- George Frideric Handel wrote the *Messiah* at fifty-six.
- Franz Joseph Haydn wrote the *Creation* at sixty-seven.
- Richard Wagner composed the opera *Parsifal* at sixty-nine.
- Merce Cunningham danced in his seventies.
- Martha Graham still choreographed in her nineties.
- Giuseppi Verdi wrote the opera *Falstaff* at eighty.
- Arthur Fiedler was active until his death at eighty-eight.
- Photographer Imogen Cunningham worked in her nineties.
- Grandma Moses retired from crocheting with arthritis around age seventy and started a new career in painting.

By using our nervous system, we grow it.

At age seventy-six, my mother-in-law moved to North Carolina from Alabama. A long-time church organist, she has found a new service niche. She is in high demand for after-dinner music and music-therapy classes at her retirement home, and she plays frequently in the musical interlude just before her church's Sunday morning service. She is well respected for her talent.

The more we use our brains as we age, the higher our performance level stays and the higher is our ratio of synapses to neurons—that is, our brains stay denser the more we use them. Nerve growth factor (NGF) is one of many trophic, or nutritional, agents that stimulate and support growth of the myelin sheath—the coating of the neural fiber—and of new synapses. NGF is released as a result of neural transmission itself. In other words, by using our nervous system, we grow it.

Applications

1   Make it a personal goal to learn something new continually. Once you've mastered it to the point where it is routine, it's time to learn something new.

2   Disuse breeds disuse. Use what you know and have. Fight idleness and boredom with all your energy. If you can't think of anything to do, offer yourself as a volunteer—there are plenty of organizations waiting for you to help out. You can be helpful to others either from the confines of your own home (e.g., telephoning, addressing, sewing, or mending) or at another site, such as an office park or hospital.

3   Strive to maintain a balanced diet from this point on. See Topic 5.2 and Appendix B.

4   Exercise caution when changing physical positions after age fifty. Be especially careful using ladders or stools to gain height—most people's sense of balance just isn't what it used to be. Leave the shower, tub, and car with a little more caution. And be sure to exercise regularly.

5   Assume that you will retain your full mental powers forever. Just because we slow down doesn't mean we have to stop! We will always have a contribution to make!

Topic 4.2 Neuronal commitment

A kind of "commitment" of neurons appears to be made in humans sometime between eight and twelve months of age. Once they are committed, the neurons ignore unfamiliar stimuli. Janet Werker, of the University of British Columbia in Vancouver, finds that babies exposed to English from birth can recognize consonants that do not occur in English from the language of the Thompson tribe (located in the Thompson and Fraser valleys of southwest British Columbia) up until eight months of age, but at twelve months they cannot discriminate between the Thompson consonants.

Application

Expose your newborn to the widest possible variety of sensory stimuli—colors, music, language, natural and mechanical sounds, touch, smell, taste—to ensure that, as an adult, he or she will have the most flexible brainpower for learning.

Topic 4.3 Irreversible damage

Generally, studies point to eight years of age as the point after which brain damage is irreversible. Neurons cannot be replaced; once they have been lost they are gone forever. However, in young children, other parts of the brain can pick up functions lost due to brain damage. The story is frequently told of a five-year-old who lost one entire hemisphere; this individual is now forty-five years old and possesses an above-average IQ. After the age of eight, such recovery appears to be impossible.

Applications

1   Buckle 'em up with seat belts and car seats every time you put your children in an automobile.

2   Have high expectations for children recovering from brain damage before eight years of age.

3   Be prepared for the possibility of permanent loss of function from brain damage that occurs after eight years of age.

Topic 4.4 Maturation and the brain

The supplies of minerals inside our bodies are critical to the formation of new synapses. Without these raw materials, we could not build new connections between neurons, which means that we could learn nothing new. Eric Lenneberg (1967), a psycholinguist, has demonstrated that there are three spurts of mineral production as we mature: (1) around age two, when we learn to walk and talk; (2) around age six, when we start to read, do math, and write; and (3) around age twelve, when we begin to reason abstractly. After the third spurt, which is associated with puberty, no more occur. Lenneberg reasons that after this third spurt, major new learnings become much more difficult. That is why, for example, it becomes harder to learn foreign languages after elementary school.

Applications

1   One reason some children learn to walk, talk, read, and so on earlier than others is that they begin their spurt of internal mineral production earlier than others. Without the minerals, they simply aren't ready. When they are ready, they will learn. Don't push children before they are ready, and don't fret or reprimand a child who appears to lag behind others. It doesn't signal that the child is lacking in ability; it just demonstrates his or her unique biological timetable.

2   The more varieties of experience children have before puberty, the more resources they have to build on as adults. Childhood experiences become the building blocks for adult accomplishments.

Topic 4.5 Old age and mental ability

Two clear trends are associated with the aging brain:

1   Between the ages of twenty and sixty, reaction time *doubles*; that is, we slow down.

2   Although the total number of neurons continues to decrease with age

at the rate of 100,000 per day, the ratio of synapses to neurons *increases* for those who continue to use their brains and *decreases* for those who stop using their brains (see Figure 4.1). Learning means new synapses, and new synapses mean higher density, which counterbalances the normal brain-weight loss. Accordingly, performance continues to improve with age among those who use their brains, while it declines among those whose brains retire when they retire from their jobs.

Figure 4.1

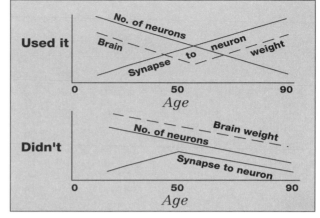

The effect of inactivity and disuse on the brain.

In a Harvard Medical School study of over one thousand physicians, Dean Whitla and Sandra Weintraub found that the ten physicians over age sixty-five with the highest performance scores on the *Assessment of Cognitive Skills,* an unpublished computer-administered test developed by Harvard's Douglas Powell (see Allison, 1991), were still actively working as physicians, while the ten physicians with the lowest performance scores were not working any longer. The working and nonworking physicians showed similar patterns of medication and illness, so the difference in performance cannot be attributed to those factors. In other words, their Physical Health scores and Mental Health scores were independent. I know that "Use it or lose it" sounds like an oversimplification, but . . .

Many reports show mental abilities declining in old age, but these reports typically fail to control for degree of brain use. Apparently the nonusers are bringing down the scores of the users! Referencing the Seattle Longitudinal Study, Warner Shaie of the Pennsylvania State University Gerontology Center finds that measurable loss in mental performance (e.g., in spatial reasoning) can be reversed with training, except for performance loss due to brain damage from drug use, disease, or trauma.

In a project funded by the University of California at Los Angeles Task Force on Psychoneuroimmunology, George Solomon and John Morley found that age does not uniformly affect the immune system (Cousins, 1989). Older healthy persons show immune levels of white blood cells, lymphocytes, granulocytes, and so on that are somewhat higher than those of comparable younger persons. In addition, older adults with "hardy" attitudes (high commitment, positive emotion, self-control, and exercise) show an even higher level of immune cells as well as of endorphins.

Applications

1 Plan for retirement. Don't become a television addict without hobbies or interests.

2   Beware, as you age, of depending on speedy performance in order to feel good about yourself. If you feel that you are overextending yourself, begin to move toward activities that are compatible with slower reaction times. You might move from driving cars and riding motorcycles to walking, riding bicycles or tricycles, and taking buses. Move from power tools to hand tools, from debate to dialogue, from reading stories to storytelling. One of the reasons that bridge, canasta, checkers, chess, Go, and many other board games are successful as intergenerational activities is that they are highly tolerant of varying speeds of individual play. Develop increasing pride in the quality of your accomplishments, decreasing pride in the speed of their execution.

> The limits of the mind's ability to positively influence health are unknown.

3   As you age, maintain high expectations for yourself, keep developing your sense of humor, take control of stress, and continue to exercise and eat right.

4   In the face of disease, "accept the diagnosis but defy the verdict," as Norman Cousins says (Cousins, 1989). Examples of recovery from "terminal" illnesses are numerous and increasing. The limits of the mind's ability to positively influence health are unknown.

Topic 4.6 Maintaining control and optimism

The principles elaborated in Topic 14.2 concerning the effect of control on stress apply equally to seniors. Specifically, Judith Rodin of Yale University (Keeton, 1992) has demonstrated that nursing home residents aged sixty-five to ninety who are allowed to take a direct planning and decision-making role in their programming:

1 Live longer		**4** Are more alert	
2 Are sick less		**5** Have less of the stress	
3 Are happier		hormone cortisol	

Also, Christopher Peterson of the University of Michigan, along with Martin Seligman of the University of Pennsylvania (see Topic 13.1), found that baseball players who were more optimistic at age twenty-five lived significantly longer.

Applications

1   If you are responsible for the care of older adults, do everything you can to include them in planning, decision making, and problem solving. Share responsibility and control with them. If you are on the staff of a community for older adults, establish committees, consult with them, and empower them by responding to their ideas, requests, and needs.

2   If you are an older adult, whether you are living alone or in a community, continue to be involved in planning your life; if you live in a community for older adults, establish committees, create suggestion boxes, ask those charged with your care to consider your ideas, and pool your resources for trips and other big-ticket items, such as lawyers, entertainment, transportation, or equipment.

Topic 4.7 Diet and aging

Evidence points toward the significant effects on longevity of restricted diets. In other words, the less you eat, the longer you live. Roderick Bronson and Ruth Lipman of the Human Nutrition Research Center at Tufts University in Boston report that reducing patients' normal food intake by 40 percent results in a 20 percent longer life span. Their report (Raloff, 1991) argues that diet restriction (1) limits deoxyribonucleic acid (DNA) damage, (2) increases enzyme-mediated repair of DNA, and (3) reduces expression of proto-oncogenes (cancer-causing genes).

Application

If living longer is more important to you than eating a lot, consider cutting back your consumption by about one-third.

For more information, contact:

Human Nutrition Research Center
Tufts University
Boston, MA 02111
617-556-3000

Topic 4.8 Exercise and aging

According to research reported in Folkins and Sime (1981), exercise programs can at least arrest and often reverse many of the degenerative physical effects of aging in older patients. One explanation of this phenomenon is that exercise promotes increased absorption of oxygen. Aerobic exercise is best. In a study conducted by researchers at the Salt Lake City Veterans Administration Hospital, three out-of-shape groups were followed: one was put on a walking regimen, another lifted weights, and the third carried on business as usual with no exercise of any kind. The walkers showed much higher scores on eight tests of mental ability, the weight lifters showed a little improvement, and the others showed no improvement.

Applications

1   Keep walking, briskly.

2   Inquire about organized and medically supervised exercise programs for seniors and join up. Senior centers have taken leadership in this area.

3   Don't stop exercising because you think you're too old. There's an aerobic exercise that's safe and beneficial for you.

Topic 4.9   Combining diet and exercise

In a study reported in Merzbacher (1979), individuals with cardiovascular disease and an average age of sixty were placed on the Pritikin diet, which includes more complex carbohydrates and fewer proteins and fats, and were assigned six to ten miles per day of jogging or walking. After completing this twenty-six-day program, subjects scored higher on intelligence tests and measurably improved their circulatory system.

Application

Don't just exercise—eat right.

Topic 4.10   Memory and aging

Although the memory processes slow down as we age, the accuracy of our memories improves. When he administered recall-and-recognition tests to youths and seniors in church fellowship halls, Paul Foos, chair of the psychology department of the University of North Carolina at Charlotte, found that the seniors, with an average age of sixty-five, consistently beat the youths. As we age, the number of items we can associate to a particular memory chunk dramatically increases. So, while we may take longer, the likelihood of accurate recall increases. In fact, there is some evidence that the rich associative network of seniors is one factor in the slowdown of their memory processes.

My eighty-two-year-old brother-in-law and I were riding through eastern North Carolina last year to a family reunion. Making small talk, I referred to a basketball player from our hometown of Kinston who had recently signed to play basketball with the University of North Carolina, calling him Shackleford. My brother-in-law commented that I didn't have the name right. I agreed and we both started searching our minds for the right name. He won the race. I asked him how he'd remembered. He said that he got an image in his mind of a retired professor friend in California named Stackhouse, flipped from that image to one of a furniture store in Goldsboro (on his route for many trips from Chapel Hill to Kinston), and came up with the right name. My effort to describe this process is captured in Kim Allman's illustration in Figure 4.2. Apparently, my brother-in-law's network of isolated memories connected in something like the following manner to give him the right answer (follow along with Figure 4.2):

- He heard "Shackleford," a relatively new auditory memory gained around age seventy, based on a well-known Kinston athlete who attended North Carolina State University, *not* the University of North Carolina at Chapel Hill.
- He associated the name Shackleford to basketball and Kinston.

Figure 4.2

My brother-in-law's memory process.

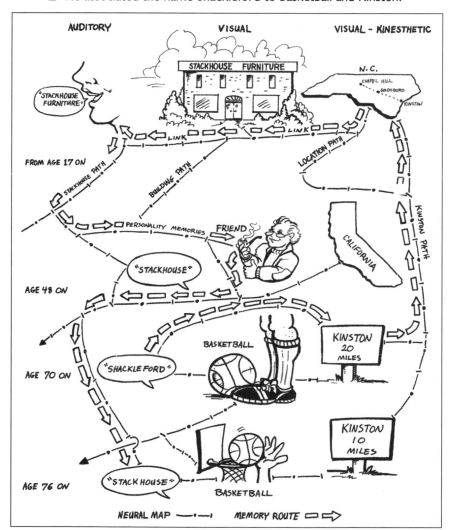

- He unconsciously and instantaneously relived his frequent trips from Chapel Hill to Kinston to visit his parents and his in-laws.
- A prominent building halfway between the two towns, Stackhouse Furniture Store, popped up ever so briefly into his consciousness.
- This submerged memory of the furniture store, firmly entrenched from about the age of seventeen, connected to another strong memory of his longstanding friendship, from about the age of forty-eight on, with a California professor named Stackhouse.
- By the time he envisioned his California friend, he became conscious that the name "Stackhouse" was the one he was looking for.

I hope that at age eighty-two my memory processes will be as abundant and effective as my brother-in-law's.

Applications

1 Slow is okay. You'll get there.

2 Don't push seniors to remember more quickly—the frustration of being pushed will interfere with the effort to remember. Give people the time they need.

Suggested readings on aging

Keeton, K. (1992). *Longevity: The Science of Staying Young.* New York: Viking.
Raloff, J. (1991, October 5). "Searching Out How a Severe Diet Slows Aging." *Science News, 140*(14).
Restak, R. M. (1984). *The Brain.* New York: Bantam.
Restak, R. M. (1988). *The Mind.* New York: Bantam.

5

Nourishment: Food for the body,

As recently as World War II, scientists as well as the general public considered diet to have little or no influence on mental functioning. Research over the last forty years, however, has revealed a close relationship between diet and the brain—so much so, in fact, that trendy brain bars are popping up that specialize in juices and foods considered to improve *mentation,* or mental activity. It is becoming clearer that our brain influences what and how we eat, and that what and how we eat influences how we think and feel. This chapter identifies various specific findings in this arena of the food-brain connection.

Topic 5.1 Recommended food balance

The National Research Council, after reviewing over five thousand studies, published a 1,300-page report in 1989 entitled *Diet and Health: Implications for Reducing Chronic Disease Risk.* A popular version of the report was published later (Woteki & Thomas, 1992). For a detailed summary of their report, see Appendix B. In general, they found that Americans eat too much fat, simple carbohydrates, and protein and insufficient amounts of complex carbohydrates (see Table 5.1). In addition, they found that dietary supplements, especially beyond the recommended daily allowance, have no benefits and may be toxic. Exceptions exist—consult your physician if you are in doubt.

Your personal almanac

fuel for the brain

Table 5.1 Imbalance in American diets

Type of food	Today's menus	Better menu
Fat	36% of calories	30% or less of calories
Cholesterol	**Men:** 435 mg daily **Women:** 304 mg daily	Less than 300 mg daily
Carbohydrates	45% of calories	At least 55% of calories
Protein	**Men:** 1.75 times the RDA[a] **Women:** 1.44 times the RDA	No more than twice the RDA

Note: Adapted from "The Latest Word on What to Eat" by Anastasia Toufexis, March 13, 1989, *Time, 133*(11), pp. 51–52.
[a]RDA = recommended daily allowance.

Applications

All of the recommendations below assume that the reader engages in a reasonably active life-style.

1 *Emphasize* fish, skinless poultry, lean meats, low-fat or nonfat dairy products, and complex carbohydrates (fruits, vegetables, and starches). Complex carbohydrates should comprise more than half the daily allowance of calories.

2 *Limit* egg yolks, organ meats, fried foods, fatty foods (pastries, spreads, dressings), animal protein (it has no known benefits and may cause cancer), alcohol, and most shellfish (there is some debate over which; scallops are apparently okay).

3 *Eliminate* dietary supplements, such as vitamins and minerals, except as recommended by a reputable doctor. Megadoses have no benefits and may be toxic. Calcium supplements, fish oil capsules, and fiber supplements provide no established benefits; these ingredients must be consumed in their normal state, in food. Megadoses of vitamin C on a regular basis *may* do some good. Consult a neuropharmacologist if you are in doubt about the effects of supplements and megadoses. Vitamin megadoses taken by expectant mothers have shown adverse effects on the spinal columns of their newborns.

4 Fat should comprise no more than 30 percent of your daily calories. As a general guide, one tablespoon of peanut butter has eight grams of fat, or ninety calories, so a daily allowance of 2,100 calories translates to the equivalent of no more than *seven* tablespoons of peanut butter per day. (Much debate centers around the recommended level of fat in the daily diet. Those with cardiovascular disease should follow a guideline that allows 10 percent of the daily calorie allowance for fat, not 30 percent.)

5 Of the fat maximum (the equivalent of seven tablespoons of peanut butter a day), no more than 10 percent (that's less than the equivalent of *one* tablespoon of peanut butter) should be saturated fat, such as coconut oil or animal fat.

6 *Limit* alcohol to the equivalent of two regular cans of beer per day or two small glasses of wine (i.e., no more than one ounce of alcohol daily). *Exception:* Expectant mothers should consume no alcohol.

7 *Limit* protein to eight grams per kilogram of body weight a day. For a 180-pound person, that would be one 8.4-ounce hamburger patty per day; for a 120-pound person, one 5.6-ounce hamburger per day.

8 *Limit* salt to about a teaspoon per day.

9   I could recite a litany of the effects of various vitamin and mineral deficiencies, such as thiamine deficiency, which causes memory loss and iron deficiency in expectant mothers and brain slowdown in their children. Suffice it to say that failure to consume a balanced diet will take its toll on brain function. If you are in doubt, consult your physician or take a reputable multivitamin (*not* a megavitamin!).

Topic 5.2   Daily calorie allowance

Russell Wilder, senior physician at the Mayo Clinic, found that *any* diet of under 2,100 calories per day is deficient in some vitamin, mineral, or trace element, unless it is tailored by a physician for a patient. After three months on a low-calorie diet, people exhibit faulty memories, increased error rates, inattentiveness, clumsiness, panic, nightmares, feelings of persecution, anxiety, hostility, and quarrelsomeness (Minninger, 1984).

Application

Do not limit yourself to fewer than 2,100 calories (adjusted for gender, body type, and age) for a sustained period without monitoring by a physician.

Topic 5.3   The munchies

In recent bulimia research, T. D. Geracioti, Jr., of the National Institute of Mental Health, and R. A. Liddle of the University of California, San Francisco, have identified a hormone that apparently controls the "munchies." In animal and human studies, higher levels of the hormone cholecystokinin (CCK) were accompanied by absence of hunger. CCK serves as an antianalgesic in animals: when a rat perceives safety, CCK is released and blocks the effect of painkillers. Perhaps bulimic patients are unable to perceive the safety required for CCK release and therefore have a constant sense of fear, threat, and hunger (Wiertelak, Maier, & Watkins, 1992). In one controlled study, bulimic and nonbulimic women were found to have equal levels of CCK before eating, yet the bulimic women had lower levels after eating. Apparently CCK is the chemical messenger that tells the hypothalamus, "Shut down the food—I'm full now." Some of us have bodies that fail to produce sufficient CCK to control our appetite.

Any diet of under 2,100 calories a day is deficient in some vitamin, mineral, or trace element, unless it is tailored by a physician for a patient.

Applications

1   Antidepressant drugs have been prescribed with some success for bulimic or binging patients. See your physician if this seems to be a promising option for you.

2   Ask your physician or a neuroendocrinologist about the research on CCK. Continuing research should yield helpful solutions to problems of binging.

3   Try other nonpharmaceutical antidepressant measures, such as exercise or escape (see Topic 14.2, Applications 3 and 4).

4   Be kind to yourself. Understand that there is a good chance that the impulse to eat is a biochemical phenomenon and you're not built like those who are immune to the munchies. Don't see yourself as psychologically deficient or weak. If you're concerned about it, do something about it, and don't blame yourself—blame nature!

Topic 5.4 The role of fat

Fat is the dietary source of acetylcholine, a neurotransmitter that is crucial to maintaining the condition of neural cell membranes. While too much fat is unhealthy, too little fat is also unhealthy; the neural cell membranes will become brittle and deteriorate over time as a result of too little acetylcholine. The result of this deterioration is memory loss and a general decrease in brain function. Dietary fat metabolizes into lecithin, which further metabolizes into choline, which then, with the help of the catalyst cholinacetyltransferase, metabolizes into acetylcholine. Some research indicates that doses of choline can improve the problem of severe memory loss.

A series of meta-analyses (DeAngelis, 1992) suggests that low-fat diets, while improving death rates from heart disease, increase death rates that result from suicides, homicides, and accidents. This apparent relationship between low-fat diets and negative affect adds emphasis to the potential dangers to the human system of too little fat.

Application

Do not eliminate fat from your diet! Aim for the recommended daily allowance (see Topic 5.3, Application 4).

Topic 5.5 Food additives

Ben Feingold of the Feingold Association has found that people, especially children, react to food additives that cause reactions to the natural salicylates in good food (Winter & Winter, 1988). Food additives include artificial sweeteners such as aspartame, flavor enhancers such as monosodium glutamate, preservatives such as nitrites, artificial colors, and artificial flavors. Aluminum-based additives appear to have especially adverse effects on the nervous system. Reactions include poor concentration, short attention span, fidgeting, aggressiveness, excitability, impulsivity, a low frustration threshold, clumsiness, and insomnia.

Applications

1 Avoid foods with additives for yourself, your loved ones, friends, and co-workers. Just don't make them available. While this subject is still being hotly debated, it would seem wise to minimize or eliminate additives in the diet, especially for expectant mothers and children exhibiting the above symptoms.

2 Read food labels to check for additives, especially aluminum.

Topic 5.6 Metabolism

Paul Moe, research leader in the Energy and Protein Nutrition Laboratory of the U.S. Department of Agriculture, reports that in their human experiments in the calorimeter (a nine-by-ten-foot chamber that measures oxygen input and carbon dioxide output with eighty thousand sensors to determine total energy expenditure), they found no differences in the efficiency with which different people metabolize food. Their conclusion was that differences in weight can't be blamed on differences in metabolism; they result from excess eating and/or deficient exercise.

William Bennett (1991) argues, however, that each body has its own "set point," or genetically programmed level of body fat. It would be a lifelong battle to attempt to maintain a lower set point. For example, if a woman's set point is 150 pounds and she decides to drop 10 pounds, her body will forever be trying to recover the lost fat. Bennett argues that, to minimize fat, we should avoid the two things that tend to raise our set point—inadequate exercise and excessive fat consumption. He's convinced that simple overeating in and of itself is not the culprit. In a study where subjects were overfed 900 calories a day for fourteen weeks, identical twins gained weight at about the same rate, while gains from $9^1/_2$ to 29 pounds were reported for unrelated people. Bennett maintains that the metabolisms of any two people at their set point would appear normal. Hence, his findings seem compatible with Moe's.

> If a woman's set point is 150 pounds and she decides to drop 10 pounds, her body will forever be trying to recover the lost fat.

Applications

1 When there's a choice, walk, don't ride.

2 When there's a choice, stand, don't sit.

3   When there's a choice, exercise or escape, don't snack.

4   Serve smaller portions. A couple in our neighborhood maintains a trim profile without exercising, yet without giving up any favorite foods. We've sworn they had to have a God-given metabolism that allowed this indulgence. Recently, however, we had them over for dinner. Because it was in front of her, the woman served the stew in bowls to the rest of us. To my consternation, I noticed that my portion barely covered the bottom inch of a bowl with a three-inch wall! I looked at my wife, who knowingly smiled back at me. Later that night, we agreed: it isn't just metabolism—it's portion size. We both grew up in homes where large portions were served. If we didn't eat large portions and ask for seconds, our mothers took it as rejection. We have to rescript ourselves to feel all right about eating smaller portions. The task is clear—and uphill!

5   When you are hungry between meals, avoid fatty snacks.

6   If you are confident that your exercise and diet levels are appropriate for you, learn to accept your set point and not feel guilty.

Topic 5.7   Body chemistry and appetite control

Sarah Leibowitz (1992, p. 74), who teaches neuropharmacology at Rockefeller University in New York City, has identified the chemical sources of urges for specific food groups, as well as the time of day during which the urges are strongest. A summary is shown in Table 5.2.

Table 5.2   The chemistry of food urges

Food group	Chemical basis of desire	Time of day desire is strongest
Carbohydrates	Turned on by norepinephrine, neuropeptide Y, cortisol; turned off by serotonin	On waking and early morning; desire decreases as the day goes on
Protein	Turned on by serotonin, opiates; turned off by neuropeptide Y, norepinephrine, dopamine, galanin	Alternates with carbohydrates in morning; rises gradually toward middle of day; peaks at dinner and evening
Fat	Turned on by galanin, opiates, aldosterone; turned off by dopamine	Desire for fat increases during middle of the day and predominates in evening

Note: Adapted from "Sarah Leibowitz (Interview)" by Fran Collin, May 1992, *Omni, 14*(8), p. 74.

Applications

1   Save fat consumption for evenings, when desire is strongest for most of us.

2   Exercise in the late afternoon or early evening (see Topic 7.3) in order to metabolize the fat more efficiently.

3   When eating an early-evening meal, minimize carbohydrate consumption and maximize protein. When eating very late, minimize protein to avoid interference with sleep.

Topic 5.8 The role of carbohydrates and proteins

The brain needs 180 grams of carbohydrates per day. Complex carbohydrates (grains, seeds, beans, fruits, and vegetables) metabolize more gradually and provide a steadier release of glucose for use by the body. Simple carbohydrates such as sugar, on the other hand, provide a quick rise in blood sugar followed by a letdown. To give you a rough idea of how much food is required to ingest 180 grams of carbohydrates, a small banana contains 21 grams. Carbohydrates yield tryptophan, which triggers serotonin, leading generally to relaxation and sleep. Proteins, especially meat and eggs, yield the amino acid tyrosine and trigger catecholamines that lead to alertness.

Applications

1   Eat or serve primarily carbohydrates and fats prior to events for which you want people relaxed and easy to please.

2   Eat or serve primarily proteins prior to events for which you want people alert and analytical.

Topic 5.9 Breakfast

Ernesto Pollitt of the University of Texas Health Science Center at Houston compared the school performance of children who skipped breakfast to those who ate a good breakfast (Pollitt, 1981). Those who ate breakfast made measurably fewer errors as the morning wore on. Other studies of both children and adults have confirmed this finding.

Application

Don't skip breakfast. If you must eat on the fly, at least grab a piece of bread that's not dredged in fat and sugar, or a banana, or a glass of milk.

Topic 5.10 Violence and sugar

Many studies report drops in violent acts when, for example, residents of detention centers are fed low- or no-sugar diets. Stephen Schoenthaler of the Social Justice Program at California State College, Stanislaus, reports from a 1980 study at the Tidewater Detention Center in Chesapeake, Virginia, that high-sugar diets promote violence this way: whenever the limbic system and the cerebral cortex have to vie for scant supplies of glucose, the limbic system always wins. In a high-sugar diet, the body is left depleted of blood sugar when a hit of dietary sugar wears off (because insulin is released to shut down the body's production of glucose); the limbic part of the brain then gobbles up the available glucose, thereby making emotional behavior dominant (the limbic system is in control) and pushing rational behavior into the background (because of a starved cerebral cortex).

Ensure that sugary foods do not replace healthy foods.

When I taught high school, I once had a violent student in my eleventh-grade homeroom. I called his parents in for a conference. The mother (the father was on the road) described a typical day. I noticed that the boy was rising at 5:30 A.M. in order to catch a 6:15 A.M. bus to school. Meanwhile, the mother stayed in bed. The son left the house without human contact or food intake, stopped by the convenience store on the way to the bus stop, grabbed a grape soda and a pack of doughnuts or cookies, and caught the bus. When he arrived at school, therefore, he was on a sugar high and was affable and demonstrative for about one hour; then, after the sugar wore off, he started hitting people. Why didn't his mother fix breakfast? Because he didn't like her breakfasts. I asked what he'd eat, if she fixed it. We agreed on a hamburger and a glass of milk, of all things. Within two weeks, his old pattern had changed, succumbing to that of a reasonably likable seventeen-year-old. I'm sure that he benefited not only from the substantial breakfast, but from having some contact with his mother before leaving home.

Application

Ensure that sugary foods do not replace healthy foods—at most they should only supplement them.

Topic 5.11 Sodium

Sodium is not just bad for hypertension and the heart. Overconsuming sodium can also lead to electrolyte imbalances and accompanying mental dysfunction. The typical body requires about 1,000 milligrams of sodium daily and about five times that much potassium. To give you a rough idea how easy it is to overconsume sodium, one tablespoon of soy sauce contains about 1,000 milligrams, or the recommended daily allowance.

Applications

1 Don't salt your food, or at least limit yourself to one shake or pinch.

2 Use a variety of spices and peppers to compensate tastewise for lessened salt intake.

Topic 5.12 Breast feeding

In *Early Development and Parenting,* Virginia Polytechnic Institute psychologist Philip Zeskind reports on an experiment with fourteen breast-fed babies and fourteen bottle-fed babies (Zeskind, 1992). He describes the nervous systems of bottle-fed babies as "engines out of tune," and those of breast-fed babies as well tuned and efficient. Breast-fed babies have overall lower heart rates and are more alert. They are also somewhat more irritable and sleep less, but Zeskind sees this as a desirable trade-off.

Applications

1 If you are the mother of a newborn, do what you need to do to breast-feed your baby as long as you can.

2 Many states have laws that make public breast-feeding a crime. Florida struck down its statute in March 1993. Help your state do the same if it has such a law.

Topic 5.13 Vitamin and mineral deficiencies

Vitamin and mineral deficiencies result from either insufficient intake or inadequate absorption. The first can be fixed by a varied and balanced diet composed primarily of fresh or frozen foods. The second can be fixed by appropriate injections administered by a physician. The consequences of a sustained deficiency are fatigue, loss of appetite, poor concentration, failing memory, depression, and insomnia. You can confirm and specify a suspected deficiency through a blood test at a laboratory qualified to test for vitamin and mineral content.

Applications

1 Vitamin supplements are best absorbed when taken with other foods. Caffeine, however, obstructs absorption, so take your multivitamins with a meal that does not include coffee, tea, or caffeinated sodas.

2   Mineral supplements are best absorbed between meals.

3   If you think that you have some of the symptoms of a deficiency, take a blood test to determine your vitamin and mineral content.

4   To get the most nutrition from your foods:
- Replace canned foods with fresh or frozen food.
- If you use canned foods, retain and use the juices in other dishes, unless you detest high sodium.
- Keep milk and bread in opaque containers.
- Don't leave food in the freezer too long.
- Use fresh juice immediately, preferably the same day it is squeezed.
- Avoid soaking vegetables.
- Choose pressure cooking, steaming, or boiling to cook vegetables, using minimum water, leaving skins on, and cooking the vegetables the shortest amount of time possible.

5   Factors that obstruct absorption, destroy nutrients, or both include:
- An excessively low calorie count
- Alcohol
- Nicotine
- Tannin
- High fiber in the diet
- Aspirin
- Medications
- Cooking

Suggested readings on diet

Katahn, M. (1991). *One Meal at a Time*. New York: W. W. Norton.

Winter, A., & Winter, R. (1988). *Eat Right, Be Bright*. New York: St. Martin's Press.

Yepsen, R. B., Jr. (1987). *How to Boost Your Brain Power: Achieving Peak Intelligence, Memory and Creativity*. Emmaus, PA: Rodale.

6

Chemicals and consequences: The

Leo Tolstoy included in his ethic of love an injunction against consuming anything that detracted from one's normal state of full alertness. Thus, he declined coffee as well as alcohol. This chapter does not make such a demand of its readers; its purpose is to summarize findings related to the impact of various kinds of drug intake on the brain.

The word *drug* comes from the Middle English *drogge* (as well as French and German forms), which means "dry." It refers to the various powders (i.e., dried forms) we know of as chemicals, or drugs. I use this word to refer to any consumable substance taken for the purpose of intervening with the normal functioning of the mind-brain.

Topic 6.1 Alcohol

Alcohol serves as a disinhibitor; that is, it "unlocks" normal inhibitions. It also serves as a depressant, or downer (often combined with coffee, whose caffeine serves as an upper). Alcohol destroys brain cells, primarily in the left hemisphere, the seat of language and logic. The number of cells killed varies according to the amount of alcohol consumed. Alcoholics and heavy drinkers kill off about 60,000 more neurons per day than their light-drinking and teetotaling friends. A Reuters release reported that people who drink heavily for thirty to forty years die with

effects of mind-altering agents

brains that weigh 105 grams less than the brains of their light-drinking friends (1,315 grams vs. 1,420 grams). If you must drink alcohol, limit the amount to one ounce per day (the equivalent of two regular beers or two small glasses of wine). Remember, you start with approximately 100 billion brain cells and lose approximately 100,000 a day anyway. How much do you want to speed up the process?

Ernest Noble, of the UCLA School of Medicine, has found that two to three drinks per day, four days per week, have an adverse effect on brain function, especially for those over forty. This level of alcohol consumption also causes premature aging. Studies of the brains of alcoholic men show reduced blood flow in the frontal lobe—the seat of memory formation, creativity, and problem solving. Alcohol makes the nerve membrane more fluid and less viscous than normal, which results in structural instability and increased susceptibility to structural change and damage.

A 1992 University of Minnesota report, based on data from 356 twin pairs, suggested that the causes of alcoholism are genetic only when it occurs in adolescent males. When alcoholism develops in adult males or in women, the evidence points to environmental causes.

> "Our body is a well-set clock, which keeps good time, but if it be too much or indiscreetly tampered with, the alarm runs out before the hour."
>
> **Joseph Hall**

Applications

1. In planning a cocktail party or reception, do not allow for more than the

equivalent of two beers per person. If individuals want to drink more, you may have it available, but make them pay for it. Don't put yourself in the position of making it easy for a person to consume more than one ounce of alcohol daily.

2   If you run a bar and are having a "happy hour" (illegal in some states), cut off special prices after the second drink. Have customers pay full price for third and subsequent drinks.

3   Provide information (posters, notices on menus, placards on tables, etc.) that cautions against consumption of more than two alcoholic drinks per day.

4   Consider medical intervention for male adolescents who show alcoholic tendencies. Counseling alone would not be sufficient to counterbalance a genetic predisposition.

5   Pregnant women ideally should not drink at all, but especially during the first four months (see Topic 6.8).

Topic 6.2 Caffeine

Caffeine serves as a stimulant, or upper. Its effect is heightened physiological arousal, which is similar to arousal caused by stress in that it results in the release of cortisol. Excessive arousal appears to result in errors of commission (e.g., typographical errors), whereas deficient arousal appears to result in errors of omission (e.g., skipping a paragraph while typing). Routine tasks are less affected by excess arousal, while more complex, unfamiliar tasks appear to suffer under high-arousal conditions, which can make it difficult to concentrate. Caffeine consumption can also trigger panic attacks.

Interestingly, the strongly introverted personality generally wakes up in a higher state of cortical arousal. If the introvert consumes caffeinated beverages upon waking, he or she will perform poorly on complex mental tasks. If the strong extravert tries a complex mental task upon waking before consuming a caffeinated beverage, he or she will perform poorly. Toward the end of the day, this pattern switches: in the evening, introverts perform complex mental tasks better with a hit of caffeine, while extraverts perform complex tasks better without caffeine.

The normal effective dose of caffeine is generally estimated at 100 milligrams, or, more precisely, at 2 milligrams per kilogram of body weight. One cup of coffee contains 75 to 125 milligrams of caffeine and is the equivalent of one cola drink, two cups of tea, two ounces of bittersweet chocolate, or twelve cups of cocoa. Physical activity will dissipate the effects of caffeine.

Consumption of 400 to 500 milligrams of caffeine per day is associated with dependence (Winter & Winter, 1988). Symptoms of caffeine dependence are diarrhea, nausea, lightheadedness, irregular heartbeat, irritability, and insomnia. One dramatic warning sign of caffeine dependence is a feeling of dizziness upon standing after having been prone (normal people experience a rise in blood pressure, while caffeine addicts experience a drop). Another symptom is the so-called Yom Kippur headache associated with fasting (and abstaining from coffee) for twelve to sixteen hours.

The arousal effects of one cup of caffeinated coffee last for approximately six hours, but vary according to the individual. I'm six feet, two inches, tall, weigh 240 pounds, and am fifty-one years old. If I drink caffeinated coffee after 5:00 P.M., I have trouble getting to sleep that night. If I drink more than two cups of strongly caffeinated coffee in a short time, I get jittery and have trouble concentrating. My limit is one cup of strong caffeinated brew (or two cups of moderate, three of weak).

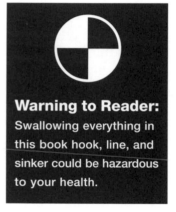

Warning to Reader: Swallowing everything in this book hook, line, and sinker could be hazardous to your health.

The myth that a cup of coffee for the road after a night of drinking counteracts the effects of alcohol is just that—a myth. At Hull University, students who consumed vodka were given two cups of coffee. Those given caffeinated coffee made twice as many psychomotor errors as those who drank decaffeinated coffee or no coffee at all. In addition, in a study of 1,500 college students, higher caffeine consumption was found to be correlated with lower academic performance.

As with most so-called laws of nature, exceptions abound.

Applications

1   Know your limit. If you are in doubt, limit yourself to one cup of strong caffeinated brew (or two moderate, three weak) every six hours (less if you are physically active).

2   Make noncaffeinated alternatives available to guests, especially for introverts in the morning and extraverts in the evening.

3   If you are responsible for a meeting, do not provide more than the equivalent of two moderately caffeinated cups of brew per person. If people ask for more, let them purchase it on their own. Don't be responsible for providing them with an excuse for less-than-effective mental activity. Switch to noncaffeinated alternatives (coffee, tea, soft drinks, juice) after the initial allotment runs out.

Chemicals and consequences   **85**

4   I've found some hotels and restaurants to be unconcerned about supplying noncaffeinated beverages for breaks. You must be specific in asking for them when you order.

Topic 6.3 Marijuana

Roy Matthew, director of the Duke Alcoholism and Addictions Program, affiliated with Duke University in Durham, North Carolina, reports that steady users of marijuana (ten joints a week for three years) show a dramatically lower (and permanent) baseline level of cerebral blood flow than nonusers. Cerebral blood flow is a measure of brain activity. Those who smoke once or twice during a three-year period show no measurable drop in baseline cerebral flow over time. However, the same nonusers and infrequent users show an immediate measurable drop in cerebral blood flow right after smoking one joint. Continued steady use of marijuana results in what Matthew calls the "amotivational syndrome"— lethargic, self-defeating behavior resulting in loss of interest in work or school, abandonment of long-term plans, and loss of pleasure in normal activity.

Maximize the use of natural highs provided by the body.

Application

If effective use of your mind is important to you, don't use marijuana.

Topic 6.4 Cocaine

When endorphin neurotransmitters jump a synapse and land on receptor sites, a pleasurable sensation ensues. Normally, the endorphins then detach from the receptor site and return to their presynaptic location. Cocaine attaches itself to the endorphins at the receptor site and prevents their return to the presynaptic site. Thus, (1) the pleasurable effect is maintained and (2) there is a shortage of endorphins when the cocaine is metabolized, resulting in strong letdown and the urge to use more of the drug.

Applications

1   *Don't!*

2   Maximize the use of natural highs provided by the body. Aerobic exercise and laughter are two good sources of natural highs (see Topic 14.2, Applications 4 and 8).

Topic 6.5 Nicotine

Nicotine interrupts the flow of oxygen to the brain. The resulting oxygen deprivation is accompanied by decreased metabolism of glucose, which translates into sluggish and faulty memory, ineffective problem solving, and lower mental output in general.

We've all heard that women should not smoke during pregnancy, but recent research suggests that stopping during pregnancy may not be enough. Michael Weitzman of the Rochester (New York) School of Medicine, in a study of mothers of 2,256 youngsters aged four to eleven, found that when mothers smoked after delivery, their children had twice the number of behavioral problems and alterations in brain function as children whose mothers did not smoke.

Applications

1 If you have excess brainpower that you don't want or need, then enjoy smoking. It's a good way to cut your brain down to a more humble performance level. Otherwise, don't smoke.

2 If you are a parent or you live or work around children, know that smoking around children has a high likelihood of causing behavioral and mental dysfunction.

Topic 6.6 Aspirin

Much has been written recently about the ability of aspirin to thin blood and about its potential positive effects on blood pressure and associated lower risk of heart attack. In addition, the right amount of aspirin can ameliorate dementia (general deterioration of mental ability): one aspirin a day will improve dementia, but two a day worsen it. After one year on one aspirin a day, demented patients showed a 17 percent improvement on tests of cognitive ability; after two years, they showed a 21 percent improvement.

Application

If you have a friend or family member suffering from dementia and the aspirin treatment has not been suggested, you might arrange to consult with the patient's physician about its appropriateness.

Topic 6.7 Prescription drugs

Nervous system depressants affect brain function. Sleeping pills, tranquilizers, muscle relaxers, and antianxiety drugs all affect the quality of brain function. Cortisone and arthritis drugs also affect brain function. Valium (diazepam) particularly affects the ability to drive safely, including staying in one's lane, maintaining constant speed, braking in a reasonable distance, recognizing signs quickly, and having peripheral awareness (Winter & Winter, 1988). Merrell Dow Pharmaceuticals identified several drugs as tending to impair performance in operating machinery (Winter & Winter, 1988):

- Painkillers
- Antidepressants
- Antihistamines
- Tranquilizers
- Sedatives
- Antipsychotics
- Stimulants
- Some antihypertensives
- Anticholinergics

The effects of these drugs are typically worsened when they are taken along with alcohol. In addition, certain combinations of these drugs can produce unpleasant or even lethal side effects.

Recently a new agency was formed to study the differences in body chemistry among ethnic groups. The Center on the Psychobiology of Ethnicity, located in Torrance, California, at the Harbor–University of California at Los Angeles Medical Center, presented its initial research reports in 1992. For further information on this agency, contact:

> *Dr. Keh-Ming Lin, Director*
> *The Center on the Psychobiology of Ethnicity*
> *Harbor–UCLA Medical Center*
> *1124 West Carson Street, B-4 South*
> *Torrance, CA 90502*
> *310-222-4266*

Applications

1   Try to find a nonpharmaceutical alternative to the prescription drugs listed above. Confer with your physician about how to identify nonpharmaceutical treatments.

2   Just as unions are sometimes considered an antidote to bad organizational management, so are pharmaceuticals an antidote to poor self-management. Ensure that you have taken charge of your life with diet, exercise, and stress elimination or reduction before you allow yourself to become drug-dependent. Read Covey (1990) and Sternberg (1988). And read on!

Your personal almanac

Topic 6.8 Effects of various agents on the embryo

During the first four months of pregnancy, brain cells in the embryo migrate from their original position to their ultimate destinations by way of glial cells, a type of supportive tissue. Alcohol appears to extend these migrations (the cells travel too far), whereas radiation appears to shorten them (they don't travel far enough). As a result, cells end up in the wrong location. The consequence is unpredictable malformation and dysfunction in the newborn infant. The effects of cocaine on the embryo are well documented in most daily newspapers, and pregnant women who consume megavitamins have children with a 25 percent greater incidence of spinal-column defects. Prescription drugs can also have damaging effects on the embryo; double- and triple-check a prescribed drug before exposing an embryo to it. The effects of nicotine are mentioned in Topic 6.5.

Make no assumptions about what is safe to consume while pregnant.

Applications

1 Make no assumptions about what is safe to consume while pregnant. Instead, consult your obstetrician. If you are not sure of your advice, consult a neuropharmacologist; if you are still not sure, do your own library research.

2 The first four months of pregnancy are especially critical. If you think there's a chance you are pregnant, assume you are and consume accordingly.

Topic 6.9 Brain nutrient drugs

Dean and Morgenthaler (1990) make dramatic claims for a new family of drugs that are not yet available on the American market—nootropics (from the Greek *noos,* or "mind," and *tropos,* or "change"). According to their research, nootropic drugs can improve mental function and arrest or even reverse some brain diseases. Most of the so-called nootropics are chemical efforts to duplicate various neurotransmitters and neuromodulators. These drugs have not been approved for use in the United States.

Applications

1 As a general rule, for the normal healthy person with no evidence of dementia, I recommend nonpharmaceutical methods for improving brain function (diet, exercise, and training in the many areas described in this book).

2 For exceptional cases where deterioration of brain function does not respond to available interventions, Dean and Morgenthaler's book can help to identify a doctor who is willing to prescribe nootropic drugs. The book itself will tell you how to become a part of the nootropic network.

Topic 6.10 A note on pain

The sources of pain vary from pressure (being hit) to puncture (being stuck), but all pain is communicated through synaptic structures called nociceptors. These receptors, which are committed to relaying pain messages, follow two pathways:

1 From the source of potential pain (e.g., a fingertip) to the spinal cord and back to the source, resulting in a reflex action (jerking the finger off a hot stove). This is a *warning* path.

2 From the source of actual pain (e.g., the burned area of the finger) to the brain and back, resulting in the sensation of pain. The inflamed area produces prostaglandins, which act on nociceptors to transmit pain messages. How much pain we feel depends on the threshold for activating our nociceptors. This threshold is a function of genetics, physical condition, attitude, and attentional focus (e.g., boxers don't really feel the pain of being hit until they stop focusing on the fight itself).

Treatments for pain include:

- Narcotic analgesics such as morphine and codeine, which actually block the pain message at the nociceptor. However, the body develops a tolerance for these drugs, so this is only a short-term solution.
- Mild analgesics such as aspirin and ibuprofen, which work at the site of the pain to reduce inflammation and block production of prostaglandins.
- Anesthetics such as novocaine and ether, which block *all* sensation, not just pain.
- Hot and cold applications such as heat lamps and ice, which activate other nerve endings that compete with the nociceptors for attention.
- Electrical stimulation such as transcutaneous electrical nerve stimulation; this works the same way as heat and cold.
- Stress reduction (see Topic 14.2).
- Patient-controlled analgesia, which is an intravenous administration.
- Biofeedback, which uses visual feedback to promote mental self-control of pain.

Applications

1 Be aware of the many possible approaches to pain treatment—pills are not the only approach.

2 For more (and free) information, write:

The Neurological Institute
P.O. Box 5801
Bethesda, MD 20824

Suggested readings on drugs

Winter, A., & Winter, R. (1988). *Eat Right, Be Bright*. New York: St. Martin's Press.
Yepsen, R. B., Jr. (1987). *How to Boost Your Brain Power: Achieving Peak Intelligence, Memory and Creativity*. Emmaus, PA: Rodale.

7

A good night's sleep: Cycles, dreams,

A good night's sleep should be declared a basic human right. This chapter reviews research findings that may be helpful in understanding both *what* a good night's sleep is and *how* we can manage to get one.

Topic 7.1 The sleep cycle

The infant averages 14 hours of sleep, the mature adult averages $7^1/_2$ hours, and the senior adult (over seventy-five) averages 6. However, studies show that the *length* of sleep is not what causes us to be refreshed upon waking. The key factor is the *number of complete sleep cycles* we enjoy. Each sleep cycle contains five distinct phases, which exhibit different brain-wave patterns. For a complete description, see *The Mind in Sleep* (Arkin, Antrobus, & Ellman, 1978) and *Biological Rhythms, Sleep, and Performance* (Webb, 1982). For our purposes, it suffices to say that one sleep cycle lasts an average of 90 minutes: 65 minutes of normal, or non-REM (rapid eye movement), sleep (see Topic 7.9); 20 minutes of REM sleep (in which we dream); and a final 5 minutes of non-REM sleep. The REM sleep phases are shorter during earlier cycles (less than 20 minutes) and longer during later ones (more than 20 minutes).

If we were to sleep completely naturally, with no alarm clocks or other sleep disturbances, we would wake up, on the average, after a multiple of 90

naps, and nightmares

minutes—for example, after $4^1/_2$ hours, 6 hours, $7^1/_2$ hours, or 9 hours, but not after 7 or 8 hours, which are not multiples of 90 minutes. In the period between cycles we are not actually sleeping; it is a sort of twilight zone from which, if we are not disturbed (by light, cold, a full bladder, noise), we move into another 90-minute cycle. A person who sleeps only four cycles (6 hours) will feel more rested than someone who has slept for 8 to 10 hours but who has not been allowed to complete any one cycle because of being awakened before it was completed. Within a single individual, cycles can vary by as much as 60 minutes from the shortest cycle to the longest one. For example, someone whose cycles average 90 minutes might experience cycles that vary in length from 60 to 120 minutes. The standard deviation for adult length of sleep is 1 hour, which means that roughly two-thirds of all adults will sleep between 7 and 8 hours.

A friend once told me, "All this stuff about cycles is a bunch of bunk. I wake up every morning when the sun rises." After talking about his sleep patterns, he discovered that he was self-disciplined in such a way that his bedtime was consistently about $7^1/_2$ hours before sunrise. He was waking between cycles, and the song of a bird, the cry of a baby, or the pressing of a full bladder could have been equally as effective as the sunrise in waking him. All it takes to awaken someone between cycles, especially if they've had sufficient sleep, is a gentle stimulus.

When my alarm goes off during the last half of my cycle, for a few hours I

> "What a delightful thing rest is! The bed has become a place of luxury to me. I would not exchange it for all the thrones in the world."
>
> **Napoléon Bonaparte**

feel as if a truck has hit me. When it goes off during the first half of my cycle, it is like waking after a 15- to 20-minute nap, and I feel refreshed. Our motor output system from the brain is completely shut down during REM sleep; that is why we dream we are moving but don't actually move, and why we feel so lifeless when we wake during REM sleep—our motor output system hasn't kicked back in yet!

Applications

1 Keep a sleep journal. Record the beginning and waking times for each natural sleep episode that is uninterrupted by an alarm or any other disturbance. Find the common multiple. For example, if your recorded sleep periods were 400, 500, 400, 200, and 700 minutes, you would conclude that your personal sleep cycle typically lasts for 100 minutes, or $1^2/_3$ hours.

2 Once you know the length of your typical sleep cycle (if you haven't kept a journal, you might assume 90 minutes), then, where possible, plan your waking accordingly. For example, my cycle is 90 minutes. If I am ready for bed at 11:00 P.M. and I know that I must rise at 6:00 A.M. in order to make a 7:00 breakfast meeting, I read for about 45 minutes to avoid the alarm going off during the last half of my cycle. Conversely, if I go to bed at midnight, I set my alarm for 6:30 A.M. and rush to get ready, rather than being interrupted toward the end of my fourth cycle.

Many of us have a body clock set for a twenty-five-hour day.

Topic 7.2 The circadian rhythm

From the Latin *circa* ("about") and *dies* ("days"), the term *circadian* simply means "about a day." We have assumed for centuries that our bodies' circadian rhythm has a twenty-four-hour cycle. Thus, we should be renewed and refreshed after every twenty-four-hour period. Recent research by Charles Czeisler of Harvard University and the Center for Circadian and Sleep Disorders at Brigham and Women's Hospital in Boston, as well as research by others, suggests that, in fact, many of us have a body clock set for a twenty-five-hour day and most of us have a natural tendency to stay up later and wake later than we do. That's why so many people play catch-up with their sleep on the weekend.

Czeisler has discovered that there is an optimum schedule when twenty-four-hour shift work is necessary, based on this twenty-five-hour rhythm. The shifts should progress from day to evening to night, each lasting several weeks, with workers going to sleep progressively later. In this manner, when workers who have worked up to an 11:00 P.M. bedtime end a day shift, they start an evening shift; they keep the 11:00 P.M. bedtime for several days and move to a midnight bedtime, then, after several days, to a 1:00 A.M. bedtime, and so on, until several weeks later they are going to bed at 7:00 A.M. and rising to start an evening shift at 4:00 P.M. This schedule takes advantage of the body's natural tendency to go to bed later and rise later—that is, to live a twenty-five-hour day. (Table 16.1 illustrates how we may take advantage of this twenty-five-hour circadian rhythm while working shifts.)

For a person working normal days, the body clock seems to be set as follows:

Time	Effect on body
6:00 P.M. to midnight	Stomach acid is high; hormone levels drop.
Midnight to 6:00 A.M.	Lowest body temperature is between 2:00 and 3:00 A.M. Body is at its lowest level of efficiency between 4:00 and 6:00 A.M. (3:00 to 5:00 A.M. for early birds, 5:00 to 7:00 A.M. for night owls)—this is an extremely high accident-prone period, characterized by low body temperature and low kidney, heart, respiratory, and mental functions.
6:00 A.M. to noon	Blood clotting activity is high. Rote memory is at its sharpest.
Noon to 6:00 P.M.	The sense of smell is better. Body temperature is at its highest between 2:00 and 3:00 P.M. Grip strength is at its highest.

The body's clock can get thrown out of kilter by disease, aging, travel, and other factors. Because the clock seems to be triggered by the daily pattern of sunrise and sunset, it can be reset by the use of bright lights. (Light treatments have also been found effective in relieving winter depression.) Czeisler reported in a May 3, 1990, press release that looking into a four-foot-square array of sixteen forty-watt bulbs according to his schedule can successfully reset the body clock up to ten hours in two days. To set a person's clock back, light treatment should be administered after the body's low-temperature point (4:00 to 6:00 A.M.); to set the body clock forward, light treatment should be administered before the low point. Light inhibits the body's release of melatonin, a neurotransmitter associated with sleep, while darkness triggers its release. Czeisler's light treatment apparently resets the body's time for shutting down melatonin release. He also recommends lightproofing the sleeping quarters of someone who must sleep during the day or in a lighted room, including use of a face mask. Sleeping in total darkness maximizes the chance of obtaining sufficient melatonin release.

Applications

1   Don't get up early (4:00 to 6:00 A.M.) to finish a project; stay up later if you must. Research documents the futility of getting up early—you're fighting your natural tendency to sleep later as well as working during the period of your body's lowest efficiency.

2   As 4:00 A.M. approaches, *go to sleep*. If you must stay awake and safety is an issue (e.g., you are driving or operating other equipment), then try to have someone to talk to. Social interaction appears to be the best stimulant. Caffeine also helps. Take breaks. Keep cool. Avoid heavy carbohydrate or fatty snacks; stick to proteins and light complex carbohydrates. Bright lights help, as does your attitude—think about something that excites you. If you know ahead of time that you will have to be up and alert during these early-morning hours, then take a nap the afternoon before. David Dinges of the University of Pennsylvania has done research that shows that people who nap before staying up all night perform better than those who don't (Dinges & Broughton, 1989).

3   With around 200 sleep clinics in the United States and many others spread throughout the world, don't accept what you perceive as a problem with sleep. Check yourself in for observation. For information on sleep programs, contact:

> *Association of Professional Sleep Societies*
> *1610 14th Street, NW, Suite 300*
> *Rochester, MN 55901*

4   See the Applications for Topic 7.6.

5   If you must sleep during daylight hours, use a face mask and earplugs to better simulate the darkness and quiet of night.

6   Dark places are associated with depression for a reason—insufficient light to shut down melatonin production. If you or a friend have a tendency to depression, avoid dairy products and choose bright, well-lighted, sunny environments (see Topic 17.2).

7   Avoid setting your alarm for before 6:00 A.M. Prepare the night before if getting up at 6:00 A.M. will cramp you: lay out clothes, prepare breakfast (bagel, yogurt, etc.), put coffee on a timer or premake it and zap it in the microwave at 6:00 A.M. Take a nap the afternoon before if you must set the alarm before 6:00.

8   If you must regularly get up before 6:00 A.M., reset your body clock by ensuring darkness and quiet for an early-to-bed schedule and waking up to bright lights. Remember, sunrise is the trigger for the typical body clock.

Topic 7.3   Sleep and exercise

Exercising tends to elicit cortical alertness, which is not what you want when going to sleep. Exercise relaxes you after experiencing stress, but good aerobic exercise generally puts your nervous system in a state of moderate arousal. In this condition, you are ideally suited for mental tasks. In order to sleep soon after a workout, you would need to consume carbohydrates and dairy products.

Sleep following alcohol consumption is not as restful as alcohol-free sleep.

Applications

1   Exercise no later than several hours before bedtime. Exercise arouses the cortex and that delays sleep onset.

2   If you must exercise just before retiring for the evening (I know a television sports announcer who exercises after a night game because he's so keyed up), try reading a relatively unemotional book in bed rather than an exciting one (e.g., Plato rather than Agatha Christie) to help you get to sleep. Also, consider the Applications in Topic 7.4.

Topic 7.4   Sleep and diet

Milk products stimulate melatonin production, which improves sleep. Simple sugars and fats decrease the oxygen supply to the brain, which decreases alertness and makes you sleepy.

Alcohol consumption reduces the relative amount of time we spend in REM sleep; therefore, sleep following alcohol consumption is not as restful as alcohol-free sleep. The more alcohol we consume, the less REM sleep we get, and the less rested we are in the morning.

Food additives in general and artificial sweeteners in particular tend to increase alertness, which interferes with sleep. And eating a large meal in the evening interferes with sleep.

Applications

1   To maximize the chances of a good night's sleep, avoid snacks with additives or artificial sweeteners before bedtime, and eat moderately.

A good night's sleep   **97**

2   To increase your chances of a good night's sleep, have a milk product or light carbohydrate snack shortly before bedtime. Warning: If you have the classic "warm milk," don't sweeten it with artificial sweetener—have it plain or with honey, sugar, or some other natural flavoring.

3   If you drink alcohol in the evening, plan to allow at least one hour for the alcohol to metabolize before you go to sleep; allow more time for more consumption. Also, alcohol dehydrates and water rehydrates, so it helps to drink water between the time you stop drinking alcohol and the time you go to bed. For example, if you've been drinking alcohol throughout an evening dinner party at your home, clean up that night, not the next day, as a way of giving the alcohol time to metabolize, and drink water while you're cleaning. Or go for a gentle walk or stroll before retiring, then read for a while—and drink water. If you want a restful night's sleep, switch to a nonalcoholic beverage before the evening is over.

4   When flying across time zones, avoid drinking caffeine and alcohol in favor of milk. (See the anti-jet-lag diet in Topic 16.3, Application 4.)

Topic 7.5 Sleep and weight

The amount of sleep we require is directly related to our body weight—that is, skinnier people require less sleep; heavier people sleep more.

Application

If you would like to require less sleep, get trim.

Topic 7.6 The effect of sleep deprivation

People who are significantly deprived of sufficient sleep engage in microsleep, a brief period in which they lose consciousness. Microsleep is not restorative—it is a warning that you have lost control. A person who has begun to microsleep is a safety hazard. It is possible to drift in and out of microsleep and not be aware of it. Torbjorn Akerstedt of the Karolinska Institute in Stockholm connected eleven railroad operators to wire monitors. He found that six exhibited microsleep (i.e., they dozed at the helm according to the electrode measurements), yet only four were aware that they had dozed. Two plowed through warning signals while asleep (Long, 1987).

The safety hazards of severe sleep deprivation—several days without sleep—can be eliminated by one night of natural, uninterrupted sleep (typically nine to ten hours).

Applications

1   If you must experience severe sleep deprivation, nap whenever possible.

2   If you have experienced severe sleep deprivation and are engaging in a safety-related activity (driving, operating large machinery), take appropriate safety precautions: alert a backup, take frequent breaks and move around, take deep breaths, or sip a caffeine drink.

3   The maximum sleep deprivation possible without posing a major safety hazard is either (a) two to three days on no sleep, (b) six days with $1\frac{1}{2}$ hours' sleep each day, or (c) nine days with three hours' sleep each day (Webb, 1982).

Topic 7.7 Sleep and medication

The sleeping pills Dalmane and Halcion, while inducing sleep, have a negative effect on brain function, causing memory loss, withdrawal symptoms, and loss of coordination. The British medical journal *Lancet* (see Dahlitz et al., 1991) reports that a pill made from melatonin (which is naturally secreted by the pineal gland) causes insomniacs to fall asleep more quickly. Jane Brody (1992) reports on research on a melatonin pill that is under way at the Oregon Health Sciences University in Portland. Researchers call melatonin the "Dracula hormone," because it simulates the effect of nighttime.

People who nap consistently live longer and show a 30 percent lower incidence of heart disease.

Application

Try natural sleep inducers before developing a dependency on medication. (See the list of examples in Topic 7.11.) If nothing works for you, make sure that your physician stays on top of melatonin research and can provide pills for you as soon as they are available.

Topic 7.8 Naps

People who nap consistently live longer and show a 30 percent lower incidence of heart disease. My eighty-seven-year-old father-in-law has taken a nap after lunch for at least the last seventy years and has outlived all the men in his family. The ideal time for a nap seems to be between noon and 3:00 P.M., at the height of the circadian rhythm, and the ideal length seems to be thirty minutes. Evening naps appear to interfere with sleep. The worst time to nap is at the bottom of the circadian rhythm, between 3:00 and 6:00 A.M. (Webb, 1982).

Rossi and Nimmons (1991) talk of "ultradian breaks" and recommend two or three twenty-minute naps a day. The urge to nap occurs in a natural rhythm, and denying this urge has a negative effect on health, productivity, and general well-being. This denial occurs most commonly among office workers who stoically resist throughout the day. The result is chronic mild arousal.

Application

When possible, take a fifteen- to thirty-minute nap in early to midafternoon to get recharged. Some people practice meditation to achieve the same effect. Minimize your reliance on caffeine for recharging. *Viva la siesta!*

Topic 7.9 Dreams

Everybody dreams. Dreaming takes place during REM sleep, which first begins around the fourteenth to sixteenth week in the womb. The REM sleep of infants occupies about 45 to 60 percent of their total sleep time, while mature and senior adults engage in REM sleep about 20 to 25 percent of their sleep time. During REM, the nervous system's sensory output, external sensory input, and inhibition or control are blocked. Physiologically, this is accompanied by a drastic drop in the production of the neurotransmitters serotonin and norepinephrine. Meanwhile, as the inhibiting effect of the serotonin and norepinephrine disappears, the neurotransmitter acetylcholine increases in the brain stem and activates a flood of internal memories and perceptions. The fact that we exert no management of these internal perceptions results in an often bizarre collage of whatever comes to the big screen during this central core dump.

Hobson (1988) has defined a theory of dreams he calls the activation-synthesis model. What this means is that dreams are made (synthesized) out of the uncontrolled internal images and perceptions that bounce off each other (are activated) during REM sleep. He argues, accordingly, that "the meaning of dreams . . . is thus transparent rather than opaque. The content of most dreams can be read directly, without decoding. Since the dream state is open-ended, individual dreams are likely to reveal specific cognitive styles, specific aspects of an individual's projective view of the world, and specific historical experiences" (p. 219). Hobson points out that the physiology and content of dreams are similar to those of mental illness. The difference, he says, is that in dreaming we don't expect to have control of our minds, whereas the mentally ill have poor or no control of their memories and images where we would expect control to exist. He also presents a highly readable, recent review of dream research, including its history, a neurobiological description of dreaming, and a discussion of interpretation of dreams.

Applications

1   Regard your dreams as a form of brainstorming, in which a flood of unevaluated and unmanaged images and ideas piggyback off each other and merge in often bizarre ways.

2   Understand that the search for latent, hidden meanings in dreams is a game with a potential for inappropriate results. I had a dream last night about trying to destroy a toy train before a Japanese woman prevented me—my wife was setting the charge as I kicked off on my bicycle. Each of these images represents something I read about recently—major rail accidents in Manhattan and South Carolina and an article in *Time* magazine about a Japanese executive who was forced to take a vacation. Don't ask *why* these images occur in your dreams; more appropriately, ask *where* they come from. Remember that bizarre combinations can result from zero management control.

> Regard your dreams as a form of brainstorming.

Topic 7.10 Nightmares

Visualization techniques have proved to be a big help in reducing or eliminating nightmares. They consist of re-creating a visual scene or episode with one's eyes closed and can include actual physical movements; watch Olympic skiers visualize a run with movements before starting. These techniques can be self-taught and self-administered, or they can be learned with the help of a therapist or dream specialist. For further discussion, see Topic 13.1, Application 5; Topic 14.2, Application 7; and Gawain (1978).

Applications

1   If you want to try teaching yourself visualization techniques for nightmare reduction, try the following:

    1 Recall your most recent nightmare in full detail.
    2 Alter a significant detail in the nightmare (change a tiger to a cat, a man to a woman, a knife to a feather).
    3 Play through the complete nightmare, substituting this new detail throughout.
    4 Continue this sequence until the nightmare stops or becomes acceptable.

2   Visit a sleep clinic for professional help. See Topic 7.2, Application 3.

Topic 7.11 Getting back to sleep

If you've awakened in the middle of the night and can't get back to sleep, it's a good bet that, somehow, you've become aroused. What you need to do is shut down your aroused state. Several of the strategies mentioned earlier in this chapter will minimize the chance of your waking. However, if the worst happens and you become wakeful, there are several ways to lower your level of arousal.

Applications

1   Often, we can't get to sleep because thoughts are racing around in our heads trying to keep from being forgotten. Keep a pad and pen beside your bed and take a mental dump by writing down all those thoughts bumping into each other. You can then sleep peacefully and deal with them tomorrow.

2   Sometimes our sleep is disturbed by an emotionally arousing disturbance, such as a phone call or a surprise intrusion. You need to come down from this state of limbic arousal—in other words, you need to get bored again. Try reading the most sleep-inducing book you can think of.

3   Get out of bed, leave the bedroom, and start a constructive but boring activity in subdued light. Getting up to a large dose of bright light will suppress melatonin production, which you don't want to happen. Associate your bed only with sleep.

4   Drink a cup of warm milk with honey.

5   Take a melatonin pill. They should be available in the United States by the time this book is published.

6   Check to make sure that your room is pitch-black; use wide, long, opaque shades that block out all light, or an eye mask.

7   Meditate.

8   If you can, simply enjoy resting.

Topic 7.12 Sleep and aging

The senior adult's sleep episodes (which can include more than one sleep cycle) are 20 percent shorter than those of younger people (6 vs. $7\frac{1}{2}$ hours), and the total time awake between initially going to sleep and getting up for good in the morning progresses gradually from around 1 percent in infancy to around 6 percent in seniors.

Applications

1   While some shortening of sleep requirements and some increase in sleep-time wakefulness is normal in senior adults, drastic changes are not. Look for pharmaceuticals, diet, illness, or lack of exercise as probable culprits.

2   Understand that you probably will not sleep as long and as continually at age seventy-five as you did at age twenty-five. Build a nap into your schedule and simply get up and do something constructive if you cannot sleep.

Understand that you probably will not sleep as long and as continually at age seventy-five as you did at age twenty-five.

Topic 7.13 Stability in sleep patterns

A study that related pilot error in landings to the interval between sleep periods (Webb, 1982) found that the more variable the interval between sleep periods, the more likely a pilot is to make an error in landing. In other words, for a five-day period, if pilot A is up for seventeen hours the first day, twelve the second, twenty the third, fifteen the fourth, and twenty-one the fifth, and pilot B is up for sixteen, eighteen, seventeen, eighteen, and sixteen hours on the same five days, pilot A will be more likely to make an error in landing (or other similar errors) than pilot B, whose intervals between sleep periods show less variation from day to day.

Application

Pilots, and others in jobs with major safety implications that require continuing alertness, should minimize the day-to-day variation in the number of hours between getting up and going to sleep.

Summary

Some of the major principles associated with getting to sleep are listed below:

Getting to sleep:
- Consume dairy products (the warmer the better).
- Avoid artificial sweeteners.
- Avoid food additives.
- Avoid caffeine within six hours of bedtime.
- Keep to a regular bedtime.
- Consume carbohydrates and fats.

- Avoid protein.
- Read or view unexciting material.
- Avoid exercise within four hours of bedtime.
- Sleep in absolute darkness (use a mask if necessary).
- Maintain quiet (use earplugs if necessary).
- Do not take naps after 3:00 P.M.
- Meditate.
- Take melatonin pills if they are available.

Getting quality sleep:
- Lose weight.
- Avoid alcohol within four hours of bedtime.
- Drink water after alcohol consumption.
- Plan sleep according to sleep cycles and circadian rhythms.
- Do aerobic exercise regularly, but not close to bedtime.

Getting back to sleep:
- Write down what's on your mind.
- Read something unexciting.
- Drink warm milk with honey.

Suggested readings on sleep

Arkin, A. M., Antrobus, J. S., and Ellman, S. J. (Eds.). (1978). *The Mind in Sleep.* Hillsdale, NJ: Lawrence Erlbaum.

Hobson, J. A. (1988). *The Dreaming Brain.* New York: Basic Books.

Webb, W. B. (Ed.). (1982). *Biological Rhythms, Sleep, and Performance.* Chichester, England: Wiley.

Webb, W. B. (1992). *Sleep: The Gentle Tyrant.* (2nd ed.). Bolton, MA: Anker.

A brain potpourri: From handedness

This chapter covers three subjects, none of which is lengthy enough to merit a chapter of its own: the significance of being left- or right-handed, the significance of exercise, and aspects of current research on disease as it relates to the brain-mind.

Topic 8.1 Handedness

About 10 percent of the population is left-handed, a proportion that appears to persist across generations, socioeconomic conditions, and race. Of these left-handers, 60 percent are male and 40 percent female. Handedness appears to be related both to our specific genetic inheritance (if both parents are left-handed, one out of two offspring is left-handed; if one parent is left-handed, one out of six offspring is; and if neither parent is left-handed, only one out of sixteen offspring is) and to the stress and trauma associated with pregnancy and birth (because the left brain is more sensitive to oxygen deprivation, functions such as handedness may be shifted to the right hemisphere, causing left-handedness).

Left-handedness is associated with right-brain qualities: lefties tend to be more creative and imaginative, better at visual-spatial tasks, and better at mathematics. Left-handedness is also associated with a higher accident and injury rate; left-handers have 20 percent more sports-related injuries, 25 percent more work-related accidents, a 49 percent higher risk of home accidents, a 54 percent

to headaches

higher risk while using tools, and an 85 percent higher risk while driving a car. This may explain why righties outlive lefties by five years (females) to ten years (males). Challenging these statistics, Stanley Coren (1992), of the University of British Columbia psychology department, says that they're based on the old days when lefties were forced to be right-handed; therefore, there are simply not as many left-handers proportionately among seniors today as there will be in several decades.

It's not easy being left-handed in a right-handed world! Interestingly, some parts of our environment favor left-handers. The standard qwerty keyboard, for example (*qwerty* stands for the sequence of letters on the left side of the top row), places the most frequently used letter, *e*, on the left side, as well as other highly popular typing letters: *a, r, t, s, d, c,* and *b*. Maybe that's why I (a rightie) have developed tendinitis in my left arm from keyboarding—I have to wear a brace on my left wrist when I'm going to be typing for more than thirty minutes.

> "Strength of mind is Exercise, not Rest."
>
> **Alexander Pope**

Applications

1   If you are left-handed, learn to shop for and use tools and equipment that are user-friendly for lefties. If you are responsible for buying things for lefties or training them, put yourself in their position before making purchasing decisions. Better yet, ask them! Too many of us make decisions affecting left-handers without assessing their strengths and weaknesses.

2 For further ideas and information, call or write:

Lefthanders International
P.O. Box 8249
Topeka, KS 66608
913-234-2177

This organization boasts thirty thousand members and publishes *Lefthander Magazine,* which is organized from back to front.

3 If you're a right-handed keyboarder, use a left-wrist brace to minimize stress on the left arm while keyboarding for long periods of time. You might also try using a Dvorak keyboard, in which the most frequently used keys are assigned to the strongest fingers, rather than a qwerty keyboard. If you're a leftie, stick with qwerty.

Topic 8.2 Exercise: Physical activity

Jean Pierre Changeux, of the Pasteur Institute in Paris, and Christopher Henderson have found that simple movement of the muscles stimulates the growth of axons, which carry messages between neurons. The number of axons is directly related to intelligence, and people (infants as well as adults) who move about more benefit from greater axonal development. Less movement results in fewer axons. Hence, the couch-potato syndrome is associated with lesser intelligence.

Applications

1 Move it or lose it.

2 Encourage physical activity from the cradle to the grave. Even people confined to wheelchairs or with limited mobility should move whatever they can. (contributed by Jane Howard)

Topic 8.3 Exercise: Aerobics

Bailey (1991) applies the term *aerobic* to exercise that meets four criteria:

1 It must be nonstop.
2 It must last for a minimum of twelve minutes.
3 It must proceed at a comfortable pace.
4 It must exercise the muscles of the lower body.

He defines "comfortable pace" with a formula: at the conclusion of exercising, your pulse should be 220 minus your age times 0.65 (or 0.8 for athletes). For me, that would mean a pulse of about 110. This formula is intended for the average person (about two-thirds of the population). For a more personal application of the formula, check pages 41–45 in Bailey (1991).

Mentally, aerobic exercise has at least three effects. First, it clearly improves speed of recall. It is not clear whether it has any effect on the quality of mental functioning or the amount of recall. Second, it releases endorphins, the neurotransmitters that relax us into a state of cortical alertness. This is not the only way to reach cortical alertness (other relaxation methods will work as well), but it is certainly one way. Third, as reported in a National Institute of Mental Health study of over nineteen hundred individuals, people with little or no recreational activity are twice as likely to have depressive symptoms as people who regularly do aerobic exercise.

Interestingly, Edwin Boyle, Jr., of the Miami Heart Institute, found that arteriosclerotic patients with memory loss improved their memory after breathing pure oxygen, with effects lasting up to six months! Aerobic exercise, of course, heightens oxygen intake.

Another series of studies concluded that hunger is inhibited when (1) the brain contains high levels of glucose and serotonin and (2) the blood contains high levels of epinephrine, norepinephrine, and dopamine. Exercise tends to raise levels of all five of these neurotransmitters.

> People with little or no recreational activity are twice as likely to have depressive symptoms as people who regularly do aerobic exercise.

Applications

1 Walk (or its equivalent—see Appendix C) for at least twenty minutes four times a week.

2 For maximum benefit, exercise *after* the most stressful part of the day is over and *before* a period in which mental alertness is required or desired. For some of us, this may have to be an either-or situation. Remember that high stress nullifies the effect of aerobic exercise. You must exercise again after a stressful episode.

3 Avoid exercising before bedtime, as it tends to interfere with sleep.

4 Don't ride when you can walk; don't sit when you can stand.

5 Learn deep-breathing exercises (breathe in for six counts, hold for four counts, expel for six counts) and isometric exercises for times when you must be sedentary for long periods.

A brain potpourri

Topic 8.4 Exercise: The importance of choice

Norman Cousins (1989) writes of studies that emphasize how choice influences the degree of health benefits of exercise. If an individual is forced to engage in an exercise against his or her will, the health benefits tend to be lessened. Cousins cites the ineffectiveness of his having been assigned to walk on a treadmill versus his dramatic improvement after he changed, by his choice, to walking on a track. Apparently the stress of engaging in exercise not of our choosing can outweigh its health benefits. As another example of this, my wife's first husband loved playing tennis, especially during hot summer afternoons. She hated it and often sustained headaches when she was pressured into playing with him. She still avoids tennis twelve years later. See Chapter Fourteen for further discussion of the importance of personal control in managing stress.

Application

Avoid engaging in an exercise for its health benefits if you don't really have a positive attitude toward it. Choose an exercise that appeals to you. I've had many friends try to encourage me to take aerobics classes. For me, personally, that is a distasteful proposition—I don't like the music many aerobics instructors use to motivate their participants. Instead, I walk. I love to walk. I could write an essay on why I like walking, but I'd better resist . . .

Topic 8.5 Exercise: Altering mood and cravings

In a study of sixteen addicted smokers and eighteen regular snackers, Robert Thayer (1989) reported that brisk ten-minute walks reduced their cravings and improved their mood. The walking smokers reported an average 50 percent increase over controls in time before craving a smoke. Those in a poor mood who walked instead of snacking reported significantly higher and longer elevations of mood over nonwalking snackers.

Applications

1   During prolonged sedentary periods or periods of stress, take a brisk ten-minute walk every couple of hours—outdoors, if possible.

2   During coffee breaks, try taking a ten-minute walk outside instead. The resulting natural arousal will equal or better the arousal you would get from more caffeine and stale office air. Walk by yourself or with a group, whichever pleases you.

Topic 8.6 Disease: Psychoneuroimmunology

Descartes's mind-body dualism has traditionally dominated medical thinking: adjust the body to fix a bodily problem and adjust the mind to fix a mental problem. However, recent research suggests that a single system exists in which mental symptoms (e.g., depression) can have either a mental cause (e.g., job loss, divorce, death of a close friend) or a bodily cause (e.g., excessive secretion of melatonin). This field is called psychoneuroimmunology (PNI); it is the study of the feedback loop, traced by Karen Bulloch of the University of California at San Diego, between the brain and the immune system—the lymphocytes (white blood cells residing in lymph), the thymus, the spleen, and marrow. In this system, lymphocytes attack and neutralize invaders, and natural killer cells (NKs) fight viruses and tumors.

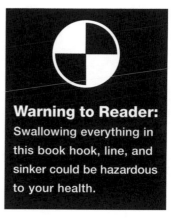

Warning to Reader: Swallowing everything in this book hook, line, and sinker could be hazardous to your health.

The loop works like this: the brain can emit chemicals under stress that depress the immune function, so that stress leads to disease, or the immune system can produce chemicals such as lymphokines in the thymus that can cause depression; in this case, disease leads to stress. Edwin Blalock, of the University of Alabama in Birmingham, discovered that the cells of the immune system can produce the same hormones as the brain, and that immune-system cells have the same receptors as brain cells. He says that immune cells act like a classic sensory organ, sending messages to the brain the way the eyes and ears do.

The original discovery of the mind's control over immune-cell levels was made by psychologist Robert Ader and immunologist Nicholas Cohen at the University of Rochester in the mid 1970s. They gave rats a saccharine solution, followed by an injection of cyclophosphamide, which induces nausea and reduces the immune function. Rats who continued drinking the saccharine solution without the cyclophosphamide injections showed a continuing drop in immune function. Ader gave the field its name: psychoneuroimmunology.

Increasing evidence suggests that emotional states affect the immune level. Sandra Levy of the Pittsburgh Cancer Institute found joy level to be the second-best predictor of survival time for patients with recurrent breast cancer. (The best predictor was the length of disease-free intervals.) She found that more than half of the fluctuation in the NK level could be attributed to psychological factors, including perceived social support and how the patient coped with stress. Other studies by Levy, Lydia Temoshok (University of California, San Francisco), and Carrie Millon (University of Miami School of Medicine) point to the high relationship between a patient's level of assertiveness and fighting spirit and his or her immune level. Temoshok studied men with AIDS and found that more assertive men had higher immune levels. Millon found that men infected with the AIDS virus had higher immune levels if they were narcissistic and strong-willed.

Ornstein and Sobel's *The Healing Brain* (1987) is a highly readable treatment of this subject. The authors relate amazing stories of the power of the mind's control over the body, including one experiment in which a placebo treatment had the equivalent pain-reducing ability of eight milligrams of morphine. They say that the brain is more of a pharmacy than a computer. Another interesting treatment is found in Norman Cousins's *Anatomy of an Illness* (1979, pp. 67–69), where he tells of the witch doctor in Albert Schweitzer's village. The two doctors had an arrangement to provide three levels of service to the villagers—bend, mend, and send. The witch doctor provided two levels: one for those with vague complaints such as stomach pain, which he treated by the traditional methods (e.g., *bending* the patient's spirits with incantations), and one for those with simple specific complaints such as cuts and bruises, which he and his assistants treated with modern first aid (e.g., *mending* with iodine). For the third level—complex specific complaints such as a broken leg—the villager was referred (*sent*) to Dr. Schweitzer.

The late Franz Ingelfinger, editor of the *New England Journal of Medicine,* wrote in his last article (Ingelfinger, 1980, p. 45) that he judged 85 percent of all human illnesses to be addressed by the immune system. Ever since Seneca, who wrote, "It is part of the cure to wish to be cured," people have debated the effect of the mind on the healing process. In fact, in many ways, this debate is at the core of cognitive science. Herbert Benson, of the Mind/Body Clinic of New England Deaconess Hospital in Boston, uses the relaxation response—the body's reaction to activities such as meditation and aerobic exercise—on patients with hypertension and reports that 80 percent are able to reduce either blood pressure or drug dosage. David C. McClelland of Boston University (McClelland, 1986, 1988) found salivary immunoglobin type A to be:

- Low among persons with a high need for power when they are stressed and out of control
- High among persons experiencing love
- High among persons who are temporarily experiencing positive emotion (as in watching a film of Mother Teresa)
- High among those with stronger senses of humor

Cousins (1989) is careful to explain that people should not abandon medical assistance in favor of exclusively concentrating on positive emotions to cure disease. He urges patients to accept medical diagnosis and treatment but to augment it by taking an active role in the healing process. He says that patients who don't deny the diagnosis but defy the verdict seem to do better than others (p. 45). This sense of "defying the verdict" is what Cousins means by "hardiness," discussed in Topic 13.2.

Your personal almanac

Applications

1 To ensure maximum functioning of your immune system during both sickness and health, maintain your sense of humor, have positive expectations (hope and trust in the medical processes), play an active role in the healing process, and stay relaxed, by removing or minimizing your stressors and dissipating stress when it occurs.

2 Several books about PNI are available for both caregivers and seriously ill patients. Start with Cousins (1989), LeShan (1989), Siegel (1987), and Simonton, Simonton, and Creighton (1980).

Increase the level of humor in your life.

3 Seek out doctors with a more holistic approach. (contributed by Rick Bradley)

4 Make a commitment for yourself and your close friends, family, and associates to be supportive of one another, spread good humor, and show appropriate optimism.

5 When faced by higher-than-expected levels of sickness at home or at work, look to stress as a possible cause. Identify the stressors and eliminate them as much as possible.

6 Encourage yourself to increase the level of humor in your life, both humor that you initiate (tell jokes, be witty, go to comedic plays and movies, be around funny people, read humorous books) and humor that you react to (let yourself belly-laugh, don't always hold back). Norman Cousins calls a good belly laugh "internal jogging."

7 Develop a sense that you are in control of your life and a fighting spirit that stays on the lookout for ways to improve your situation. Remember the Alcoholics Anonymous version of the Serenity Prayer: "God, grant me the serenity to accept the things I cannot change today, the courage to change the things I can today, and the wisdom to know the difference." To accept too much negativity in your life is to be personally responsible for lowering your own immune level. (See more on motivation in Chapters Thirteen through Fifteen.)

8 Kiecolt-Glaser and Glaser (1992) identify eight specific behavioral strategies for improving immune function:
   1 Aerobic exercise
   2 Relaxation
   3 Social support
   4 Learned control, such as biofeedback

5 Classical conditioning

6 Cognitive training

7 Therapy

8 Self-disclosure (talking or writing about one's problems)

Topic 8.7 Disease: Caregivers

Those who fall into the role of providing long-term care (e.g., to Alzheimer's patients) develop health problems of their own. The emotional and physical pressures associated with around-the-clock caregiving often lead to the kinds of diseases normally associated with prolonged stress. Periodic temporary relief that allows the caregiver to get away for a couple of hours at a time appears to minimize such health complications.

Applications

1 Two interventions have been found to be effective in helping caregivers maintain their immune level: teaching them relaxation and other stress-reduction methods and providing them with relief when they feel they need it, so they can get out and go to a movie, go shopping, or just walk.

2 If you are a caregiver, or if you know one, find a support group of people you can call on for short-term relief. Most cities have a clearinghouse that will put you in touch with providers of respite care. Don't be a martyr—it's not healthy.

3 See Topic 8.6, Application 2, for suggested readings.

Topic 8.8 Disease: Treatments for nervous system disorders

Progress is being made daily in finding pharmaceutical, surgical, and other interventions for the various nervous system disorders. Recent breakthroughs include:

- Sumatriptan for migraines
- Deprenyl and embryonic adrenal tissue transplants for Parkinson's disease
- Substance P, cycloserine, and monoclonal antibodies for Alzheimer's disease
- Bright lights, sleep deprivation (resetting the body's clock), and serotonin reuptake inhibitors (e.g., Prozac, tricyclics, and monoamine oxidase inhibitors) for depression
- Antidepressants such as Anafranil for obsessive-compulsive disorder, which is caused by a serotonin malfunction

- Benzodiazepines and buspirone for generalized anxiety
- Carbamazepine for manic depression
- Antidepressants and benzodiazepines for panic
- Nitric oxide for penile-erection problems
- Reducing serotonin levels to relieve suicide proneness
- Clozapine and risperidone for schizophrenia

As recently as the spring of 1992, Samuel Weiss and Brent Reynolds of the University of Calgary (Canada) Faculty of Medicine discovered reserves of immature brain cells in adult mice that could be coaxed into dividing into new cells. This phenomenon had been thought possible only in embryos. The implications for humans are now under study.

Applications

1   Don't accept the limitations of last year's prognosis. Your physician may or may not be completely up to date on treatment possibilities for a disorder of interest to you. Continue to do your own research and to consult with specialists.

2   Write for current information on disorders of interest to you. Obtain the addresses of specific foundations from your librarian.

3   Try coupling pharmaceutical treatment for nervous system disorders with some form of psychotherapy. Medicine seems to be more effective when it is accompanied by appropriate psychotherapy. In his book (Cavett, 1992), Dick Cavett tells how he recovered from depression through psychopharmacology combined with talking therapy.

> Don't accept the limitations of last year's prognosis.

Topic 8.9 Disease: Headaches

Gallagher (1990) provides a comprehensive treatment of types of headaches and their remedies. A few principles drawn from his book are appropriate:

- Most headaches can be limited or eliminated by pharmaceutical methods or by nonpharmaceutical methods such as diet or biofeedback.
- Most headaches are associated with vasoconstriction (tightening of the blood vessels).
- Vasoconstriction can be offset or prevented by limiting consumption of foodstuffs with tyramin, an amino acid believed to be associated with vasoconstriction. (See Table 8.1 for a list of migraine-precipitating foods.)

- Once a headache begins, dietary methods are ineffective—it's time for drugs.
- Menstrual migraines can be eliminated by finding the precipitating foods from the list in Table 8.1 and avoiding them starting several days before the onset of menses and continuing until it is over. One friend has successfully eliminated her menstrual migraines by cutting out sugar two to three days before the expected onset of menses, another friend by eliminating alcohol consumption two to three days before.
- For nonmenstrual migraines, one would simply eliminate a suspected food until a migraine occurred, then assume that the food wasn't the cause of the headache and eliminate another food.

Table 8.1 Migraine-precipitating foods

Meat and fish

Pickled herring
Chicken livers
Sausage
Salami
Pepperoni
Bologna
Hot dogs
Marinated meats
Aged, canned, or cured meats

Vegetables

Fava beans
Lima beans
Navy beans
Pea pods
Sauerkraut
Onions

Baked goods

Fresh baked breads
Sourdough

Fruits

Canned figs
Raisins
Papaya
Passion fruit
Avocado
Bananas
Red plums
Citrus fruit
(limit to $1/2$ cup per day)

Dairy

Aged and processed cheese
Yogurt (limit to $1/2$ cup per day)
Sour cream

Desserts

Chocolate

Beverages

Alcoholic
Caffeine
   (limit to 2 cups per day)
Chocolate milk
Buttermilk

Other

Soy sauce
MSG
Meat tenderizer
Seasoning salt
Canned soups
TV dinners
Garlic
Yeast extracts
Nuts

Note: From *Drug Therapy for Headache*, edited by R. Michael Gallagher, 1990, New York: Marcel Dekker. ©1991 by Marcel Dekker, Inc. Extracted from the National Headache Foundation Diet, Chicago, IL. Reprinted by permission.

Applications

1   Experiment: systematically eliminate different foods from the list in Table 8.1 before expected headaches. If a headache happens, resume that food and next time try eliminating another. Or try combinations of foods.

2   Consult with your physician for pharmaceutical assistance. If this produces no results, read Gallagher (1990) and discuss some of his recommendations with your physician.

3   For further information, call the National Headache Foundation at 800-843-2256.

Suggested readings on handedness, exercise, and disease

Bailey, C. (1991). *The New Fit or Fat*. Boston: Houghton Mifflin.

Coren, S. (1992). *The Left-Hander Syndrome: The Causes and Consequences of Left-Handedness*. New York: Free Press.

Cousins, N. (1979). *Anatomy of an Illness*. New York: W. W. Norton.

Cousins, N. (1989). *Head First: The Biology of Hope*. New York: Dutton.

Ornstein, R., and Sobel, D. (1987). *The Healing Brain*. New York: Simon & Schuster.

Part three

The brain and your personality:

Emotions, traits, and intelligence

The brain and your personality:

Emotions, traits, and intelligence

9

The nature-and-nurture debate:

I think it is appropriate, when we talk about personality issues, to recall Paul Valéry's comment: "Seeing is forgetting the name of the thing one sees." Valéry is talking about the tendency to substitute labels for the thing itself. He urges us to beware of labels. Labels originate at the point where a careful observer has arrived at a single word or phrase to express a complex set of attributes that is under observation. Those who come upon the label at a later time must choose whether to reexamine the attributes before accepting the label or to simply accept the label on faith. If the stakes are high, it pays to reexamine the real thing, rather than automatically accepting the label. Here are two simple examples:

1   I label my feelings for my wife as love, but rather than simply repeating "I love you" to convey my feelings, I should reexamine my behavior from time to time to see if it is still saying what I mean by love. The Neil Diamond song "You Don't Send Me Flowers Anymore" is evidence of a label that has lost touch with its origins.

2   A death occurred in a major medical center because of excessive trust in labels. An inaccurately labeled drug container was sent from the pharmacy to the operating room, and because of assumptions by a pharmacist's technician and a surgeon that the label was correct, a patient died. A closer look or whiff would have prevented this unnecessary loss of life.

The pendulum swings

But with this warning I must still insist that labels are a necessary shortcut. We simply do not have the time or energy to look freshly at everything; we must be selective. And the fact that our world is full of differences requires a language to talk about them. We could take pains to describe everyone we meet with the objective, descriptive detail of an anthropologist, but then we'd all have to be anthropologists. Indira Gandhi reportedly commented on the subject of diversity with the observation that an orchestra of one hundred violins does not hold our interest with anywhere near the power of the multi-instrument orchestra. Having acknowledged that we are different, let us proceed with learning a language to describe those differences.

Some (e.g., Mischel, 1968) complain that we should avoid the use of labels, maintaining that there are simply not enough labels to go around to describe the billions of people on the Earth. Others, such as Hans Eysenck (Eysenck, 1967, 1970, 1981; Eysenck & Eysenck, 1985), have defended the use of personality labels. In the study of color, we find 340,000 discriminable points, each of which can be defined as a unique intersection of the three variables of hue, tint, and saturation. Likewise, if we were to propose ten personality variables, each with ten degrees of variation, that would be sufficient to describe ten billion unique individuals. This is more than enough to label everyone presently on this planet with no need for repetition. Our labels will be words like *extravert* and *agreeable*.

> "Should one tell you that a mountain had changed its place, you are at liberty to doubt it; but if anyone tells you that a man has changed his character, do not believe it."
>
> **Muhammad**

Each label can vary in strength: just as we can have a 30 percent or 90 percent solution of hydrochloric acid, we also can have differing degrees of extraversion and agreeableness. One recent school of thought, as expressed in the literature surrounding the *Myers-Briggs Type Indicator* (Myers & McCaulley, 1985), has seen labels like *extravert* as bipolar—in other words, one either is or is not extraverted. I, and many of the researchers cited in this chapter, reject that dichotomization as simplistic and inadequate to describe the abundant diversity of our species.

The equalizer model

I hereby propose the "equalizer" model of personality description. You know what an equalizer is—a series of knobs that go up and down to create different qualities and quantities of sound production. Imagine a huge equalizer designed to create multisensory experiences. The machine would have five channels—Sight, Sound, Touch and Motion, Smell, and Taste—and each channel would have several component controls. Sight would have three components (hue, tint, and saturation); Sound four (pitch, rhythm, volume, and timbre); Touch and Motion six (shape, size, texture, temperature, direction, and speed); Smell seven (minty, floral, ethereal, musky, resinous, foul, and acrid); and Taste four (salty, sweet, sour, and bitter). See Ackerman (1990) for a readable and complete description of the senses.

Figure 9.1

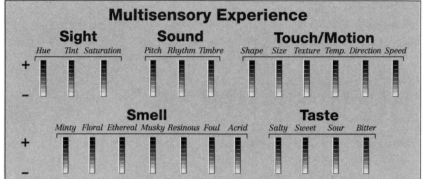

An equalizer for multisensory experiences. Every multisensory experience can be described by determining the point on each scale that fits the experience.

Some of the components might be subdivided further; for example, shape could be divided into curve, length, and other subcomponents. By varying the control knobs, we could create a specific multisensory experience, such as "having wine and cheese in the late afternoon at an outdoor café on the Champs-Elysées." If we were to add another channel—Language—we could even have conversation in the background and foreground. The illustration in Figure 9.1 tries to capture such an equalizer.

Now take the same idea and apply it to personality. The channels would be Intelligence–Domains, Intelligence–Components, Traits, Values, and Motivators. Each channel would have components: Intelligence–Domains would have seven (linguistic, musical, logical and mathematical, spatial, interpersonal, kinesthetic, and intrapersonal); Intelligence–Components would have three (production, creativity, and problem solving); Traits would have five (resilience, extraversion, openness, agreeableness, and conscientiousness), each with six different subcomponents; Values would have six (spiritual, aesthetic, financial, physical, social, and political); and Motivators would have three (personalization, pervasiveness, and permanence). The illustration in Figure 9.2 tries to capture this personality equalizer.

The difference in the two equalizers is crucial: while the multisensory-experience machine is hooked up to wires, microchips, lights, and amplifiers, the personality equalizer is hooked up to the central nervous system, the circulatory system, the endocrine system, and the muscular-skeletal system, all of which, in turn, are hooked up to the external environment. This invites a logical question—to what degree are we free as individuals to modify the position of our knobs? Or, as parents, teachers, therapists, managers, or friends, to what degree can we modify the position of the knobs of our children, spouses, students, patients, subordinates (and bosses!), and friends? That leads us to a discussion on the genetics of personality.

Figure 9.2

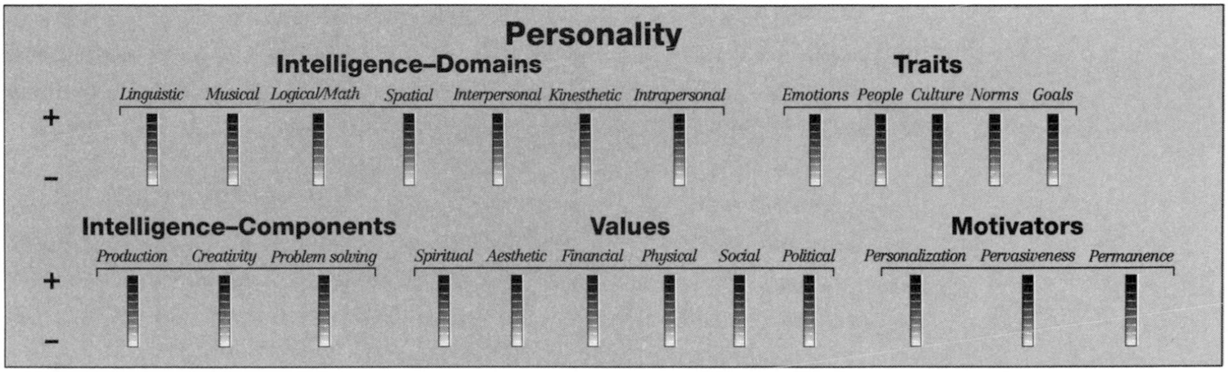

An equalizer model of personality. Each person can be described by reference to points on each of the scales of the equalizer.

The evidence for a genetic basis of personality
Consider the following cases, which show evidence of the heritability of behavior in organisms as simple as single-celled planaria and as complex as humans.

Planaria
In the dark corners of the biology lab, a young research assistant exposed a batch of planaria in a petri dish to a flash of light. He immediately followed this with an electric shock. The planaria "scrunched up," in an attempt to protect themselves from the shock. After several repetitions of the light-shock-scrunch sequence, the assistant discontinued the shocks. The planaria, now conditioned to associate the light flash with the shock, scrunched up as soon as the light flashed. Smart cells!

The research assistant proceeded to phase 2. The trained planaria were ground into a slurry, which was fed to a new group of planaria who had been exposed to neither shocks nor flashes. After this group had "digested" the slurry, the curious research assistant flashed the light on them. They scrunched up! Ingesting the genetic material of trained planaria was as good as having received the training directly.

Honey Bees

"Foul brood" is an infectious disease of honey bees that afflicts larvae in the cells of their honeycomb. Certain hygienic strains of bees fight the disease by locating cells with the disease, opening the wax cap, removing the larvae, and moving them out of the hive. W. C. Rothenbuhler (Dawkins, 1989) discovered that the behavior of the hygienic bees was governed by two distinct genes—one gene for uncapping the cell and a second gene for dragging out and disposing of the diseased larva. Unless both genes were present in a worker bee, the hygienic behavior didn't happen. If a bee possessed only the uncapping gene, it would gleefully fill its day uncapping the disease-containing cells but would not remove the afflicted larvae. Alone, without any of the uncapping bees around, bees with the removal gene would do nothing. However, if Rothenbuhler himself removed the wax caps, these removal bees would gladly spend their days dragging diseased larvae out of the hive. (This reminds me of a friend who loved to wash dishes: when we went camping with the Boy Scouts, I would always cook, and he would always wash. He didn't cook, and I didn't wash.)

Genetics plays a far more significant role than was thought up to now.

Male children

Two days after their birth, a group of male children were circumcised. Some would cry from pain and stress, while the others would contentedly suck on their pacifiers. Donald Cohen (Neubauer & Neubauer, 1990) concluded that, because these different behaviors occurred so soon after birth with no opportunity for parental influence, the two extremes of vulnerable and invulnerable behavior were genetically determined.

Twins

Citing material from twin studies in Minnesota, Britain, Scandinavia, and Australia, researchers (Neubauer & Neubauer, 1990; Eaves, Eysenck, & Martin, 1989; Tellagen et al., 1988) are coming to the unavoidable conclusion that genetics plays a far more significant role than was thought up to now. Most researchers currently studying this nature-nurture relationship are calling it a fifty-fifty ratio, attributing half the variation in behavior to genetics and half to environmental influence. For example, if your IQ is 20 points above the mean, or about 120, then roughly 10 of the points are attributable to genetic influence and the other 10 to environmental influence. The general conclusion of most behavioral genetics researchers, however, is that environmental influence serves as an enhancer or preventer of genetic predispositions and, therefore, that environment can't create dispositions for which no genetic basis exists. This current research is a confirmation of the ancient saw that you can't make a silk purse from a sow's ear.

Just how do twin studies lead us to this conclusion? Monozygotic, or identical, twins, who develop from one single egg, have identical genetic coding. Some sets of twins are separated from one another at birth—for example, they may be given up for adoption, with one twin moving to California, the other to Georgia. Other pairs grow up together. To the degree that environmental influences shape behavior, identical twins reared together would be expected to be more similar than those reared apart. That, however, is not the case; the similarity between identical twins does not increase if they are reared together. Separated identical twins show strong similarities, even including religious feelings and vocational preferences. Neubauer and Neubauer (1990, pp. 20–21) relate two striking examples of this persistence of genetic material:

1   Two monozygotic twin girls were separated at birth and placed in homes far apart. About four years later, researchers interviewed the adoptive parents of each girl. The parents of Shauna said, "She is a terrible eater— won't cooperate, stubborn, strong-willed. I can't get her to eat *anything* unless I put cinnamon on it." The parents of Ellen said, "Ellen is a lovely child—cooperative and outgoing." The researcher probed, asking, "How are her eating habits?" The response was: "Fantastic—she eats anything I put before her, as long as I put cinnamon on it!" (p. 20).

2   Two monozygotic twin boys were separated at birth and placed in homes far apart. They were interviewed twenty-seven years later. Both had turned out to be obsessive-compulsive neatniks, scrubbing their separate homes frequently and constantly picking up and making things neat and clean. When they were asked to explain their compulsion for neatness, one attributed it to his reaction to an adoptive parent who was a slob, while the other attributed it to his upbringing by an adoptive parent who was a neatnik!

Topic 9.1 Inherited personality traits

Neubauer and Neubauer (1990, pp. 38 ff.) write of the research on genetic origins of personality traits. Among the traits for which strong evidence of an inherited basis exists are the following (see Topic 3.9 for information on the heritability of sexuality):

- Aggressiveness
- Alcoholism (see Topic 6.1)
- Autism
- Depression
- Empathy
- Engageability (aggressive pursuit of one's needs)
- Excitability
- Imagination
- Language facility

The nature-and-nurture debate   **125**

- Leadership
- Maturation rate
- Obsessions
- Person-versus-object orientation
- Quickness to anger

- Shyness
- Susceptibility to addiction
- Traditionalism
- Vulnerability to stress
- Weakness of will

Continuing research is aimed at determining both the makeup and the degree of heritability of personality factors: which factors seem to be especially influenced genetically, and to what degree. Among the environmental factors that Neubauer and Neubauer identify as tending to have the most impact on personality development are:

- The quality and quantity of language the child is exposed to
- The amount of play the child has
- Expressed affection
- Availability of toys
- The presence of parents
- The presence of other children
- The natural expression of emotion in the household
- Intellectual expectations (riddles, questions, problem solving, etc.)
- Control, limits, and discipline (deprivation and excess have a negative effect)

In summary, genetics would appear to be like a flower, with environment more like fertilizer, rain, or soil. Or, as Neubauer and Neubauer say, genes appear to set limits for the range of development. They are not a blueprint that fully defines the final product; instead, they establish the range of possible variation.

Applications

1   As a parent, you can only do what your informed judgment suggests is appropriate. Realize that some traits will emerge in your offspring that you do not share. To deny the validity of these traits can lead to guilt and frustration on both your part and your child's. Develop the habit of taking your child's strengths and helping them develop. As Goethe wrote: "That which he has inherited has been made his own."

2   If you are a therapist, manager, coach, or other "people developer," you will find that the people you deal with will exhibit some traits that relate well to a job they are trying to do and some that do not. It is reasonable to hold people accountable for their relevant strengths, but it is unreasonable to browbeat them for their weaknesses. For example, if you coach a boy's basketball team and a player shoots well but shies away from the responsibility of calling plays, work on his shooting. Don't make him play point guard and browbeat him for not being more of a playmaker. If you must make him play point guard, praise his shooting and be knowingly supportive of his efforts to make plays. Say, "I know that playing you at point guard is not using your strengths to your advantage, but for now you're the best person for the job. I won't expect you to perform as well as you do as a shooting guard, but I will support you in every way that I can to make the best of the circumstances."

3 In hiring or choosing a person to do a job, make the selection on the basis of relevant strengths. Don't make the mistake of choosing employees because their credentials are generally impressive; hire them because their credentials are job-related. For example, a common mistake is to hire a creative, innovative person for a routine job. This will lead to a higher-than-necessary error rate and eventual turnover. If you must hire a creative person to do a routine job, make sure you both know that the routine job is only temporary and that a better job fit will come soon. Then manage the employee with understanding and support in the routine job. Say, "We both need to be aware that the time you spend as a bank teller will be boring much of the time, and as a result, you will be more error-prone than other tellers. Let's figure out what we can do to minimize error and keep you motivated during this rotation. When your next assignment comes along, your creativity will be more challenged. But for now, let's figure out a survival strategy."

Don't try to change people. Learn to build on what they are and compensate for what they are not.

4 As a general rule, don't try to change people. Learn to build on what they are and compensate for what they are not. I'll never love the chore of managing family finances, but I've made it bearable by figuring out a way to make it more interesting. I've done this by learning a computer program. I know people who have entered into marriage with the confidence that they would ultimately be able to change the less desirable traits of their future spouse. This typically leads to frustration and resentment as the change strategies prove to be ineffectual.

5 Don't confuse personality traits with learnable skills. There are many bodies of knowledge and specific skills that I could learn if I wanted to. In that respect, you could "change" me by teaching me a skill or a body of knowledge. But that learning doesn't mean that a personality trait will change as a result. I have an architect friend who once hated to make presentations before groups. He is an introverted, idea-focused person. He knew he would never love presentations, but he decided he would at least be good at it. He took Ty Boyd's public seminar and learned the skills involved in making effective presentations. Now he gets good marks for his presentations, even though he still doesn't like doing them and prefers being creative in the privacy of his office. But he is less anxious about his presentations because he knows the tricks of the trade.

6 With respect to adopted children, Eysenck and Kamin (1981, p. 51) write, "At no time do adopted children and foster parents correlate more than .10, and adopted children do not grow to resemble their adopting parents." I have friends who have taken it hard that their incorrigible adopted children haven't developed the kind of loving, nurturing, thoughtful behaviors the adopting parents have shown them. This should not be seen as a personal failure. The parents should continue to provide support and encourage skill and social development, but they need to encourage their adopted children to build on their strengths, rather than trying to force them into a path alien to their nature.

Topic 9.2 Genetics and disease

Figure 9.3

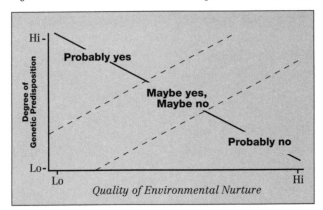

The nature-nurture paradigm for incidence of genetically based disease.

Figure 9.3 illustrates the relationship between environmental nurture and genetic predisposition for genetically based diseases. Generally, the relationship is interactive—the better the nurture and the lower the genetic predisposition, the better the chances are of not contracting a genetically based disease. The poorer the nurture and the higher the predisposition, the better the chances are of contracting the disease. High nurture combined with a high predisposition and low nurture combined with a low predisposition are each more of a toss-up—high nurture will not guarantee suppression, and low nurture will not guarantee expression of a genetically predisposed disease.

Applications

1 The best nurture can only minimize the chances of avoiding a disease toward which you are genetically predisposed. When you contract a disease following good nurture, assume a genetic predisposition; don't feel as if the nurture was somehow inadequate. Continued good nurture will facilitate recovery. (See Topic 8.6 for a related discussion of psychoneuroimmunology.)

2 Conversely, don't assume that avoiding a disease is the result of excellent nurture; you may simply be genetically resistant.

Suggested readings on nature, nurture, and personality

Dawkins, R. (1989). *The Selfish Gene.* (2nd ed.). Oxford: Oxford University Press.

Eaves, L. J., Eysenck, H. J., & Martin, N. G. (1989). *Genes, Culture and Personality.* London: Academic Press.

Neubauer, P. B., & Neubauer, A. (1990). *Nature's Thumbprint: The New Genetics of Personality.* Reading, MA: Addison-Wesley.

10

Are personality traits for real?

Do personality traits really exist? It is beyond the scope of this book to present the many points of view on this topic. I encourage you to begin with Walter Mischel's *Personality and Assessment* (1968) for a well-reasoned warning against the use of traits. Mischel's argument runs something like this: Say that procrastination is offered as a trait. Well, there are literally thousands of situations in which we may or may not procrastinate: mailing holiday gifts, depositing paychecks, cooking dinner, reading a professional book, scheduling a physical examination, writing a letter . . . The list could go on indefinitely. In addition, each item on the list could be subdivided: procrastinating at cooking dinner for unwanted guests, for our boss, for our lover, and so on. And even these could be subdivided: procrastinating at cooking dinner for our lover when a breakoff is desired, when we want to impress our lover with culinary flamboyance, when we want the chance to work closely together in the kitchen, when we hope that cooking will be abandoned in favor of dining out, or when we hope that if there is no food it will lead to quicker sex—with food following! What Mischel means to say is that people act differently in different situations and never (well, hardly ever) exhibit a single behavior in every possible situation that could elicit it. Therefore, says Mischel, to label someone a procrastinator (here we go with labels again) is not only irresponsible; it is impossible to prove. We would have to enumerate thousands of situations,

The Big-Five model

with subdivisions, in order to say with confidence that a person is a procrastinator. Personality tests that attempt to measure the degree of a person's tendency toward a particular trait only ask a sample of ten to fifteen questions out of the universe of tens of thousands in order to make a statement like "Fran Doe is a procrastinator about 82 percent of the time." Says Mischel: "Poppycock!"

I and others who argue for the existence of personality traits, which are also called temperaments (see Buss, 1989, for an excellent summary), will grant that it is risky to use a dozen or so questionnaire items to form a conclusion about the degree of a particular temperament in a person. However, we can minimize that risk by careful selection, choosing only questions that all people can identify with in some way, such as "People tell me that they can depend on me to finish things when I say I will." In addition, by presenting two statements and asking which is more like the person most of the time (e.g., "I am late to many appointments" and "I enjoy parties with lots of people"), we can ask the respondent to subjectively rewind the tape of his or her recent life and form a judgment as to which statement is a better fit. By using carefully selected items and question formats, we can obtain valid and reliable estimates concerning how a person will tend to respond across situations that invite behaviors related to a particular temperament.

> "If there be light, then there is darkness; if cold, then heat; if height, depth also; if solid, then fluid; hardness and softness; roughness and smoothness; calm and tempest; prosperity and adversity; life and death."
>
> **Pythagoras**

A history of temperament theory

Western civilization has operated under the paradigm of four personality temperaments since the early Greeks enumerated the four elements of air, fire, earth, and water, along with their associated personality traits (see Kuhn, 1970, for a discussion of paradigms). The fixedness of this paradigm in the minds of Western thinkers is evident in Table 10.1, which lists the various manifestations of the four temperaments over the last several thousand years. I have tried to group the four labels from each source in the column with which, in my opinion, each seems most closely linked.

Table 10.1 The four temperaments from early Greece to the present

Source	Air	Fire	Earth	Water
Mythology	Apollo	Hermes	Zeus	Dionysus
Hippocrates	Phlegmatic	Melancholic	Sanguine	Choleric
The Elizabethans (Also Galen & Wundt)	Phlegmatic	Melancholic	Sanguine	Choleric
Native American	East/Eagle	West/Bear	South/Squirrel	North/Buffalo
Herrmann (1989)	Cerebral left	Cerebral right	Limbic left	Limbic right
Lefton, Buzzotta, & Sherberg (1985)	Q2, Submissive-Hostile	Q1, Dominant-Hostile	Q3, Submissive-Warm	Q4, Dominant-Warm
Hersey & Blanchard (1976)	S-1, Telling	S-4, Delegating	S-2, Selling	S-3, Participating
LIFO[a] (Atkins, 1978)	Conserving/Holding	Adapting/Dealing	Controlling/Taking	Supporting/Giving
AVA[b] (Clark, 1956)	V3, Stability	V4, Structure	V1, Dominance	V2, Sociability
DISC[c] (Marston, 1987)	Dominance	Influence	Steadiness	Compliance
Keirsey & Bates (1978)	Troubleshooter	Visionary	Traditionalist	Catalyst
Social Styles (Merrill & Reid, 1981)	Analytic	Expressive	Driver	Amiable
Jung (1971)	Thinker	Intuitor	Sensor	Feeler
MBTI[d] (Myers & McCaulley, 1985)	Extravert/Introvert	Sensor/Intuitor	Thinker/Feeler	Judger/Perceiver
Kolbe (1990)	Follow through	Quick start	Implementor	Fact finder

[a] LIFO = life orientations.
[b] AVA = activity vector analysis.
[c] DISC = dominance, influence, steadiness, compliance.
[d] MBTI = *Myers-Briggs Type Indicator*.

This four-factor model of temperament still persists. The most compelling argument to support it is made in Hans Eysenck's *The Structure of Human Personality* (1970). Eysenck presents the psychological dimensions of extraversion

Figure 10.1

and neuroticism as the basis of the four-factor model (Figure 10.1). Each of the two dimensions forms an axis of a two-by-two grid, with the vectors that emerge from each of the four quadrants defining the four temperaments. But even Eysenck's work shows this four-factor model breaking down. In subsequent writings (Eysenck & Kamin, 1981; Eysenck & Eysenck, 1985), he portrays three dimensions (the third being psychoticism) and their various combinations.

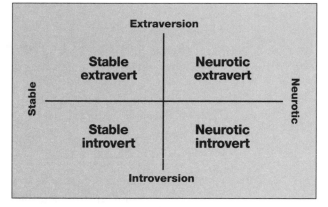

Eysenck's four-factor model.

Consensus appears to be emerging in the community of personality scholars that five, not four, factors best account for the broad categories of variability in human personality. As early as 1963, W. T. Norman defined these five factors based on his careful factor analysis as Emotional Stability, Extraversion, Culture, Agreeableness, and Conscientiousness (see Topic 10.1). An excellent summary of the research leading up to the definitions of what we now know as the Big Five, or the Five-Factor Model, can be found in John, Angleitner, and Ostendorf (1988). Digman and Inouye (1986, p. 116) summarize this trend in personality research as follows: "A series of research studies of personality traits has led to a finding consistent enough to approach the status of law. The finding is this: If a large number of rating scales is used and if the scope of the scales is very broad, the domain of personality descriptors is almost completely accounted for by five robust factors."

It is interesting to note an increasing convergence of Eastern and Western intellectual traditions. My introduction to this convergence was back in the 1960s when I read the works of F.S.C. Northrop—*The Logic of the Sciences and Humanities* (1947) and *The Meeting of East and West* (1946)—and, more recently, when I read Fritjof Capra's *The Tao of Physics* (1984). Now, while writing this chapter, I am reading Daniel Reid's *The Tao of Health, Sex, and Longevity* (1989), in which Reid argues for the Eastern view of five elements (*wu-hsing*)—wood, fire, earth, metal, and water. He proceeds to show how all of human existence, according to the Tao masters, is organized around these five elements, not the four of Western intellectual tradition. Can you sense the paradigm shifting underfoot?

The most important difference between the four-factor model as measured by the *Myers-Briggs Type Indicator* (*MBTI*) (Myers & McCaulley, 1985) and the Five-Factor Model is that the *MBTI* provides no direct measure of the first factor, Emotions (Norman's Emotional Stability, Costa & McCrae's Neuroticism).

Yet, after Extraversion, it is the most extensively documented factor. McCrae and Costa (1989) have written an excellent article explaining the differences in the two models.

Topic 10.1 The Big Five

The most popular version of the Big Five is the one developed by Costa and McCrae (1992). The five dimensions are labeled Resilience, Extraversion, Openness, Agreeableness, and Conscientiousness.

The Resilience dimension

The Resilience dimension of the Five-Factor Model is really about one's degree of experience with negative emotions. At one extreme we have the *Sedate*, who tends to experience life on a more rational level than most people and who sometimes appears rather impervious to his or her surroundings. I think, for example, of my choir director, who didn't miss a beat during a dress rehearsal when the podium on which he was standing collapsed forward. He simply placed his feet at an angle like a snowplow and kept his baton moving. Of course, all the singers and instrumentalists broke out laughing at this classic example of nonre-activity. He's unflappable. This extreme is also the foundation for many valuable social roles—from air traffic controllers and airline pilots to military snipers, financial managers, and engineers.

On the other extreme, we have the *Reactive*, who experiences more negative emotions than most people and who reports less satisfaction with life than most people do. This is not meant to place a value judgment on Reactives, however; a susceptibility to negative emotions and discontent with life provide the basis for filling extremely important roles in our society, such as social scientists and academicians.

Along the continuum from Reactive to Sedate is the *Responsive*, who has a mixture of the qualities of both the Sedate and the Reactive. Responsives are more able to turn behaviors from both extremes on and off, according to what seems appropriate to the situation. Typically, however, a Responsive cannot maintain the calmness of a Sedate for as long a period of time or sustain the nervous edge of alertness of a Reactive (as, for example, would be typical of a stock trader during a session).

The Extraversion dimension

The Extraversion dimension is about the degree of one's preference for being actively engaged with other people. On one hand, the *Extravert* tends to exert more leadership, to be more physically and verbally active, and to be more friendly and outgoing around others than most people. This extraverted profile is the foundation of many important social roles, such as salespeople, politicians, artists, and social scientists.

On the other hand, the *Introvert* tends to be more independent, reserved, steady, and comfortable being alone than are most people. This introverted profile is the basis of such varied and important social roles as production managers and physical and natural scientists.

In between these two extremes is the *Ambivert,* who is able to move comfortably from outgoing social situations to the isolation of working alone. The stereotypical Ambivert is the player-coach, who moves easily from the leadership demands of a coach to the personal production demands of a player.

The Openness dimension

The Openness dimension refers to the degree to which a person is curious about his or her inner and outer worlds. On one hand, the *Explorer* has broader interests, is fascinated by novelty and innovation, would generally be perceived as liberal, and reports more introspection and reflection. Explorers are not unprincipled, but they tend to be open to considering new approaches. The Explorer profile forms the basis for such important social roles as entrepreneurs, architects, change agents, artists, and theoretical scientists (social and physical).

The *Preserver* has narrower interests, is perceived as more conventional, and is more comfortable with the familiar. Preservers are thought of as being more conservative, but not necessarily more authoritarian. The Preserver profile is the basis for such important social roles as financial managers, performers, project managers, and applied scientists.

In the middle of the continuum lies the *Moderate.* Moderates can explore the novel with interest when necessary but consider too much novelty to be tiresome; on the other hand, they can focus on the familiar for extended periods of time, but eventually develop a hunger for novelty.

This trait does not relate to intelligence—Explorers and Preservers both score well on traditional measures of intelligence. Instead, it helps to define creativity, since openness to new experience is an important ingredient of creativity.

The Agreeableness dimension

The Agreeableness dimension is a measure of altruism versus egocentrism. At one end of the continuum, the *Adapter* tends to subordinate personal needs to those of the group and to accept the group's norms rather than insisting on his or her personal norms. Harmony is more important to the Adapter than, for example,

The strereotypical Ambivert is the player-coach, who moves easily from the leadership demands of a coach to the personal production demands of a player.

broadcasting a personal notion of truth. Galileo, in recanting his Copernican views before the Inquisition, behaved like an Adapter. The Adapter profile is the core of such important social roles as teachers, social workers, and psychologists.

At the other end of the continuum, the *Challenger* is more focused on his or her personal norms and needs rather than on those of the group. The Challenger is more concerned with acquiring and exercising power. Challengers follow the beat of their own drum, rather than getting in step with the group. The Challenger profile is the foundation of such important social roles as advertising executives, managers, and military leaders.

In the middle of the continuum is the *Negotiator,* who is able to move from leadership to followership as the situation demands. Psychoanalyst and author Karen Horney (1945) described the two extremes of this trait as "moving toward people" (Adapter) and "moving against people" (Challenger). In the extreme, tender-minded Adapters become dependent personalities who've lost their sense of self; tough-minded Challengers become narcissistic, antisocial, authoritarian, or paranoid personalities who've lost their sense of fellow feeling. In one sense, this trait is about the dependence, or altruism, of the Adapter, the independence, or egocentrism, of the Challenger, and the interdependence, or situationalism, of the Negotiator.

The Conscientiousness dimension

The Conscientiousness dimension concerns self-control in the service of one's will to achieve. On one hand, the *Focused* person exhibits high self-control, resulting in a consistent focus on personal and occupational goals. In its normal state, this trait is characterized by academic and career achievement, but when it turns extreme, it results in workaholism. Focused people are difficult to distract. This profile is the basis for such important social roles as leaders, executives, and, in general, high achievers.

On the other hand, the *Flexible* person is more easily distracted, less focused on goals, more hedonistic, and generally more lax with respect to goals. Flexibles are easily seduced from the task at hand by a passing idea, activity, or person; that is, they have weak control over their impulses. They do not necessarily work less than Focused people, but less of their total work effort is goal-directed. Flexibility facilitates creativity, inasmuch as people remain open to possibilities longer without feeling driven to closure and moving on. This profile is the core of such important social roles as researchers, detectives, and consultants.

Toward the middle of this continuum is the *Balanced* person, who finds it easier to move from focus to laxity, from production to research. Balanced people would make ideal managers for either a group of Flexibles or a group of

Focused people because they have some of both qualities. They can keep Flexibles reasonably on target without alienating them, and they can keep Focused people cautious enough to prevent them from jumping to conclusions and relaxed enough to prevent them from suffering a coronary.

Summary

The five dimensions fit onto a bipolar continuum, which is a progression with graduated changes between two extreme and contrasting characteristics. For example, temperature is a bipolar continuum that is defined by the two extremes of hot and cold. I generally report a person's profile by placing the five scores in one of three zones in each bipolar continuum: high, medium, and low. A Big Five Feedback Form is included as Appendix D. Table 10.2 shows the Big Five traits with anchor words that describe extreme scorers. Midrange descriptors would consist of relatively equal anchors from each of the two extremes. For example, extreme extraverts are usually talkative and sociable and extreme introverts are usually quiet and private, while ambiverts might see themselves as equally talkative and private.

Table 10.2 The Big Five personality dimensions with anchors for extreme scorers				
Factor	**Resilience**	**Extraversion**	**Openness**	**Agreeableness**	**Conscientiousness**
High score	Sedate	Extravert	Explorer	Adapter	Focused
	High-score descriptors				
	Content	Sociable	Curious	Accepting	Productive
	Controlled	Optimistic	Liberal	Team player	Decisive
	Secure	Talker	Variety-seeking	Trusting	Organized
	Stress-free	Happy	Dreamer	Agreeable	Dependable
Midscore	**Responsive**	**Ambivert**	**Moderate**	**Negotiator**	**Balanced**
	Low-score descriptors				
	Tense	Reserved	Efficient	Questioning	Spontaneous
	Alert	Writing	Practical	Competitive	Chaotic
	Fast	Private	Conservative	Self-interested	Permissive
	Anxious	Inhibited	Habits	Direct	Unfocused
Low score	**Reactive**	**Introvert**	**Preserver**	**Challenger**	**Flexible**

Application

Two tests are commercially available for measuring the Big Five: the *NEO Five Factor Inventory* and the *NEO-PI-R* (Costa & McCrae, 1992). The first is shorter (60 questions) and is self-scoring. The second is longer (240 questions) and provides six "facet" scores for each of the five factors, for a total of thirty-five scores (five factors and thirty facets of these factors). The longer test has self-scoring and computer-scoring versions.

Topic 10.2 Facets of the Big Five

In developing a test to measure the Big Five, Costa and McCrae (1992) have found six facets that help in defining each of the five factors; they are listed in Table 10.3.

Table 10.3 The facets of the Big Five personality traits

Resilience	Extraversion	Openness	Agreeableness	Conscientiousness
Calmness	Warmth	Fantasy	Trust	Competence
Even temperament	Gregariousness	Aesthetics	Straightforwardness	Order
Contentment	Assertiveness	Feelings	Altruism	Dutifulness
Poise	Activity	Actions	Compliance	Achievement-striving
Self-control	Excitement-seeking	Ideas	Modesty	Self-discipline
Hardiness	Positive emotions	Values	Tender-mindedness	Deliberation

Note: From the *NEO Personality Inventory: Revised Professional Manual* by P. T. Costa, Jr., and R. R. McCrae, 1992, Odessa, FL: Psychological Assessment Resources. © 1978, 1985, 1989, 1992 by PAR, Inc. Reprinted by permission of Psychological Assessment Resources, Inc., Odessa, FL 33556. Further reproduction is prohibited without permission of PAR, Inc.

Complete definitions of the thirty facets are available in Costa and McCrae (1992). Here are brief definitions:

Resilience facets:

R1 *Calmness.* The absence of worry and fear about how things will turn out.

R2 *Even temperament.* How slowly one comes to feel anger and bitterness.

R3 *Contentment.* One's resistance to sad and hopeless feelings.

R4 *Poise.* Keeping cool in awkward public situations.

R5 *Self-control.* The tendency to resist temptation.

R6 *Hardiness.* One's resistance to panic in emergency or stressful situations.

Extraversion facets:

E1 *Warmth.* One's capacity for affection, friendliness, and cordiality.

E2 *Gregariousness.* A preference for being around other people.

E3 *Assertiveness.* The tendency to express oneself forcefully and without reluctance.

E4 *Activity.* Level of energy; the tendency toward a fast-paced life-style.

E5 *Excitement-seeking.* An appetite for the thrills of bright colors and noisy settings.

E6 *Positive emotions.* One's capacity for laughter, joy, and love; optimism; happiness.

Openness facets:

O1 *Fantasy.* The ability to create an interesting inner world through imagination and fantasy.

O2 *Aesthetics.* A wide and deep appreciation for art and beauty; sensitivity.

O3 *Feelings.* The ability to value and experience a wide range of positive and negative emotions.

O4 *Actions.* A preference for novelty and variety over the routine and familiar.

O5 *Ideas.* Intellectual curiosity; openness to new and unconventional ideas.

O6 *Values.* The willingness to examine social, political, and religious values; lack of dogmatism.

Agreeableness facets:

A1 *Trust.* The tendency to regard others as honest and well intentioned; lack of skepticism.

A2 *Straightforwardness.* Proneness to candor and frankness; tendency not to be deceptive or manipulative.

A3 *Altruism.* Generosity, consideration, willingness to help others.

A4 *Compliance.* Proneness to submit to the will of others; cooperativeness as opposed to competitiveness; inhibition of aggressive feelings.

A5 *Modesty.* Humility; lack of arrogance or narcissism.

A6 *Tender-mindedness.* The ability to feel concern, pity, and sympathy for others.

Conscientiousness facets:

C1 *Competence.* The tendency to feel prepared and capable; high self-esteem; an internal locus.

C2 *Order.* A tendency to feel well organized and methodical; neatness; a tendency toward compulsiveness.

C3 *Dutifulness.* Strict adherence to one's conscience; reliability.

C4 *Achievement-striving.* The ability to set high goals and focus on them; a tendency toward workaholism.

C5 *Self-discipline.* The capacity to motivate oneself to get the job done and resist distractions.

C6 *Deliberation.* The ability to think something through before acting on it.

Applications

1 Remember that pure personality traits do not exist. For example, while extraverts usually exhibit dominance, sometimes they don't, and sometimes introverts do. The five families of traits are merely an attempt to capture the more frequently occurring combinations of subtraits. This sort of classification is helpful in understanding trends and probabilities, but we must always look freshly at individuals to see where they differ from the norm.

2 In using personality traits as an aid for team building and group development, it is important to understand that there is no one right way to be. The task is to understand how best to use what you have learned about personalities to help you get work done more effectively. Most groups need to be cautioned about teasing one another when they first encounter differing personality traits.

Topic 10.3 Relationships versus self-development

McCrae and Costa (1990) identify the second and fourth factors (Extraversion and Agreeableness) as the two traits particularly important in developing relationships. The Extraversion dimension reflects the quantity of relationships, while the Agreeableness dimension reflects their quality. The other three factors—Resilience, Openness, and Conscientiousness—refer more to the development of the self, regardless of the relationship context.

Application

Understand that, in building a relationship, it is important to continually communicate with one another, particularly on issues related to Extraversion and Agreeableness. See Costa and McCrae (1992) and McCrae and Costa (1990) for further discussion and some examples.

Topic 10.4 Changes over time

McCrae and Costa (1990), in their work with the Baltimore Longitudinal Study of Aging, have looked for changes in temperament over time. They found that up through the early twenties, the tendency is to score lower on Agreeableness, Conscientiousness, and Resilience than on the other two factors. They attribute this to the preoccupation of young people with identity formation (people who are low on Agreeableness are Challengers) and with their low career commitment (those who are low on Conscientiousness are Flexible). By age thirty this difference has lessened, due to increased Agreeableness, Conscientiousness, and Resilience and moderation of the Extraversion and Openness attributes. Another way of saying it is that as we enter adulthood and the world of work, we become a little more goal-oriented, a little easier to get along with, somewhat less sociable, more emotionally stable, and a little more conservative (see Figure 10.2).

Figure 10.2

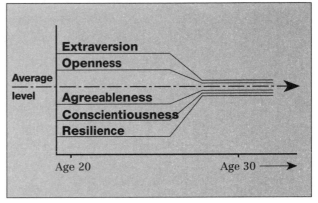

Development of stability in adult personality.

Applications

1 Be reasonably accepting of selfishness and impulsivity among youth, knowing that—with understanding parents and societal nudging—the tendency is for people in their twenties to move toward a more cooperative and goal-focused adulthood.

2 Conversely, be reasonably accepting of the higher emotionality, minimal time with self, and complaints of boredom of young people, for this too will change with time.

Topic 10.5 Sex differences in the Big Five

Virtually no differences exist between men and women on the Extraversion, Openness, Agreeableness, and Conscientiousness dimensions. Costa and McCrae (1992) report some small differences on specific facets within these dimensions. However, women do tend to score lower on the Resilience dimension. On only one of the Resilience facets—even temperament—do women score the same as men. We do not know whether this difference on the Resilience dimension is due to real differences in emotional control, or whether women are simply more forthcoming in reporting their feelings. More research is needed.

Are personality traits for real?

Application

As a group, females tend to be more reactive—that is, they tend to make more overt responses to "good news, bad news" situations. This is not to say that males, who are less reactive, do not have internal reactions—they simply tend to show them less. Remember that this control can be either an asset (as in maintaining composure in stressful situations) or a liability (as in failing to show the intensity of a reaction to one's partner).

Suggested readings on personality

Costa, P. T., Jr., & McCrae, R. R. (1992). *NEO PI-R: Professional Manual.* Odessa, FL: Psychological Assessment Resources.

McCrae, R. M., & Costa, P. T. (1990). *Personality in Adulthood.* New York: Guilford Press.

11

The psychobiology of emotions:

The word emotion *comes from the Latin* exmovēre (ex = out of, *movere* = to move), which means to move out of or agitate. The etymology of the word is closely related to that of *motivation*. Both suggest action, a state that is the opposite of standing still or being calm and laid-back. This action is related to goals: motivation is action in pursuit of a goal, while emotion is action resulting from situations that enhance or threaten a goal. Hence, to the degree that I'm motivated, I'm pursuing a goal. To the degree that I'm emotional, I'm perceiving either a threat to my goal (negative emotion) or significant progress toward my goal (positive emotion).

Emotions weren't the subject of serious study by cognitive scientists until recently. This field of study is still young, and several theories compete for followers. I have taken the material that appears to be most compatible with the overall direction of cognitive research.

Topic 11.1 A model for emotions

A review of several major recent works on the theory of emotions (Lazarus, 1991a; Plutchik & Kellerman, 1989; J. G. Thompson, 1988) suggests a five-step model to describe what might happen to someone during an emotional situation:

1   *The event.* Something happens (a remark, a gesture, an accident, etc.) that potentially relates to one of the person's goals as either a threat or an enhancer.

More than ecstacy and terror?

2 *Perception of the event.* The individual becomes fully aware of the event (through seeing, hearing, or reading, etc.).

3 *Appraisal of the perceived event.* The person determines whether or not the event relates to a goal. The value of the goal will directly affect the strength of the emotion.

4 *Filtering the appraisal.* The status of the person's body (sleepy, alert, etc.) influences the intensity of his or her appraisal (e.g., very threatening or only mildly threatening).

5 *Reaction to the appraisal.* The person channels his or her appraisal into some form of coping (from the Middle French *couper,* to strike or cut). The strength of the reaction is a direct function of the value of the goal concerned and the degree of certainty that the event will thwart or enhance goal attainment.

Applications

1 The reaction to the appraisal (step 5 above) can be either cognitive or emotional. Normally, when goals appear to be thwarted or enhanced by an event, emotions precede cognitions. These emotions can last for less than a second or for a

> "Anger raiseth invention, but it overheateth the oven."
>
> **George Savile,**
> **Marquess of Halifax**

> "Emotion turning back on itself, and not leading on to thought or action, is the element of madness."
>
> **John Sterling**

lifetime, partly depending on whether we will the cognitive part of the reaction to ultimately subdue the emotional part. See Seligman's ABCDE technique (Topic 15.2) for ways to cognitively short-circuit a disturbing emotional event.

2   Analyze events and filters, and look past situations for patterns. (contributed by Rick Bradley)

3   Put up these mottos:

"We are disturbed not by things, but by the views we take of things."
Epictetus, *The Encheiridion*

"There is nothing either good or bad, but thinking makes it so."
William Shakepeare, *Hamlet*

Topic 11.2 The molar approach to emotions

Most of the research on emotions has occurred at the molar, or behavioral, level. Many efforts have been directed toward listing the primary emotions. Various

Table 11.1 Emotional states and parallels

Biological regulatory process	Behavioral expression	Adaptive function	Subjective state	Personality trait expression
Avoid	Withdraw	Protection	*Fear*	Timid
Approach	Attack	Destruction	*Anger*	Quarrelsome
Fuse	Mate	Reproduction	*Joy*	Affectionate
Separate	Distress signal	Reintegration	*Sadness*	Gloomy
Ingest	Eat	Incorporation	*Acceptance*	Trusting
Eject	Vomit	Rejection	*Disgust*	Hostile
Start	Examine	Exploration	*Expectation*	Demanding
Stop	Freeze	Orientation	*Surprise*	Indecisive

Note: From *The Measurement of Emotions,* edited by R. Plutchik and H. Kellerman. 1989, San Diego, CA: Academic Press. © 1989 by Academic Press, Inc., Orlando, FL 32887. Reprinted by permission of the author and publisher.

studies have worked with anywhere from five hundred to several thousand words that describe emotions. Most of these studies have tended to accept two primary dimensions of emotion: *evaluation* (e.g., pleasure or pain) and *activity* (e.g., alertness or sleepiness). Lazarus (1991a) points out that pleasure and pain, rather than being emotions, are some of emotions' raw materials. The "circumplex" model locates each of the emotions on an *X-Y* coordinate system based on these two dimensions. Anger, for example, would be located in the area suggesting negative evaluation and high activity. Sadness would be located in the area of negative evaluation and low activity, excitement in the area of positive evaluation and high activity, and so on. A good current discussion of the circumplex method of listing and differentiating emotions is available in Plutchik and Kellerman (1989).

Some have maintained that there are only three pure emotions—ecstasy, terror, and despair—with all other emotions simply combinations of those three (see Schlosberg, 1954); however, most researchers seem to list somewhere between six and eight primary emotions. The clearest listing of these emotions that I found was in Plutchik and Kellerman (1989). In Table 11.1, I have italicized the column labeled "Subjective State," which contains the terms we commonly refer to as the emotions. But from glancing through the other columns, you can readily see that there are many ways of describing emotional activity.

Diagnostic extreme	Ego-defense regulatory process	Coping style	Social control institution
Anxious	Repression	Avoidance	Religion
Aggressive	Displacement	Substitution	Police, war, sports
Manic	Reaction	Reversal	Marriage and family
Depressed	Compensation	Replacement	Religion
Hysterical	Denial	Minimization	Psychiatry, shamanism
Paranoid	Projection	Blame	Medicine
Obsessive-compulsive	Intellectualization	Mapping	Science
Borderline	Regression	Help-seeking	Games, entertainment

Applications

1   Use Table 11.1 to become aware of your emotional patterns. If you find a pattern that is dysfunctional for you, make up your mind to deal with it either through learning a self-control skill on your own (such as Seligman's ABCDE model, described in Topic 15.2) or through engaging in a therapeutic relationship with a counselor.

2   For serious emotional disorders that leave someone unable to hold a job or a relationship, consult a neurosurgeon, psychiatrist, or neuropharmacologist.

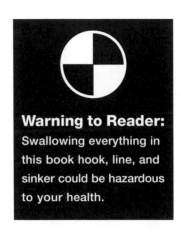

Warning to Reader: Swallowing everything in this book hook, line, and sinker could be hazardous to your health.

Topic 11.3 The molecular approach to emotions

Compared to other aspects of brain research, the emotions have suffered from relative inattention. Much of the research on emotion has been conducted at the molar level and has been centered on the researchers' ubiquitous play toy—factor analysis.

At the time of this writing, very few molecular, or microscopic, findings are etched in stone. For example, while the region of the brain called the amygdala has been strongly positioned as the "rage" center, the actual research findings have been inconsistent. Although surgical removal of the amygdala can eliminate rage, bizarre eating patterns and sexual behaviors sometimes follow. The inconsistency of the results is attributed to two factors: the first is the redundancy principle, which suggests that because of duplication of function it is impossible to pin any one function to a single location in the brain, and the second is the difficulty of absolute surgical precision, which makes it impossible to perform two procedures precisely alike—that is, without invading a neighboring area that was previously intact or leaving an area intact that was removed in a similar operation.

Nonetheless, some general principles are emerging:

- A pleasure center seems to exist called the median forebrain bundle, which runs parallel to the pain center.
- A pain center seems to exist called the periventricular system, which runs from the hindbrain or medulla to the forebrain, parallel to both the median forebrain bundle and the RAS (see Chapter Two).
- Stimulation of the posterior hypothalamus excites the sympathetic nervous system (fight-or-flight response).
- Stimulation of the anterior hypothalamus excites the parasympathetic nervous system (relaxation response).
- Damage to the parietal, temporal, or occipital lobes results in no appreciable change in emotional activity.

- Damage to the frontal lobe can result in major increases or decreases in emotionality.
- The left frontal lobe houses positive and negative emotional processes, while the right frontal lobe houses only negative processes.
- If the same site in one human's brain is stimulated at different times, different emotions can be produced.
- Hormonal levels influence the intensity of emotional response.
- Levels of specific neurotransmitters affect one's propensity toward specific emotions; for example, high melatonin leads to depression, low melatonin to high sexual appetite, high epinephrine to elation, high prolactin to anxiety. For more on this topic, see Kolata (1976, 1979).
- Each emotion seems to have unique physiological responses; for example, anxiety leads to greater phasic increases in systolic blood pressure, anger to greater phasic increases in diastolic blood pressure, fear to vasoconstriction (the skin pales), anger to vasodilation (the skin flushes). Progress is slow in describing these unique responses because of the difficulty of eliciting one single emotion and measuring its accompanying processes (J. G. Thompson, 1988).
- The physiological responses to emotion (cardiovascular, muscular-skeletal, thermoregulatory, respiratory, gastrointestinal, urinary, and reproductive) can result in related disorders, such as headache, stomach pain, blushing, sweating, Raynaud's disease (vasoconstriction in the digits of the hands and feet), muscular tightness, and diarrhea.
- These physiological disorders seem to be mutually exclusive: people who sweat don't blush and people who blush don't have chronic headaches.
- One emotion elicits different attacks in different individuals: anger can elicit headache in one person, sweat in another.
- Physiological disorders are only partially connected to conscious awareness of one's emotional state.

Applications

1 Develop an appreciation for the fact that emotional responses, whether weak or strong, have complex origins. They may be attributed to brain structure, body chemistry, stress, habit, or personal cognitive intention. Do not assume you know the causes of someone's emotionality. If knowing the cause is important, consult with a variety of specialists, such as neurosurgeons, neuropharmacologists, or psychiatrists. Never forget that, while many emotions can be controlled by personal will, some people's emotions are held captive by aberrant biochemical forces.

2   Become aware of your own physical reactions to emotional situations. Control emotions through responding to physical reactions and vice versa. (contributed by Rick Bradley)

Topic 11.4 The appraisal filter

When we receive "news" from our environment, it is neither good nor bad until our appraisal process has passed judgment.

The notion that the mind serves as a kind of gatekeeper for emotional behavior is at the core of the cognitive theory of emotions. The opposing theory, developed earlier in this century, is that a person reacts automatically, without mental intervention, whenever certain emotion-evoking stimuli appear. Today, a consensus is emerging that embraces the notion that events with the potential to elicit emotional responses must first pass the appraisal activity of the mind. This appraisal activity is typically rapid. It may have several components and may be sequential or simultaneous, but researchers agree that it takes place between stimulus and response. When we receive "news" from our environment, it is neither good nor bad until our appraisal process has passed judgment.

The clearest and most recent description of this appraisal process (Lazarus, 1991b, p. 827) identifies six ingredients:

1   *Goal relevance:* Does this news relate to one of my goals or values?

2   *Goal congruence or incongruence:* Does this news serve to enhance or thwart my goal or value?

3   *Goal content:* How is my ego involved? (The answer helps to tap the relevant emotional response—for example, anger versus guilt.)

4   *Source of blame or credit:* Who's responsible, me or thee?

5   *Coping potential:* Can I handle the consequences of this news or event?

6   *Future expectations:* Will things get better or worse?

Lazarus calls the first three elements primary appraisal and the last three secondary appraisal. Note the similarity of Lazarus's secondary appraisal elements to

The brain and your personality

Seligman's three elements of learned optimism: personalization, pervasiveness, and permanence (see Topic 13.1).

These six mental-appraisal interventions control the gate that determines whether or not a perceived event leads to an emotional response. In reading this manuscript, Rick Bradley commented that no one could use this process without a personal commitment to truth.

Applications

1   Commit your goals to writing. Document situations that promote or thwart goal attainment. Analyze for patterns. (contributed by Rick Bradley)

2   Make a personal commitment to truth. (contributed by Rick Bradley)

3   Make a list of your personal hot buttons, words, phrases, actions, or situations that cause you to become angry or emotional. Determine in advance what you will do to alter your normal response the next time one of your hot buttons is pushed.

Topic 11.5 Emotion's home: The body as catalyst

J. G. Thompson (1988) identifies four ways in which biological mechanisms can influence emotion-related neurotransmitter levels. These mechanisms can influence the degree to which an emotion gets expressed, depending, of course, upon the prior or simultaneous appraisal process. It's as though these four mechanisms serve as a kind of catalyst, influencing the degree but probably not the kind of emotional response. They are:

1   *Genetic vulnerability:* This is a very complex issue. See Topics 9.1 and 9.2 for discussion of this topic.

2   *Diet:* Many of the chemicals that block or facilitate the development and transmission of emotion-related neurotransmitters can, at this point, only be manufactured within the body. See Kolata (1976, 1979) for a more complete treatment.

3   *Hormonal level:* In the complex interaction of hormones with neurotransmitters, hormonal levels that are too high or too low can sometimes have a dramatic impact on the intensity of emotional response. Research seems to be stuck at the chicken-and-egg syndrome here—do hormones control neurotransmitter levels or vice versa? While it is not clear how the causal relation works, it is clear that hormonal levels are related to emotional response. As an example, we know that estrogen levels are directly related to left-brain activity (Kimura & Hampson, 1990).

4 *Circadian rhythm:* The degree to which one is able to satisfy the sleep-wake cycle and the twenty-five-hour day can affect hormonal and neurotransmitter levels, intensifying emotional response. That is why we may be more testy, tearful, or giggly during sleep deprivation or jet lag.

Applications

1 The single most effective way to keep emotional responses comfortable is to stay in good physical condition, using the right diet (see Chapter Five), aerobic exercise plan (see Topics 8.3 and 8.4), amount of sleep (see Chapter Seven), and stress management program (see Topic 14.2).

2 If the previous application doesn't work satisfactorily, consult appropriate cognitive scientists, such as neurosurgeons, psychiatrists, or neuropharmacologists.

Topic 11.6 Coping mechanisms

Once we have appraised a situation as threatening or enhancing our well-being, we tend to follow one of four coping styles (J. G. Thompson, 1988):

1 *Verbal:* This left-hemisphere response suggests, for example, an individual who responds with vindictive thoughts but without any accompanying physiological arousal.

2 *Nonverbal:* This right-hemisphere response suggests, for example, an individual who feels upset but doesn't know why; that is, he or she doesn't relate the upset to an event or emotion but instead may think it is the flu.

3 *Both verbal and nonverbal:* This style is characterized by a high cognitive response (left hemisphere) and a high somatic response (right hemisphere), as when someone thinks, "I'm really letting my anger get me down."

4 *Neither verbal nor nonverbal:* With this style, a person chooses to see the event as neutral (neither threatening nor enhancing) with respect to his or her goals and values; therefore, no cognitive (mental) or somatic (physical) coping is required. Note the similarity of this

The brain and your personality

coping style to the one in Seligman's ABCDE technique (see Topic 15.2). With respect to this style, I like to recall Graham Greene's comment that hatred is a failure of the imagination.

Applications

1 Understand that positive emotions are responses to events perceived as enhancing attainment of one or more of our goals. Positive emotions are healthy; they promote a feeling of satisfaction with life. We can increase the experience of positive emotions by changing our goals if not enough enhancing events happen, changing our environment (see Sternberg's three problem-solving strategies in Topic 12.1), or changing our interpretation of events (we may be seeing events as threats when, in fact, they are enhancers, even if they are only weak enhancers).

2 The emotion of angry hostility places us in a double-bind: both holding it in *and* venting it are bad for the heart (Ironson et al., 1992) and the immune system. The secret to dealing with anger is to express it without getting angry. Get it out, deal with it, and get over it.

> The secret to dealing with anger is to express it without getting angry. Get it out, deal with it, and get over it.

Topic 11.7 A note on deception

In two recent major works on the problem of deception (Ekman, 1985; Rogers, 1988), the results are clear: we cannot reliably determine whether another person is lying. To quote Paul Ekman (1985, p. 97): "*No clue to deceit is reliable for all human beings,* but singly and in combination they can help the lie catcher in judging most people."

The most common technique for detecting lies is to observe whether or not a person exhibits stressful symptoms while answering questions about which he or she has or could have "guilty knowledge"; this might be done by polygraphy, interviews, film analysis, or other methods. So, for example, if I answer "No!" when I'm asked whether I ate the last piece of cake, then my skin turns pale, I develop a nervous twitch in my shoulder, and I look away, normally you would suspect that I'm lying. Ekman has identified, however, two common exceptions to this. He calls one the Brokaw hazard, which consists of judging a person's responses without baseline data (named after NBC's Tom Brokaw, who interpreted circumlocution in an interview as a sign of lying, not allowing for the fact that many people both tell the truth and use circumlocutions). If I *always* respond with a paling of the skin, a twitch, and a glance out the window, that behavior pattern would not indicate any more stress than usual; hence it is no clue to deceit. Ekman calls the second exception the Othello error; it reflects the fact that some people can lie without exhibiting stress, and some can exhibit stress symptoms without lying. A low voice can lie and a high voice tell the truth. My stress symptoms could appear as a result of my fear of not being believed, rather than of getting caught.

The bottom line is that stress symptoms reveal only one thing—stress. Stress is not deceit. The polygraph is not a lie detector. It is a *stress* detector and should be called that. For a good discussion of the severe limitations of the polygraph as a lie detector, see Ekman (1985) or Rogers (1988).

Applications

1 Don't rely on polygraphs as an employment screening device.

2 Ekman (1985) provides an appendix that lists thirty-eight questions to use in assessing the probability that a person is lying. If you must frequently render judgments on whether people are lying, use Ekman's list as a guide.

Suggested readings on the emotions

Ekman, P. (1985). *Telling Lies*. New York: W. W. Norton.

Lazarus, R. S. (1991a). *Emotion and Adaptation*. New York: Oxford University Press.

Plutchik, R., & Kellerman, H. (Eds.). (1989). *The Measurement of Emotions*. (Vol. 4 in R. Plutchik & H. Kellerman (Eds.), *Emotions: Theory, Research, and Experience*). San Diego, CA: Academic Press.

Rogers, R. (Ed.). (1988). *Clinical Assessment of Malingering and Deception*. New York: Guilford Press.

Thompson, J. G. (1988). *The Psychobiology of Emotions*. New York: Plenum.

12

The three faces of intelligence:

When people speak of IQ (Intelligence Quotient, or mental age divided by chronological age times 100), they typically are referring to a score on some test of verbal and numerical reasoning—those scoring above 100 are seen as having an above-average IQ, those scoring under 100 a below-average IQ. The problem is that these test scores are not really based on any generally accepted theory of intelligence, nor do they help predict success in life (Epstein & Meier, 1989). The tests originated in France as an academic screening device, and today, for the most part, they continue to be primarily an academic screening device. At the beginning of *The Triarchic Mind*, Robert Sternberg (1988) provides a stimulating history of IQ measurement. Among the problems with current IQ measures that he has suggested are the following:

- Inappropriate use of the stopwatch
- Cultural bias
- Academic bias
- The assumption of a fixed quantity of IQ
- The lack of a generally accepted theory of intelligence
- The narrowness of verbal and numerical reasoning as indicators of intelligence
- The assumption that verbally intelligent people read everything for details

Process, content, and structure

In this chapter, we will discuss three different kinds of definitions of intelligence: *process, content,* and *structure.* The *process* definition is that of Robert Sternberg (1988), who describes the various processes at work during intellectual activity. The *content* definition is that of Howard Gardner (1983), who maintains that different kinds of intelligence exist within an individual, and that an individual has differing degrees of ability in each kind of intelligence. These two definitions complement each other: Gardner identifies several different unique domains, or playing fields, whereas Sternberg identifies the basic self-managing processes that operate regardless of domain. Using the industry of resort management as an analogy, Gardner describes domains as being rather like different kinds of resorts, such as golf or tennis resorts, theme parks, tropical paradises, luxury hotels, beaches, arts centers, cruise ships, campgrounds, and sports camps. Continuing with this analogy, Sternberg's processes are rather like the management principles that apply to all resorts regardless of content, such as those involved in information systems, sales and marketing, people management, long-range planning, financial systems, and research and development.

The third definition—*structure*—is that of Hans Eysenck. Continuing with the resort management analogy, his structural definition of intelligence is much like the physical facility itself—buildings, grounds, staff, equipment, supplies, and infrastructure—and the persons who take care of it—construction workers,

> "Can there be any doubt that walking on the street involves intelligence?"
>
> **Robert J. Sternberg,**
> *The Triarchic Mind*

maintenance crews, inspectors, groundkeeping crews, food service workers, and sanitation workers. Eysenck's description of the biological structure of intelligence applies regardless of content or process. It is molecular, while Gardner's and Sternberg's descriptions are molar. Figure 12.1 shows the relation of the three definitions to each other.

Figure 12.1

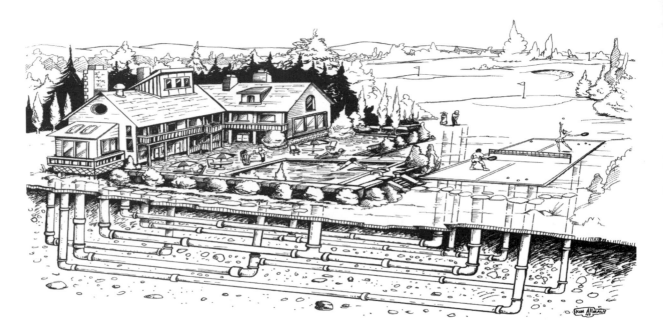

The three aspects of intelligence as illustrated by a resort. The domains of intelligence (Gardner) are represented by the tennis court, golf course, and swimming pool, three separate and distinct areas of expertise; the structure of intelligence (Eysenck and others) is represented by the underground pipes and the structures with which they communicate; and the process of intelligence (Sternberg) is represented by the administration building at the top left.

Topic 12.1 Sternberg's process definition of intelligence

Sternberg defines intelligence as the capacity for mental self-management. This definition obviously includes more than the traditional word, number, and space problems of current IQ tests. Figure 12.2 attempts to visualize how the mind manages itself according to Sternberg. Sternberg sees three large, inclusive domains in which self-management is necessary: the componential, experiential, and contextual domains.

I like to call the *componential* domain of intellect the production function; it researches, plans, and executes a mental effort. The typical example of the componential function at work is the college research paper. Gazzaniga (1985) describes the Interpreter as seated in the left hemisphere of the brain; Sternberg's componential and contextual functions would appear to be a more detailed analysis of how this Interpreter works.

I call the *experiential* domain the creativity function. This function engages in the quest for originality—novelty, uniqueness, innovation, insight, and so on.

The brain and your personality

(See Chapters Twenty-One and Twenty-Two for further elaboration.) The experiential function appears to provide the basis of what Gardner (1983) calls domains (see Topic 12.2). I think that Gardner's theory is compatible with Sternberg's in the sense that the experiential function could have a variety of contents; six of them are identified by Gardner. Sternberg identifies two aspects of dealing with

Figure 12.2

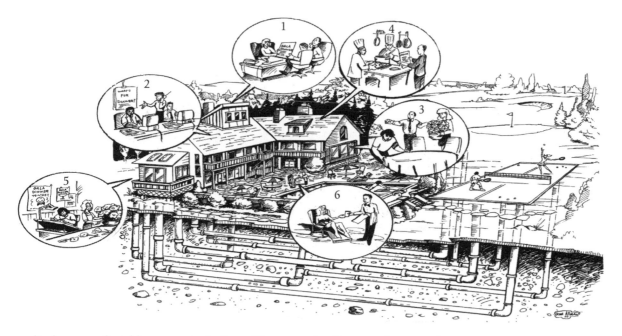

novelty: how comfortable we are in dealing with new, unfamiliar experiences and how readily we understand these experiences and are able to make them a part of our normal routine, or routinize them.

The *contextual* domain is the problem solver, or, as Sternberg says, the "street-smart" function. Whereas the componential function deals with the efficiency of the mental effort and the experiential function deals with the originality of the effort, the contextual function deals with the rigidity of the effort. To the degree that a person always chooses the same strategy to solve problems, he or she is less intelligent than the person who calls upon different strategies that are appropriate to different occasions. The three main problem-solving strategy types are:

Sternberg's components of intelligence. 1. Goal formation; **2.** research; **3.** strategizing; **4.** tactics; **5.** creativity; **6.** implementation.

1 *Altering yourself:* Maybe what I'm doing is causing the problem. Hence, if I change my behavior, I can solve the problem.

2 *Altering others:* Maybe what others (my spouse, boss, co-workers, friend) are doing is causing the problem. Hence, if I can change them, I can solve the problem.

The three faces of intelligence

3   *Altering the situation:* Maybe some features of the environment surrounding the problem (the workplace, home, organizational chart, etc.) are causing the problem. Hence, if I can change them, I can solve the problem.

To illustrate the three contextual problem-solving strategies, let us say that you experience a problem in your marriage. You could try changing your behavior (altering yourself), your spouse's behavior (altering others), or divorcing (altering the situation). The more intelligent (more mentally flexible) person will vary these three strategy types as problems arise. The less intelligent (more mentally rigid) person will tend to persist with the same strategy type. These rigid persisters become known as martyrs or doormats (always altering themselves), control freaks (always altering others), or quitters (always altering the situation).

Applications

1   In Figure 12.2, step 6 (implementation) is the aspect of intelligence usually referred to. The ability to use a great many words, numbers, and objects with masterful understanding, as measured by any of a myriad of IQ tests (Wunderlich, Schlosson, Wesman, California, Stanford-Binet, Wechsler, etc.), has served personnel and hiring managers, university admissions officers, counselors, and researchers for decades in their effort to distinguish the more intelligent from the less intelligent. In truth, all they have done is distinguish the more fluent in numbers, words, and object manipulation from the less fluent. And this is only the tip of the intellectual iceberg.

If you truly wish to identify the more intelligent, for whatever reason, you need to look for more than what we are here calling fluency of execution. Intelligence is not skin-deep. You must look for the ability to establish goals for a complex project and administer it (step 1), to find information relevant to a problem through appropriate research (step 2), to be flexible in selecting a strategy to solve a problem (step 3), to plan the steps of that strategy (step 4), and to be appropriately creative in the design of the strategy (step 5). Steps 1, 2, and 4 are perhaps best measured through interviews and reference checks. Step 3, flexible strategy selection, can be measured directly by one of two tests: the *Tacit Knowledge Inventory,* published by The Psychological Corporation, San Antonio, Texas, under Sternberg's guidance, and *AccuVision,* a video-based metric distributed by Electronic Selection Systems Corp., Maitland, Florida. Flexible strategy selection can be measured indirectly through various Authoritarianism scales such as the combination of scores on the Challenger and Preserver traits on the *NEO-PI-R* (Costa & McCrae, 1992). (See also

Chapters Nine and Ten.) The various situational leadership instruments from Blanchard Training & Development, Escondido, California, also provide an indirect measure. Step 5, creativity, can be assessed by tests (see Amabile, 1983), portfolios, and interviews.

Appendix E is a guide to use in evaluating tests, interviews, references, portfolios, and so on as a way of assessing the overall intelligence of a person.

2 If you are trying to hire someone, you may decide that not all of the six components of intelligence are important, or at least not equally important. In that case, you may hire someone who has less overall intelligence, but who can do a special job well. Generally, those who demonstrate mastery in all six areas rise to positions of greatest responsibility.

3 If you sense that you are lacking in one of these six areas, you can make up for that lack in one of two ways: either develop your ability through various educational opportunities or delegate tasks to others who excel in areas where you feel deficient. For example, if you tend to be rigid in selecting problem-solving strategies, then identify one or more co-workers with whom you can consult and who will be flexible in advising you to alter yourself, others, or the situation. Perhaps you are a person who consistently tries to alter the situation as a way of solving problems (spending money, reorganizing, rearranging, firing or transferring people, discontinuing products or services). Identify people who can advise you how to develop other, perhaps more effective, strategies, such as altering yourself (changing habits, increasing communication, learning or improving a skill or body of knowledge, changing an attitude, reordering priorities) or altering others (coaching and counseling, training, disciplining).

Recruit individuals for management or leadership positions who exhibit flexibility in their problem solving.

4 Abandon the traditional management style (the so-called Theory X of Douglas McGregor) that alters others, seeing employees as the root of all evil. Total Quality Management puts a heavy emphasis on altering the situation; it sees most errors as process-related, not people-related. (contributed by Rick Bradley)

5 Check yourself against the list of intelligent behaviors found in Appendix F.

6 Recruit individuals for management or leadership positions who exhibit flexibility in their problem solving and a willingness to attack process issues. (contributed by Rick Bradley)

7 Provide training in problem-solving techniques. (contributed by Rick Bradley)

Topic 12.2 Gardner's content definition of intelligence

Gardner (1983) has established eight criteria for identifying a domain of intellectual content:

1 Isolation by brain damage

2 The existence of prodigies in that domain

3 A core set of operations

4 Developmental uniqueness

5 Evolutionary plausibility

6 Validation from experimental psychology

7 Validation from psychometrics

8 The existence of a unique symbol system to communicate its content

He proposes that six domains of intellectual content satisfy these criteria, as outlined and justified in his book, *Frames of Mind* (1983). I have summarized them as follows:

1 *Linguistic:* Isolated in the left hemisphere, the linguistic domain performs the primary operations of semantics, grammar, phonology, and rhetoric.

2 *Musical:* Isolated in the right hemisphere, the musical domain performs the primary operations of pitch, volume, rhythm, and timbre.

3 *Logical-mathematical:* Isolated in the right hemisphere for males and present in both hemispheres for females, the logical-mathematical domain performs the primary operations of long chains of reasoning, the capacity for abstraction, and calculation.

4 *Spatial:* Isolated in the posterior right hemisphere, the spatial domain performs the primary operations of correct object perception and the ability to transform and rotate objects in the mind.

5 *Bodily-kinesthetic:* This domain is isolated in the left hemisphere in

The brain and your personality

right-brain-dominant people and the right hemisphere in left-brain-dominant people. It performs the primary operations of controlling the body and manipulating objects.

6 *Personal:* Isolated in the right frontal area for males and the bilateral frontal area for females, the personal domain performs the primary operations of intrapersonal understanding (knowing one's own feelings) and interpersonal understanding (knowing the moods, feelings, and needs of others).

Gardner maintains that these six domains are independent; high performance in one domain is not necessarily accompanied by high performance in another. Outstanding performance in two or more domains by one person is rare. While William and Henry James are both known as great writers (linguistic domain), Henry's novels are said to read like psychology texts (logical-mathematical domain) and William's psychology texts are said to read like novels (personal domain).

Recognize the domain of excellence in each child and encourage development in it.

Applications

1 School curricula should include each of the six domains and teachers should be prepared to assist students in developing in their strongest domain. In the early school years, children should be encouraged in all domains so that strengths and natural talents become apparent. Gardner's *The Unschooled Mind* (1991) describes curricular applications of his theory.

2 Employers should expect high performance in one domain only and accept high performance in two or more domains as the exception. For example, to expect a human resources expert (personal domain) to be a financial expert (logical-mathematical domain) is like expecting a starting quarterback (bodily-kinesthetic domain) to be a best-selling writer (linguistic domain).

3 Parents should attempt to recognize the domain of excellence in each child and encourage development in it. All too often, a parent will encourage development in one domain (say, musical) even though the child's domain of strength is in another (say, bodily-kinesthetic). As in Application 1 above, parents should encourage their young children in all six domains with their goal being to identify one or more for special encouragement. For a parent to expect a child to have strengths in a particular domain just because the parent does is to fail to acknowledge the role of genetics in human development (see Chapter Nine).

Topic 12.3 Eysenck's structural definition of intelligence

In a direction of study that will proliferate as we approach the twenty-first century, Hans Eysenck has explored the neurobiological correlates of intelligence. He has identified three correlates of IQ: *reaction time, inspection time,* and *average evoked potential* (AEP) (Eysenck & Kamin, 1981; Eysenck & Eysenck, 1985). Clearly the first two, which are observed behaviors, are less biological than the third, which is a description of brain waves, but they have a common thread in their effort to identify the biological basis of intelligence.

In experiments on both auditory and visual reaction times, the reaction time of subjects with lower IQs—as measured by what Sternberg calls performance measures, such as the Wechsler and Stanford-Binet tests and Raven's matrices—*increases* as more stimuli are added. On the other hand, the more complex the stimulus, the faster the reaction of higher-IQ subjects (this is known as Hick's law). In other words, brighter people take progressively less time to react to progressively more complex stimuli. In addition, they show less variability in their reaction time. They not only are quicker; they are more consistent.

When asked to inspect a stimulus and provide a specific response, higher-IQ subjects take less time. An inspection test might have the following pattern: if you see a blue dot, press the button on the right; if you see a green dot, press the button in the center; if you see a red dot, press the button on the left.

The AEP is measured by the amplitude (height) of an electroencephalogram (EEG) wave, the frequency of the wave (length of time in milliseconds between waves), and the complexity (irregularity) of the wave. According to AEP studies:

- The more intelligent the subject, the more complex the wave.
- The less intelligent the subject, the more variance there is across 100 tests.
- In studies of high- and low-income children, the AEP has been shown to be more culture-free, with smaller differences between classes, than the *Wechsler Adult Intelligence Scale.*
- Facing familiar stimuli, higher-IQ brains fire fewer neurons. Richard Haier, of the Brain Imaging Center at the University of California, Irvine, has found that positron emission tomography scans show higher brain activity while a subject is learning a game (for example, the Russian game Tetris, which has been adapted by Nintendo and Spectrum Holobyte) and less activity later, with activity decreasing as scores increase. He also confirms that the higher the IQ, the less brain activity there is.
- Facing novel, unfamiliar stimuli, higher-IQ brains fire more neurons (i.e., bring more resources to bear).

The brain and your personality

Figure 12.3 shows the different patterns of higher-IQ and lower-IQ subjects performing two tests of reaction time—an auditory test and a visual test.

Figure 12.3

Applications

1 Where culture-free measures of IQ are critically important, consider using either an auditory-reaction-time test with a supplementary visual-reaction-time test (auditory tests are more reliable) or an EEG.

2 IQ is less job-related when a worker is dealing with repetitive, familiar tasks. As tasks become more complex, IQ becomes more job-related. Don't look for bright candidates for routine work.

3 Dietary, exercise, sleep, and other factors can affect the purity of the synaptic gap and the durability and firing efficiency of neurons (see Chapter Two). Don't let poor habits create a drag on your intellectual functioning.

4 In your daily approach to life, consciously try to improve reaction time and inspection time on tasks of greatest relevance to your career and lifetime goals.

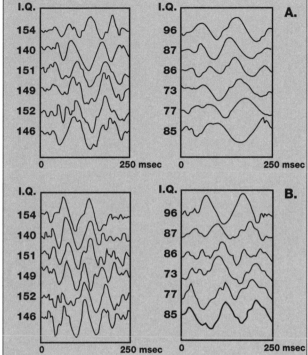

A comparison of evoked potential brain waves in high- and low-IQ subjects.

A. *Auditory stimulation:* evoked potential waveforms for (left) six high-IQ and (right) six low-IQ subjects. **B.** *Visual stimulation:* evoked potential waveforms for (left) six high-IQ and (right) six low-IQ subjects. Reprinted from Eysenck and Eysenck (1985) with permission of Plenum Publishing Corp. and the authors.

Suggested readings on intelligence

Armstrong, T. (1993). *Seven Kinds of Smart: Identifying and Developing Your Many Intelligences.* New York: Plume.

Brody, N. (1992). *Intelligence.* (2nd ed.). San Diego, CA: Academic Press.

Eysenck, H. J., & Eysenck, M. W. (1985). *Personality and Individual Differences: A Natural Science Approach.* New York: Plenum.

Eysenck, H. J., & Kamin, L. (1981). *The Intelligence Controversy.* New York: Wiley.

Gardner, H. (1983). *Frames of Mind: The Theory of Multiple Intelligences.* New York: Basic Books.

Sternberg, R. J. (1988). *The Triarchic Mind: A New Theory of Human Intelligence.* New York: Viking.

Part four

People at work:

Using mind-brain research for continuous performance improvement

People at work:

Using mind-brain research for continuous performance improvement

Optimism and hardiness: Two sides

The word motivation *derives from the Latin* motivus, a form of *movēre*, which means "to move." The difference between being motivated and unmotivated, then, is whether or not the subject in question is moving. A classic example of an unmotivated person is the so-called couch potato, who sits or lies unmoving while watching seemingly endless hours of television. The remote-control zapper is the only thing that moves.

Generally, motivation is described as goal-oriented behavior. The vast literature on the subject of motivation revolves around two aspects of goals: how an individual rates his or her chances of attaining a goal successfully and how he or she rates the value of the goal itself. The problem with motivation comes when individuals who have a good chance of success choose not to pursue a highly valued goal.

For most of us, when life is going well—whatever that means to us individually—we are motivated. It is adversity that knocks us down. The motivated get back up and get on with life. The less motivated tend to become resigned to their fate and to accept what life hands them. You've heard the expression "When the going gets tough, the tough get going." I think that statement refers to motivation. In this and the following two chapters we will take a careful look at the difference between those of us who find it easier to bounce back and those who find it harder. In addition, we will explore ways to compensate for that difference.

of the motivation coin

For a textbook definition of motivation, here is one by Geen, Beatty, and Arkin (1984, p. 3): "Motivation is the study of the intrapersonal processes which direct, activate, and maintain behavior."

As we scan the current writing on motivation, two closely related approaches rise to the surface: Seligman's work on optimism and Cousins's work on hardiness.

> "Action may not always bring happiness; but there is no happiness without action."
>
> **Benjamin Disraeli**

Topic 13.1 Seligman: Optimism versus helplessness

Martin Seligman, in his book *Learned Optimism* (1991), describes how rats and humans learn to be helpless. When either rats or humans experimentally learn that they have no control over their environment, they give up trying to exert control. Whether the bothersome stimuli are electroshocks or noise, unsuccessful attempts to stop them are followed by defeatist despair. Seligman has found three ingredients of this learned helplessness among humans, which he contrasts to learned optimism. The three ingredients are personalization, permanence, and pervasiveness. (See the related discussion in Topic 11.4.) Depending on how we typically respond to success or adversity along these three dimensions, we are described as optimistic or pessimistic. In Table 13.1, I have summarized the healthy, more motivated explanatory style and the less healthy, unmotivated explanatory style.

Seligman concludes from his research that the optimistic explanatory style is associated with high motivation, success, achievement, and physical and mental health, while the pessimistic explanatory style is associated with the opposite traits. In addition, he finds that certain pessimistic people who constantly ruminate about their misfortune in life and brood about the pessimistic aspects of personalization, permanence, and pervasiveness are at high risk for depression.

Table 13.1 Seligman's explanatory styles

Explanation of adversity

Optimist	Pessimist
It's someone else's fault (external personalization)	It's my fault (internal personalization)
It's only temporary (not permanent)	It's gonna last forever (permanent)
It won't affect other areas of my life (limited pervasiveness)	It'll affect every area of my life (universal pervasiveness)

Explanation of success

Optimist	Pessimist
I made it happen (internal personalization)	Someone else made it happen (external personalization)
This is one in a line of many successes (permanent)	It'll never happen again (not permanent)
The effect will ripple throughout my life (universal pervasiveness)	It won't help me in any other areas of my life (limited pervasiveness)

Notice that the preferred explanatory styles are opposite in their response to success or adversity: the more healthy (optimistic) explanatory style for success (internal, permanent, and pervasive) is in fact unhealthy (pessimistic) as a way to explain adversity. Conversely, the more unhealthy (pessimistic) way to explain success (external, temporary, and limited) is in fact the healthy (optimistic) way to explain adversity. Figure 13.1 illustrates this model as a flowchart.

Benjamin Libet, a neurophysiologist at the University of California, San Francisco, has demonstrated that brain activity precedes consciousness. Hence, he concludes, intentions are spontaneous and actions are intentional. We choose our actions based on a spontaneous set of alternatives, so there is a point in time before an emotional reaction during which we can select a more optimistic, as opposed to a more pessimistic, response. See Restak (1991).

Applications

1 Get a copy of Seligman's *Learned Optimism*. It is an easy read, intended for the layperson. He provides both an adult's and a child's version of his Explanatory Style Questionnaire, from which you can obtain a sense of how you compare to the rest of the population with respect to optimism and pessimism. The questionnaire also includes much research on the ability of the explanatory style to predict job or sports success, and it has a fascinating section on psychohistory—the ability of

Figure 13.1

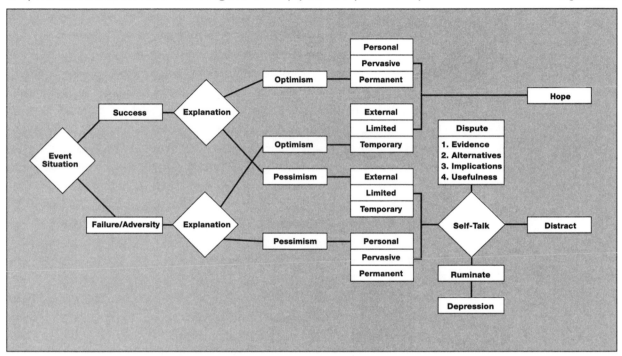

the explanatory style to predict the future (specifically, presidential elections). A computer-scored version of the Explanatory Style Questionnaire is available from Dr. Seligman or his associate, Peter Schulma, at 215-898-2748 in Philadelphia.

Optimism-pessimism flowchart. (Designed by the Center for Applied Cognitive Studies, based on the work of Martin E. P. Seligman in *Learned Optimism*, 1991).

2 Learn to use Seligman's ABCDE model (see Topic 15.2). Seligman has found that pessimistic people can learn to use a more optimistic style by employing this model. Teach the ABCDE model to teams and groups of people who have to work together. The phenomenon called groupthink, in which a group arrives at a quick, uncritical consensus, can have devastating effects on a group; it can be prevented by an understanding of the ABCDE model.

3 If you or someone you know would like assistance in developing a more optimistic style, select a psychotherapist who practices cognitive therapy, a directive therapy aimed at changing the way a client perceives his or her environment, which is closely allied with Seligman's research.

4   If you are a ruminator, then you need to learn more than just a more optimistic explanatory style. You need to learn how to jerk away from the hold that pessimistic thoughts have on you. Seligman suggests several distracting techniques in his book, including wearing a rubber band on your wrist (snap it when you start ruminating) and creating physical distractions (such as slapping the wall or doing isometric exercises), as ways to pop the pessimistic preoccupation out of your mind.

5   For some people, visualization techniques are effective both for removing pessimistic thoughts and for encouraging optimistic ones (see Gawain, 1978). Here is an example. First, get a clear picture of the unpleasant thought in your mind, with your eyes closed. Then, as though you were turning a television control knob, make the image lighter and lighter until all you see is white light. Slowly bring it back into view, continuing to make it darker until all you see is blackness. When the unpleasant image reappears, take control of it and reduce it to whiteness or blackness, whichever you prefer. You can do the same with sounds in your head that are unpleasant and stressful, such as parental scripts: try turning up the imaginary volume knob until they are so loud that they sound like static, then gradually turn them down until they are inaudible.

6   Seligman has developed a technique by which you can assess the attributional style of a public figure (your mayor, coach, etc.) by studiously watching television clips and reading newspaper and magazine accounts. If you send $3.00 (as of this writing), Seligman will send you the necessary instructions to conduct a CAVE (content analysis of verbatim explanations). Mail to:

> *Dr. Martin Seligman (or Peter Schulma)*
> *Department of Psychology*
> *University of Pennsylvania*
> *3815 Walnut Street*
> *Philadelphia, PA 19104-6196*

7   Michael Lewis of the Robert Wood Johnson Medical School (formerly Rutgers University Medical School) in Piscataway, New Jersey, reports that most girls grow up with a pessimistic explanatory style. Parents and teachers tend to lavish more praise on boys. Be aware of this tendency and be sure to encourage young girls to attribute their successes to their ability and their failures to bad luck.

Topic 13.2 Cousins: The four ingredients of hardiness

Norman Cousins (1989), who himself has recovered from three life-threatening illnesses, has become the primary popularizer for the new field of psychoneuroimmunology (see also Topic 8.6). Cousins summarizes a large body of research and experience with a quote from Seneca: "It is part of the cure to wish to be cured." This attitude—wanting to play an active role in curing oneself—is the essence of the motivated person. Cousins calls it hardiness and says it is composed of four ingredients. I have summarized them as follows:

1 *Positive expectations* (vs. negative expectations): Expecting successful outcomes for oneself and others

2 *Relaxation* (vs. stress): Dissipating stress through appropriate methods

3 *Positive emotions* (vs. negative emotions): Maintaining a sense of humor and joyfulness

4 *Active role* (vs. passive role): Being a doer, not just being done unto.

> "It is part of the cure to wish to be cured."
> **Seneca**

Applications

1 Rosenthal and Jacobson (1968) lit the torch on the power of the self-fulfilling prophecy, or the Pygmalion effect. Their lesson is simple: expect bad things, and bad things tend to happen; expect good things, and good things tend to happen. See also Topic 15.3.

2 Topics 14.2–14.6 provide abundant information and suggested applications on ways to dissipate stress.

3 Check out the bibliography on laughter in the back of Cousins (1989). Give yourself permission to perform the whole range of laughs—from the robust belly laugh to the social titter. Laughter is healthy. Cousins reports that laughter can improve sleep. See Topic 13.1, Application 8, and the Applications in Topic 8.6 for more ideas.

4 Focus on positive emotions. See fewer horror films, more inspirational films; listen to music in a major key. In one study, students randomly assigned to watch films of Mother Teresa had higher levels of salivary immunoglobulin A, a measure of the level of immune-system functioning, after viewing than did students assigned to watch films of Nazis.

5 The Society for the Preservation of Barbershop Quartet Singing in America has documented the positive effect of singing on health. Call 800-876-SING for more information. (contributed by Jack Wilson)

6 Give a damn! Robert Sternberg (see Topic 12.1) says that there are three basic strategies we can use to affect the world around us: change me, change thee, and change the situation. Use them. Don't stick with a strategy type that's not working. If you do what you've always done, you'll always get what you've always gotten!

7 The Eastern concept of Chi is defined as the force we feel when our life is in balance. A study of Eastern philosophy, science, and literature will lead us in the direction of self-control, which is the essence of optimism and hardiness.

In the next two chapters, we will explore some other issues related to motivation. First, in Chapter Fourteen, we will look at some of the molecular approaches to motivation; then, in Chapter Fifteen, we will look at the molar approaches. All of these approaches are, in essence, different ways of exploring what Cousins and Seligman call hardiness and optimism.

Suggested readings on optimism and hardiness
Cousins, N. (1979). *Anatomy of an Illness*. New York: W. W. Norton.
Cousins, N. (1989). *Head First: The Biology of Hope*. New York: Dutton.
Petri, H. L. (1991). *Motivation: Theory, Research, and Applications*. (3rd ed.). Belmont, CA: Wadsworth.
Seligman, M.E.P. (1991). *Learned Optimism*. New York: Knopf.

Stress and burnout: The neuro

Motivation can be seen with the zoom focused close-in, as in the dulling effects of excess fat and lactic acid, or far-out, as in the concept of learned optimism. This chapter presents what we know about the close-in, or molecular, nature of motivation; Chapter Fifteen will present summaries of the molar approaches.

Topic 14.1 The neurobiology of motivation

How can we define motivation physically? One way is by describing the physical correlates of the psychological state. Therefore, we ask this question: What are the physical correlates of optimism and hardiness? At the risk of oversimplifying, here is the answer:

- Optimal functioning of the immune system
- Optimal functioning of the cerebral cortex (cortical alertness)
- Moderate activation of the limbic system (moderate stress)
- Optimal diet and exercise
- Effective functioning of the "pleasure center" of the brain

Applications

1   The immune system is discussed in Topic 8.6 and the limbic system in Topics 14.2–14.4.

biology of motivation

2   Cortical alertness is described in Chapter Two.

3   Diet is described in Chapter Five, and exercise is described in Chapter Eight.

4   The pleasure center of the brain is mentioned in Topic 11.3.

> "He who has health, has hope; and he who has hope, has everything."
>
> **Arabian proverb**

Topic 14.2 Stress: What is it and how do you relieve it?

If motivation is action, then the study of motivation is the study of why some people act while others don't. Biologically, the definition of inaction is death; those who are alive but not active might best be described as burned out (see Topic 14.5). What is burnout? Most simply, it is the result of unrelieved stress; it can be reached through one of two routes: more intense, shorter-term stress or less intense, longer-term stress (Golembiewski, 1988).

What is stress? Jeffrey Gray (1971) defines stress, along with fear and anxiety, as one of the emotions. An emotion is a reaction to an actual, expected, missing, or removed reinforcing event (a reward or a punisher). Fear is a form of emotion associated with the desire to terminate, escape from, or avoid a dangerous event, which might be internal or external. Anxiety differs from fear in that fear deals with actual or threatened dangers, whereas anxiety deals with

Stress and burnout

imagined or unreal dangers (Campbell, 1989). Because it includes both fear and anxiety, stress may be defined as the emotion that results from the desire to terminate, escape from, or avoid a real or imagined, current or imminent, negatively reinforcing event. This negatively reinforcing event is usually referred to as a *stressor*. Stressors can be anything from fear-arousing enemies to anxiety-arousing fantasies.

Stressors are not only negative and hostile, as when we are evicted from a home; they may also be positive and friendly, as when we move into a new home. In both cases, prolonged stress can be harmful, causing us to feel the need to get away from the stressor.

When stress occurs, our bodies mobilize for one of the three F's: freeze, fight, or flee (the fight-or-flight syndrome). This mobilization includes:

■ Dilation of the pupils, for maximum visual perception even in darkness
■ Constriction of the arteries, for maximum pressure to pump blood to the heart and other muscles (the heart goes from one to five gallons pumped per minute)
■ Activation of the adrenal gland, for pumping cortisol, which maintains pupil dilation and artery constriction by stimulating the formation of epinephrine and norepinephrine, sensitizing adrenergic receptors, and inhibiting the breakdown of epinephrine and norepinephrine
■ Enlargement of the vessels to the heart to facilitate the return flow of blood
■ Metabolism of fat (from fatty cells) and glucose (from the liver) for energy
■ Constriction of vessels to the skin, kidney, and digestive tract, shutting down digestion and maximizing readiness for the fight-or-flight syndrome

Control of this process lies in the hypothalamus, which acts as a control console: stimulation of the front part of the hypothalamus calms the emotions (the parasympathetic nervous system response), while stimulation of the back section activates the mobilization processes (the sympathetic nervous system response)—this is known as the general adaptation syndrome (GAS). The term *general adaptation syndrome* originated with Hans Selye (1952); a complete and more technical, but highly readable, description of it can be found in R. Williams (1989).

Normally, stress comes and goes, like the tides. Fears and anxieties, for most of us, subside shortly after onset. Ira Black (1991) reports that sympathetic nervous system stimulation of thirty to ninety minutes can result in a 200 to 300 percent increase in enzyme and impulse activity for twelve hours to three

> When stress occurs, our bodies mobilize for one of the three F's: freeze, fight, or flee.

days, and, in some cases, for up to two weeks. But what happens when fears and anxieties don't subside? What happens when stressors don't go away and the feelings of fear and anxiety persist over time? During this sustained period of GAS, when the posterior hypothalamus is active, the performance of the immune system (see Topic 8.6) is seriously impaired. Minor results of this stress-related impairment include colds, flu, backaches, tight chest, migraine headaches, tension headaches, allergy outbreaks, and skin ailments. More chronic and life-threatening results can include hypertension, ulcers, accident-proneness, addictions, asthma, colon or bowel disorders, diabetes, kidney disease, rheumatoid arthritis, and mental illness. Killers that can result include heart disease, stroke, cancer, and suicide. In addition, chronic stress can result in energy depletion, depression, insecurity, impotence or frigidity, apathy, emotional withdrawal, insomnia, chronic fatigue, helplessness or hopelessness, anxiety, confusion, lack of concentration, and poor memory.

How do we prevent stressors from occurring or stop them once they begin? The simplest answer lies in the word *control*. If we resign ourselves to the inevitability of long-term stress, it will continue to ravage our bodies. However, if we decide that we have some degree of control and can limit or prevent stressors, the effects of stress can be minimized or even eliminated.

Applications

1 If any of the disorders listed above affect you or those close to you, confirm with your physician the possibility that they are stress-related. Then identify and list the stressors that cause you to continue to feel tightness in the chest, rapid heartbeat, acid stomach, and so on. Consider specific ways you can control each stressor, using the techniques in the following Applications. You might also seek the assistance of a psychotherapist who is trained in stress-reduction strategies.

2 *Relax:* Meditation, hypnosis, deep breathing, napping, saunas, and just resting quietly—all these and other methods are equally effective. Research says that meditation techniques are no more effective than other relaxation techniques (see Druckman & Bjork, 1991). I'm reminded of a favorite saying of mine: "Meditation is not what you think." The state of mind during hypnosis is no different from that of the normal, awake, alert mind. See an excellent summary of research on hypnosis in *The Harvard Health Letter,* April 1991, 7(10), 1–4. Hypnosis is a guided form of conscious selective attention and dissociation characterized by suggestibility. Even the best subjects do nothing under hypnosis that they wouldn't do otherwise.

3 *Escape:* Do anything that "takes your mind off" the stressors, such as reading, watching television, listening to music, pursuing hobbies and crafts, or cooking. When our minds are filled with such activities, limbic arousal shuts down and cortical arousal takes over. As we take part in a totally absorbing activity, any activity in the posterior hypothalamus moves to its forward area and to subsequent parasympathetic arousal.

> Ten minutes of belly laughs can provide two hours of pain-free sleep.

4 *Exercise:* Although any exercise is helpful in relieving stress, aerobic exercise is best. The simplest definition of aerobic exercise is any physical activity that keeps the heart pumping at elevated levels continuously for twelve to thirty minutes. Jogging, swimming, and brisk walking are aerobic, for example, while tennis, golf, and basketball are not (unless they are played nonstop). For further discussion, see Covert Bailey's excellent, newly revised *New Fit or Fat* (1991). See Chapter Eight for more discussion on this topic.

5 *Don't rely on sex:* Sexual orgasm releases the sympathetic nervous system's grip and leads to a parasympathetic response. But because sex drive and stress levels are inversely related, a person under extreme stress probably would not find sexual activity the release that others might. Instead, those who are experiencing extreme stress should probably try some other strategy, such as those in Applications 2–4 and 6–12, before trying sex. When high stress levels have been reduced, sexual activity can arise more spontaneously.

6 *Eat and drink moderately:* Ingestion of moderate amounts of food or nonalcoholic beverages assists in dissipating stomach acids and returning stress levels to normal.

7 *Visualize:* Richard Restak (1991) relates an Eastern three-step technique for relieving "monkey mind," otherwise known as jumpiness or jitteriness. First, stare at an object, such as a plant. Then close your eyes and visualize that same object. Finally, open your eyes to confirm your visualization. This form of meditative observation, by focusing your attention, is calming. (For more information on visualizing, see Topic 13.1, Application 5.)

8 *Laugh:* Cousins (1989) reports that ten minutes of belly laughs can provide two hours of pain-free sleep. Laughter appears to be an especially important ingredient in recovering from life-threatening illness. Cousins reports that even a few moments of laughter can reduce the sedimentation rate, which is a measure of inflammation. Specifically, laughter results in enhanced respiration, an increased number of immune cells, an increase in immune-cell proliferation, a decrease in cortisol, an increase in endorphins, and an increase in salivary immunoglobulin A concentrations. Tests of problem-solving ability yield better results when they are preceded by laughter. Laughter has a way of turning off posterior hypothalamic activity and freeing the cerebral cortex for stress-free activity.

9 *Seek relief:* Arrange ways to get away from stressors. Have lists of babysitters, substitute caregivers, and temporary help. Use your creativity and the creativity of others to develop ways to relieve stress, such as neighborhood dinner co-ops and babysitting co-ops. Research says that simply knowing that relief is available is relaxing in and of itself. Air traffic controllers are more relaxed if they know they can call on relief when they need it. Usually, when flextime is initiated in organizations, few people use it; just knowing that it is an option is comfort enough. In one experiment, subjects taking a test were randomly assigned to one of two conditions: both groups had noise outside their room, but only one group was told they could shut the door if the noise became bothersome. The group given permission didn't close the door, yet they scored higher than the group without permission.

10 *Reframe the stressor:* Find a new way to explain your stressor so that it becomes less stressful. See Seligman (1991) and Bandler and Grinder (1982).

11 *Consider medication:* For severe long-term stress situations, you might consult a physician for pharmaceutical relief when other measures prove to be ineffective. Medication could be aimed at:

- Blocking alpha and beta receptors for adrenergic neurotransmitters to prevent sympathetic arousal
- Shutting down cortisol production (e.g., alprazolam and ketoconazole) in the adrenal gland
- Inhibiting the release of epinephrine and norepinephrine (the neurotransmitter GABA inhibits production of epinephrine and norepinephrine; Valium is one of the catalysts for GABA)
- Increasing cholinergic neurotransmitters (e.g., acetylcholine) and sensitizing muscarinic receptors, resulting in the release of cyclic guanosine monophosphate, which stimulates a parasympathetic response (the heart slows, pupils contract, digestion is stimulated)

Drugs can help prevent or shut down a sympathetic response and bring on a parasympathetic response. One result of failure to shut down sympathetic arousal is Type A behavior. See Topic 14.4 for more information on this behavior.

12 *Pets:* Handling pets is a great stress reliever, which explains the popular practice of taking pets to rest-home patients. (contributed by Rick Bradley)

Topic 14.3 Stress and arousal

Although there is evidence that many kinds of arousal exist, including both limbic and cortical arousal, research over the years has proceeded as though there were only one general type. One of the more popular examples of this research has come to be known as the Yerkes-Dodson law (Figure 14.1). It has two aspects. First, there is an optimum level of arousal. Too low a state of arousal, as when you are sleepy, appears to result in errors of omission, while too high a state of arousal, as when you are jittery from too much caffeine, results in errors of commission. In other words, when you are underaroused, you may leave things out, skip things, and be forgetful; when you are over-aroused, you may hit the wrong key while typing, act impulsively, and lose proper restraint. The second aspect is that the optimum point of arousal for complex tasks is different from the optimum point for simple tasks. Higher arousal (e.g., that extra cup of coffee) is more conducive to performing simpler tasks, while lower arousal is more conducive to performing more complex tasks (see Topic 6.2).

Redford Williams (1989) has identified a hierarchical relationship among three different forms of arousal. The kind of arousal described above and by the Yerkes-Dodson law might be described as *normal cortical arousal*. Williams describes two other forms of arousal that can suppress cortical arousal, regardless of whether an individual is under- or over-aroused cortically. The first is what he calls *focused attention and aggression*, such as that exhibited in athletic competition or military observation duty. Focused attention and aggression is a form of arousal accompanied by higher-than-normal levels of testosterone and characterized by partially suppressed cortical arousal; therefore, creativity and problem-solving ability are reduced. The other kind of arousal is what we have called the *general adaptation syndrome* (GAS) (see Topic 14.2), or fight-or-flight syndrome. During GAS, high cortisol levels are accompanied by virtually total suppression of cortical arousal. The four states are shown in Table 14.1, based on concepts developed by Redford Williams (1989).

Figure 14.1

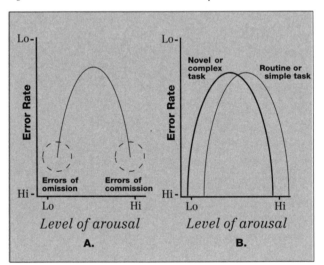

The Yerkes-Dodson law.

A. Normal optimal level of arousal. **B.** Simple, routine tasks require a somewhat higher level of arousal than complex, novel ones.

Table 14.1 The four states of arousal

Sleep	Normal arousal	Focused attention and aggression	Fight-or-flight syndrome
Typical behaviors during this state			
Rest, dream	Solve problems and be creative	Productivity, routinized behavior	Automatic pilot survival mode
Active neurotransmitters			
Melatonin	Acetylcholine, dopamine, serotonin	Testosterone	Epinephrine, norepinephrine, cortisol
Condition during normal arousal			
Partially suppressed	Active	Accessible	Accessible
Condition during focused attention			
Almost totally suppressed	Partially suppressed	Active	Accessible
Condition during fight-or-flight			
Almost totally suppressed	Almost totally suppressed	Almost totally suppressed	Active

Applications

1 If you happen to let yourself get overstimulated, for example, by drinking too much of a caffeinated beverage, switch to a task that is simpler and more repetitive than the task at hand (e.g., switch from writing to cleaning up). You will make fewer errors and the increased energy level required will help dissipate the high arousal. Otherwise, go exercise!

2 If you must perform a particularly complex task, such as writing an involved report or reviewing a complex set of numbers, switch to a noncaffeinated drink, limiting yourself to approximately one heavily caffeinated beverage every six hours. (For me, one cup of strong, home-dripped coffee equals two to three cups of standard commercial brew, with respect to its caffeine effect.) See Topic 6.2 for additional information on caffeine.

3 If you are concerned that focused attention and aggression is or will be interfering with your mental self-management, try aerobic exercise to calm you down before the big presentation, meeting, or date. The exercise will lower your testosterone level and its accompanying aggression.

Note: Based on ideas in *The Trusting Heart: Great News About Type A Behavior* by R. Williams, 1989, New York: Times Books.

Topic 14.4 Williams: Type A research

Redford Williams, in his book, *The Trusting Heart: Great News About Type A Behavior* (1989), defines Type A behavior as a cyclical form of hostile behavior that originates with cynicism, progresses into anger, culminates in an outburst of aggression, and recycles whenever the original cause of the cynicism recurs. Williams defines the onset of Type A behavior as the fulfillment of negative expectations. He contrasts cynicism with trust: cynicism expects the worst and has a toxic effect on the body, while trust expects better and has a non-toxic effect. What makes the Type A and Type B responses different is that, while both types can be cynical and hostile, Type A has a physiological defect that prevents restoration of the parasympathetic response following sympathetic arousal.

Cynicism expects the worst and has a toxic effect on the body, while trust expects better and has a nontoxic effect.

In his research at Duke University Medical School and elsewhere, Williams has learned that Type A personalities' brain-wave patterns take longer to return to normal after sympathetic arousal, because their parasympathetic response is sluggish. This is also known as parasympathetic antagonism. It is directly related to their lower production in the neuron of cyclic guanosine monophosphate, which directly triggers parasympathetic responses. Williams accounts for about 50 percent of Type A cases by postulating a low-endorphin gene that results in prolonged sympathetic arousal. For the other 50 percent, Williams points to childhoods with low trust and low touch. Far less Type A behavior exists in Japan; Williams accounts for this by pointing to the reputation of the Japanese for unconditional love in child rearing. While American kids average $17\frac{1}{2}$ seconds to resume crawling toward a toy after an "angry mother" comment, Japanese children average 49 seconds—they are less accustomed to angry comments and as a result the comments have a stronger impact.

Williams suggests that Type A personalities can use three kinds of strategies to gain control over their uncontrolled sympathetic response: religion, behavior modification, and medicine.

Applications

1 *Religion:* In Jerusalem's Hadassah Hospital, heart disease is four times higher among "secular" Jews. In Evans County, Georgia, churchgoers show lower blood pressure than nonchurchgoers. Williams suggests that religion typically urges individuals to be less concerned with love of self, more with love of others. Such behavior, followed consistently, would short-circuit the whole Type A response by breeding trust, not cynicism. An exception was seen in a study of 2,850 North Carolinians led by Keith Meador of the psychiatry department at

Vanderbilt University Medical Center in Nashville. He found that Pentecostal Christians (Church of God and Assembly of God) exhibit an incidence of depression three times higher than that of other religious groups.

2 *Behavior modification:* In addition to various communication skills available from books and workshops, such as assertiveness, conflict management, and negotiation skills, Williams suggests his Twelve-Step approach, which I summarize as follows:

1 Monitor your cynical thoughts.
2 Confess your hostility and seek support to change.
3 Stop cynical thoughts.
4 Reason with yourself.
5 Put yourself in the other person's shoes.
6 Laugh at yourself.
7 Practice the relaxation response.
8 Try trusting others.
9 Force yourself to listen more.
10 Substitute assertiveness for aggression.
11 Pretend that today is your last.
12 Practice forgiveness.

3 *Medicine:* See Topic 14.2, Application 11.

Topic 14.5 Golembiewski:
Burnout—the ultimate state of demotivation

Robert Golembiewski of the University of Georgia has developed a phase model for burnout (Golembiewski, 1988). The eight phases (see Table 14.2) are defined by levels of depersonalization, sense of personal achievement, and emotional exhaustion. Phase 1 exhibits little or no depersonalization, a reasonable sense of success and job worth, and little or no emotional fatigue, whereas phase 8 exhibits high depersonalization (people are seen as objects without innate value), absence of a personal sense of accomplishment or worth, and emotional exhaustion (a sense of being unable to cope anymore).

In a sample of over ten thousand people, 43 percent scored in phases 1 to 3 (no burnout), 13 percent scored in phases 4 and 5 (borderline burnout), and 44 percent scored in phases 6 to 8 (from moderate to extreme burnout). Physical measures of cholesterol, uric acid, blood pressure, number of sick days used, weight, smoking, drinking, and so on appear to increase uniformly along this

Table 14.2 Golembiewski's phase model of burnout

Factors of burnout	Phases							
	1	2	3	4	5	6	7	8
1. Depersonalization	Lo	Hi	Lo	Hi	Lo	Hi	Lo	Hi
2. Personal achievement[a]	Lo	Lo	Hi	Hi	Lo	Lo	Hi	Hi
3. Emotional exhaustion	Lo	Lo	Lo	Lo	Hi	Hi	Hi	Hi

Note: From *Phases of Burnout* by R. T. Golembiewski, 1988, New York: Praeger. Reprinted by permission of the author.

[a]Reversed: A low score equals a higher sense of personal achievement.

model. For example, phase 1 shows lower levels of cholesterol, with levels getting progressively higher through phase 8.

We have defined burnout as the result of prolonged stress. Golembiewski gets more specific by defining it as a sense that we and others have no worth, with no energy to do anything about it. Notice the similarity of his definition of burnout to Seligman's definition of pessimism (personal, pervasive, and permanent helplessness) (Seligman, 1991). Seligman's research focuses on depression and Golembiewski's focuses on burnout, but the working mechanisms appear to be similar. Burnout appears to be the organizational form of depression.

Golembiewski's research has two findings that are particularly important in dealing with the results of burnout. First, he found that burnout did not occur randomly throughout organizations. Instead, it seemed to occur in clusters of workers with a common supervisor. His conclusion was that the quality of the supervisor is responsible for the lion's share of burnout in organizations. Second, he found that people appear to use two different styles to deal with their stress: active and passive. When they reach the stage of burnout, passives have to take extended vacations or personal leave in order to restore their emotional resources and sense of worth, while actives might benefit more from workshops, self-help materials, and wellness programs.

Applications

1 If you are a human resources administrator, you should use employee surveys, Golembiewski's survey, or good common sense (sick-leave patterns, for example) to determine where the actual or potential pockets of burnout are in your organization. Then determine whether you need to train or replace the supervisors in those pockets. Some organizations are experimenting with eliminating the role of supervisor by developing self-directed work teams. For Golembiewski's survey, write to:

> Dr. Robert Golembiewski
> Department of Political Science
> Baldwin Hall
> University of Georgia
> Athens, GA 30602
> 404-542-2970

2 Provide seminars, self-help materials, wellness programs, and employee counseling resources to assist highly stressed employees in learning ways to cope more effectively.

3 For more passive styles of dealing with burnout, the strategies in Application 2 won't work. For passives, you may need to be prepared to offer extended leave followed by transfer to a new work unit upon return.

Topic 14.6 The two sides of the brain

Volumes of research have documented the specialization of function in the two hemispheres of the brain, and this topic has captured the imagination of the reading public. Yet the practical, day-to-day implications are few. In addition, many of the findings are exaggerated, with fantastic conclusions drawn from scant data. We do know that the left brain is the seat of language, logic, interpretation, and arithmetic, while the right brain is the seat of geometry, nonverbal processes, visual pattern recognition (faces, lines), auditory discrimination, and spatial skills. We know that the left hemisphere governs activity on the right side of the body and the right hemisphere governs activity on the left side. We know that people of all ages inwardly exhibit measurable left-brain activity when they outwardly engage in approach behaviors, cheerfulness, and other such positive emotions. Avoidance behaviors and negative emotions, on the other hand, are associated with activity in the right brain (Fox, 1991). Many excellent summaries of this research are available (e.g., Gazzaniga, 1985).

Applications
1 There is some evidence that talking, in and of itself, promotes positive emotions. If you know people who need cheering up, find ways to engage them

in conversation, either actively or passively: go to a movie or carry on a conversation with a sick friend. (Rick Bradley suggests that if you can't go in person, send a video- or audiocassette.)

2   There is some evidence that artistic activity serves as a vehicle to express negative emotions. If you know people who need to deal openly with negative emotions or experiences, try artistic, nonverbal modes of expression. Gestures (pantomimes, etc.) are a right-brain activity, hence a good vehicle for expressing emotions (which are also centered in the right brain).

3   Certain drugs, such as imipramine, are able to increase activity in the left hemisphere and hence relieve some depressive states.

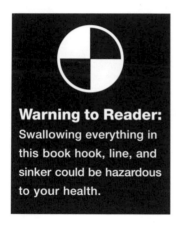

Warning to Reader:
Swallowing everything in this book hook, line, and sinker could be hazardous to your health.

Topic 14.7 Testosterone and the achievement syndrome

Moir and Jessel (1991) summarize research on the relationship between testosterone level and what might be called the achievement syndrome. They find that automized behaviors—repetitive behaviors that require little mental or physical effort yet drop off over time because of fatigue or boredom—are stronger in people with higher testosterone levels (they make fewer mistakes and don't tire as quickly). Examples of such behaviors are math computation, walking, talking, keeping balance, maintaining observation, and copying. In several controlled studies, subjects injected with testosterone showed significantly less decline in skill performance as time passed. Those who were not injected showed an increase in mistakes and fatigue. No level of testosterone is directly related to degree of persistence, which is defined as a combination of focus and energy.

Applications
1   Testosterone level can be increased by participating in a competitive sport and winning. So if you feel you need a boost in testosterone and resist the idea of injections, try finding a tennis opponent you can beat before automized behavior is required.

2   Remember from Redford Williams's research (R. Williams, 1989) that two kinds of arousal can be generated by the mind's reaction to the environment: energy to focus and concentrate, which results from increased testosterone production, and energy to fight, flee, or freeze, which results from increased cortisol (from the epinephrine-norepinephrine chain). The latter suppresses the former;

People at work

in other words, as cortisol production increases, testosterone decreases. So if automized behavior is important to you, you need to dissipate the cortisol, or stress, in your body.

Suggested readings on molecular approaches to stress

Gazzaniga, M. S. (1985). *The Social Brain*. New York: Basic Books.

Golembiewski, R. T. (1988). *Phases of Burnout*. New York: Praeger.

Selye, H. (1952). *The Story of the Adaptation Syndrome*. Montreal: Acta.

Williams, R. (1989). *The Trusting Heart: Great News About Type A Behavior*. New York: Times Books.

15

Getting an attitude: Reframing

In the previous chapter, we discussed the physiological, or molecular, side of motivation. It is important to remember that, in all probability, 50 percent of the variance in motivation can be accounted for by our genetic inheritance. Therefore, our levels of testosterone, cortisol, and guanosine monophosphate; the constitution of our endorphin gene; the distribution of the various kinds of immune cells in our system; and our hemispheric dominance—all of which affect our motivation, or level of action—are essentially set from conception. The research indicates that we primarily influence these levels downward. This means, for example, that the pursuit of hardiness allows us to fully utilize our genetic endowment of natural killer cells but probably does not increase our normal level. On the other hand, allowing stress, pessimism, and negative feelings to dominate our minds can actually lower our motivational resources.

The degree to which we see ourselves or others as more or less motivated can be accounted for by either attitude or physical makeup. We can't change physical makeup without resorting to pharmaceuticals, surgery, or genetic engineering. In a serious case, we might wish to consult a team consisting of a neurosurgeon, a psychiatrist, a neuropsychologist, and a genetic engineer to explore the possibilities of getting fixed. Otherwise, we must explore more molar, or environmental, approaches. If we choose not to tamper with nature, we can at least maximize what we've got by ensuring that our nurture is as good as it can be.

The next several sections explore the molar approaches to motivation.

strategies for a healthier outlook

Topic 15.1 Empowerment:
Extrinsic versus intrinsic rewards

The apparent consensus of current thinking on motivation revolves around the question of who sets a course of action: *external* (or *extrinsic*) *motivation* refers to courses of action set by others, while *internal* (or *intrinsic*) *motivation* refers to courses of action set by oneself. Listed in Table 15.1 are some examples of motivational situations (those in which an individual is expected to act in some way), with both external and internal versions of the motivational stimulus.

Table 15.1 External versus internal motivation

Call for action	External version	Internal version
Sales goals	Manager or company sets goals for representatives	Manager and representative set goals together and mutually agree
Incentives	Company announces incentives	Employees negotiate incentives
Child discipline	Parent determines consequences of misbehavior	Child and parent together negotiate appropriate consequences
Class award	Teacher announces award before competition, presents award afterward	Award is announced only after work is completed
Work design	Management designs and monitors	Workers design and management supports

Consistently, internal motivators yield higher performance than external motivators. Amabile (1983) notes one exception: when clear guidelines are presented that call for essentially rote performance, then external motivators yield superior results. She also identifies a variation on this principle: rewards that convey competency information, as in "A panel of art experts mistakenly judged the copy of the Van Gogh you painted to be the original." External motivators are more effective with algorithmic, or step-by-step, tasks, while internal motivators are more effective with heuristic, or experimental, ones. I am reminded of a now-discontinued (I hope) incentive program of an NFL team in which thousand-dollar bonuses were allegedly handed out after each game for every player on the opposing team who was put out of commission (e.g., if a tackler broke the leg of a pass receiver).

Consistently, internal motivators yield higher performance than external motivators.

Caine and Caine (1991) point out that under continuous stress, internal motivation becomes more and more difficult to generate. People begin to see themselves as fulfilling only goals formed by others. Amabile (1983) extensively documents the harmful effects of extrinsic motivation on creativity and problem solving. Gazzaniga (1985) has found that people learning to perform a skill under external conditions tend to perform that skill only when the reward possibilities continue to be presented. Give a person a day off for a job well done, and future good performance will tend to become tied to continuing rewards. Give what you've always given, and you'll get what you've always gotten. Stop giving, and you stop getting. Research supports mutually discussing possible rewards, rather than paternalistically doling out what you think people want.

Internal motivators are developed by *participation* in goal setting and problem solving, as opposed to allowing others to set your goals, make your decisions, and solve your problems. In the summer of 1990, my wife and I were walking down the coast of Sunset Beach, North Carolina, and we asked each other what bothers could be removed to make life more enjoyable. Jane's top bother was feeling guilty about not providing her share of the caregiving for her parents, who were living six hours away (by car) in Opelika, Alabama. I suggested that she make a conference call with her two sisters—one in Alabama, the other in Minnesota—and discuss the problem. I remember that we emphasized the wisdom of trying to figure out a solution before her parents experienced another crisis (her mother had recently broken a hip) and our options became severely limited and, in fact, thrust upon us.

The call and subsequent research resulted in several options that were mutually agreeable with the three sisters. Jane, as spokesperson, called her parents to discuss the options, one of which was to maintain the status quo. They were also invited to identify other possible options. As it turned out, her parents became very excited about one particular option: to move to a retirement community in Charlotte located about five minutes from our home, with the two sisters retiring to our region (one to the mountains, the other to the beach) within five or so years. My wife's mother brightly queried, "When do we leave?"

While the move and settling in did not happen without some sadness, regret, and fear, now, two years later, both parents are well adjusted, with new friends and new church homes. My wife's mother, a former church organist, is playing more piano than ever and entertains almost daily in the parlor after dinner. Recently, at the age of seventy-seven, she gave a one-hour organ recital for over forty residents of the retirement community. The health and vigor of Jane's parents have improved by this change, and Jane's guilt has disappeared. If our hand had been forced by a crisis, like a massive stroke, it is highly possible that guilt would have been transmogrified into resentment and anger. I see this episode as a testament to participation in internal motivation.

Gazzaniga (1985), Caine and Caine (1991), Amabile (1983), and Seligman (1991) all call for an end to external motivators. We have been operating under the paradigm of the behavioral contingency model of externally imposed rewards and punishments since the 1940s. Now the time has come to eliminate them, to encourage the new paradigm of empowerment through self- or mutually developed action planning. Gazzaniga goes so far as to decry bureaucracy and institutionalization as the enemy of internal motivation. He sees institutional relief of the symptoms of social ills as the opposite of caring: "I am claiming that a culture becomes more caring and humane the more its citizens feel themselves to be part of the problems that beset their lives. The only sure way to bring them close to such problems is to structure a culture where they deal with the problems at a personal level" (1985, p. 198).

From a societal perspective, what these researchers are saying is consistent with the current preoccupation of many social philosophers with treating root causes, not symptoms. In a recent task force on our aging population, the group coalesced around the need to address causes, but agreed that we can't ignore symptoms. For example, to ensure that each senior citizen gets at least one hot meal a day, we need to back up and treat the causes of malnutrition among that population. But our inability to provide such meals is actually both a symptom and a cause—a symptom of poor public transportation and a cause of malnutrition. The resources are there, but access is limited. So we must fix the infrastructure.

Applications

1 If you are a parent or a teacher, don't assume that you always know the right rewards and punishments. When appropriate, consult with your children or students. Read works by William Glasser and Richard Dreikurs for ideas (Glasser, 1990; Dreikurs & Cassel, 1972).

2   If you are a manager who is responsible for the performance of others, talk with them to learn what's important to them and what their career goals are. Don't assume that you know the best way to reward them or the best direction for them in their careers. A former manager of mine assumed that I was motivated by the desire to earn more and more money, even after I explained that I was more motivated by challenging projects than by big bucks. My ultimate departure from that company was largely based on his failure to abandon his externally imposed rewards for me (higher salaries) and accept my need for challenging and interesting projects. Bucks don't always have bang!

Help people understand dilemmas rather than "fixing things" for them.

3   Build an empowered work force. As part of a management team, take time to explore ways to give people increasing responsibility and opportunities to solve their own problems, make their own decisions, formulate their own plans, establish their own goals, negotiate their own rewards, and even describe their own jobs. Mutually agree on goals, then get out of their way. Don't be an *intervener* with your people, coming down like an avenging god. Instead, be a *supporter,* and be there when they need you for resources and consultation. For further ideas on empowerment, read Peter Block's *The Empowered Manager* (1987) and D. C. Kinlaw's *Developing Superior Work Teams* (1990).

4   As a spouse and friend, help people understand dilemmas rather than "fixing things" for them. Long term, these externally imposed solutions tend to lose their power. If your friend or spouse can participate in formulating his or her own solutions, these internally generated solutions are more likely to hold their power. Be more of a consultant than a boss. "Teach a person how to fish and . . ."

5   Do not protect alcoholics or other addictive personalities from the consequences of their binges. Such protectors used to be called patsies and are now called enablers. A considerable literature has emerged on this subject as a part of the Adult Children of Alcoholics movement. Write for information, a bibliography, catalogs, and reading material to:

National Association for Children of Alcoholics
31582 Coast Highway, Suite B
South Laguna, CA 92677
714-499-3889

or

Adult Children of Alcoholics
P.O. Box 3216
Torrance, CA 90505
213-534-1815
Send a stamped, self-addressed envelope for a schedule of meetings.

6 Amabile (1983) identifies several indicators for judging whether or not a person is intrinsically motivated. I summarize four of them as follows:

- The individual is curious or stimulated by the task.
- The individual gains a sense of competence from the task itself.
- The individual perceives the task as free of strong external control.
- The individual feels as if he or she is at play, not at work.

7 In one corporation where I am currently consulting, management doles out recognition cards as rewards. Employees then exchange the cards for a gift of their choosing. Many employees have confided that they would much rather receive a verbal recognition statement specifying what they did well and the impact it had on the company. Stay close enough to the people close to you to know what rewards they really value.

Topic 15.2 Learned optimism: Seligman's ABCDE model

In Topic 13.1, I presented Martin Seligman's concept of the explanatory style, which is based on optimism versus pessimism. Optimism is linked to positive moods and achievement, whereas pessimism is linked to depression. Optimism results from personal, pervasive, and permanent explanations of success and external, specific, and temporary explanations of adversity. Pessimism results from external, specific, and temporary explanations of success and personal, pervasive, and permanent explanations of adversity.

Seligman has found success in teaching a form of learned optimism to people with a pessimistic explanatory style, using the ABCDE approach. ABC refers to how we react negatively to success or adversity, while DE refers to how we can rethink the pessimistic reaction into an optimistic one. The letters are defined as follows:

- *A (Adversity).* Recognize when adversity hits. For die-hard pessimists, successes are a form of adversity; they say, "It won't last," "I was just lucky," or "Too little, too late."

- *B (Beliefs).* Be aware of what you believe about the adversity.

- *C (Consequences).* Be aware of the emotional and other consequences of your belief about that adversity.

- *D (Disputation).* Question whether your beliefs are the only explanation. For example, ask:
  - What is the evidence for my beliefs?
  - What are other possible explanations for what happened?
  - What are the implications of my believing this way, and do they make it worth holding onto my beliefs?
  - How useful are my beliefs? Do I or others get any benefits from holding onto them? Would we get more benefits from holding other beliefs?

- *E (Energization).* Be aware of the new consequences (feelings, behaviors, actions) that do or could follow from a different (and more optimistic) explanation or set of beliefs.

Here is an example of the ABCDE model as I applied it to a specific situation. My train of thought went like this:

1   I didn't finish this chapter by the end of the Thanksgiving holiday as I promised my wife and myself I would do. (*Adversity*)

2   I'm an incurable procrastinator who'll never meet my goals. (*Beliefs: a personal, pervasive, and permanent explanation, which is therefore pessimistic*)

3   I might as well abandon this project and settle for a life of less ambitious projects. That way, my wife won't be disappointed with me when I miss deadlines. (*Consequence*)

4   Wait a minute! Lots of writers set unrealistic deadlines. Besides, my wife and I did several things together and with her parents that had a very positive impact on our relationship. And if sticking to my schedule were so all-fired important to her, she could have insisted on doing some of those things without me. (*Disputation*)

5   I'll talk about my schedule with her and get her input on whether the remainder of the schedule is important to her. If not, I'll push my deadlines back. If so, I'll ask her assistance and cooperation in finding ways to make more time for writing. I really don't want to give up this project—it's exciting, even if it is a little off-schedule. (*Energization*)

Applications

1   Seligman (1991) presents a series of examples showing how the DE steps help to dispute and break up the negative effects of the ABC part. He also recommends keeping a journal of adverse events using the ABCDE structure for each entry.

2   Each time you are aware of negative feelings following a specific event, follow it up immediately with questions aimed at disputing your pessimistic explanation: look for evidence, alternatives, implications, and usefulness. If you can't dispute your feelings because of the circumstances of the moment, make it a point to do it later in the day during a moment of quiet and reflection. Always ask, Is there another explanation for what happened that is more useful and more pleasing? Emphasize the personal, pervasive, and permanent features of your successes, and the external, specific, and temporary features of your adversities.

> Emphasize the personal, pervasive, and permanent features of your successes, and the external, specific, and temporary features of your adversities.

Topic 15.3 The Pygmalion effect: Rosenthal and the self-fulfilling prophecy

Many regard Robert Rosenthal as the prophet of the Pygmalion effect (also known as the self-fulfilling prophecy). According to the myth, Pygmalion created a female statue and treated it with such affection that, through Aphrodite's intervention, the statue came to life and responded to him. Such is the essence of the self-fulfilling prophecy: what we expect tends to come true. In a famous report (Rosenthal & Jacobson, 1968), Rosenthal describes a case in which a researcher told teachers that a testing program had identified some students as having high potential and others as having low potential. In fact, the students had been picked randomly and assigned to one of the two groups. The results after a year in school: the so-called high-potential group showed significant gains in achievement and ability as measured by standardized tests.

Rosenthal's initial report has been followed by twenty years of research exploring the limits of the self-fulfilling prophecy. The thinking today is that, while we can't think a statue into coming alive, we can certainly influence our level of performance and that of others by the level of our expectations. Cousins (1989) includes positive expectations as one of the four key ingredients of hardiness as it relates to psychoneuroimmunology. The concept of the self-fulfilling prophecy is also very close

Getting an attitude   **197**

Table 15.2 Rosenthal's six methods for communicating expectations

Communication method	Positive versions	Negative versions
1 Expressing confidence in my ability to help you	"I know I can train you" "Stick with me—I make winners" "I've got the Midas touch"	"I'm not sure I know how to train you" "I'm not very good at training"
2 Expressing confidence in your ability	"I know you can do it"	"I'm not sure if you can do it"
3 Nonverbals: tone of voice, eye contact, energy level	Smile, nod, pat, eye contact, upbeat energy	Looking away, tentative tone of voice, distant
4 Feedback: specific and ample; mentioning good with the bad	"Good coverage, yet a couple of technical flaws"	"Try harder" "All wrong" "Reread it; you'll see what I mean"
5 Input: amount of information given to person	"Let's go over it in detail"	"I don't have time to go over it"
6 Output: amount of production encouraged	"Here's a new challenge"	"Better try the same thing again"

to Seligman's concept of the optimistic explanatory style; in some ways, Seligman's research has subsumed Rosenthal's. Rosenthal identifies six ways to communicate expectations. I have summarized them and provided examples in Table 15.2.

Applications

1   Be aware that negative expectations of yourself or others are likely to produce negative results. While positive expectations ("I think I can" or "You can do it") cannot guarantee success, they certainly increase its chances.

2   Think of a particular person in your life who performs at a lower level than you'd like to see. Examine the six communication methods in Table 15.2 and see if you may be communicating negative expectations without meaning to. Work on being as positive with this person as you can in each of the six ways. Write out a script for yourself with sample comments in each of the six areas.

3   View the 1987 award-winning video, *Productivity and the Self-Fulfilling Prophecy* (CRM Films, 2215 Faraday Avenue, Carlsbad, CA 92008). Check with your regional media distributor for ordering information. Discuss its implications for your situation. A video with implications for race relations is 1970's *The Eye of the Storm* (produced by the American Broadcast Company, distributed by the Center for Humanities, Inc., P.O. Box 1000, Mt. Kisco, NY 10549). It shows how the self-fulfilling prophecy works in conjunction with prejudice.

4   Keep the idea of a self-fulfilling prophecy in mind when you are working with teams. Be positive in your approach to problem solving and work toward win-win situations or compromises. Keep the team asking "How can we make this work?" There are many situations in which one positive person can turn the entire team around. (contributed by Jane Howard)

Topic 15.4 Neurolinguistic programming: Establishing rapport

The most readable treatment of neurolinguistic programming (NLP) is Genie Laborde's *Influencing with Integrity* (1983). NLP originated when some psychotherapists began to wonder how the great therapists—Fritz Perls, Virginia Satir, Milton Eriksen—worked their magic with patients. They concluded that these outstanding therapists demonstrated the ability to consciously or unconsciously establish a deep rapport with their patients, leading to trust, disclosure, openness to change, and receptivity to the therapist. Through extensive observation, the researchers concluded that this rapport was established when the therapists matched content and paced tempo with the client.

Matching content has been made popular through the VAK concept of visual, auditory, and kinesthetic matching. In visual matching, the patient says, "I can't *see* what she means," and the therapist responds, "What she wants is *hazy* to you." By matching the visual imagery contained in the patient's language, the therapist builds rapport. If the patient's language contains auditory imagery ("I *hear* what you're saying"), the therapist can respond with an auditory image ("I'm coming through to you *loud and clear*"). Kinesthetic matching—"I'm *struggling* to understand you"—might be answered with "You're trying to *grasp* what I mean." Pacing involves matching the tempo of the patient's speech, movements, and breathing: the therapist talks more slowly when the patient does, synchronizes his or her breathing, and matches fidgeting with fidgeting. Figure 15.1 is a guide to the many possible ways to match and pace as a way to establish rapport.

I do need to point out, and not assume that it is obvious, that matching and pacing are situational and not continuous. To continue to match and pace hour after hour, day after day, would be inauthentic and unhealthy. Hans Selye has more to say about this problem in Topic 15.5.

Applications

1   Pick a person you need to influence. Peruse Figure 15.1 and identify one or more channels through which you might try to establish rapport in an acceptable way.

2   Read Laborde's *Influencing with Integrity* (1983) and *Fine Tune Your Brain* (1988). In addition to ample explanatory material, Laborde provides an excellent bibliography.

Figure 15.1

The elements of rapport.   **3**   Observe and model yourself after an influential person.

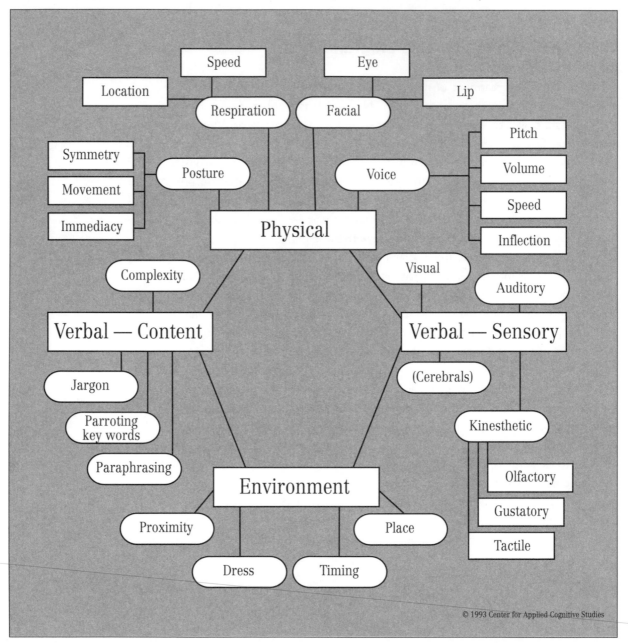

© 1993 Center for Applied Cognitive Studies

4   Watch for demonstrations of rapport that you have established with someone you have been talking with. If one of you shifts position and you notice that the other one shifts too, you have probably established rapport. (contributed by Jane Howard)

Topic 15.5 Hans Selye and trait dissonance

Hans Selye once wrote of the rabbit and the turtle. Some of us approach life more like a rabbit, running from place to place, nibbling when we can, shooting off in all directions. Others approach life more like a turtle, proceeding methodically from point to point with careful attention to detail, taking things one at a time. Both extremes are healthy. What is unhealthy, or stressful, is when we try to be different from our nature. For example, the rabbit spouse says to his or her turtle companion, "You never want to go anywhere or do anything." The turtle, feeling guilty, decides to become a rabbit for the night and go bar-hopping with the rabbit spouse. That, according to Selye, is what causes stress.

    Well, at least it is *one* cause of stress!

Applications

1   To what degree do you expect others to be like you—to use your vocabulary, to walk at your speed, to talk as fast or slowly as you do? Do you feel that others are inferior to you because they talk more slowly than you do (a classic source of misunderstanding between a New Englander and a Southerner)? Be aware of these judgments, and don't let such surface behaviors be mistaken for indicators of ability. (Rick Bradley recalls a former manager whose perception of a co-worker was that he was "slow" because he had an unhurried gait.)

2   When you feel pressured to change your personality to meet with a spouse's, friend's, or boss's approval, it's time to sit down with that person and talk it through. If you are unsuccessful, you may need to bring in a third party (counselor, consultant, friend) to help establish the necessity of maintaining your differences in personality and behavior. Don't ignore the conflict—that will only lead to resentment and may rupture the relationship.

What is motivation and how can we increase it?

What calls us to act? What motivates us? Put most simply, it is the perception that we are in charge of our lives. When we feel that we are out of control it is usually because we perceive real or imagined deficiencies in our physical or mental makeup—we feel we are not strong enough, not fast enough, not insightful enough. These deficiencies can be addressed by specific strategies for improvement. At the risk of appearing to oversimplify the motivation problem, I have listed in Table 15.3 the state of research with respect to the likely causes of low motivation and possible remedies.

Above all, take charge! Cheerfully!

Table 15.3 Causes and remedies for low motivation

Likely causes	Possible remedies
Physical	
Low testosterone	Testosterone injections; competitions at which you can win
Parasympathetic antagonism	Drugs that perform acetylcholine's function of sensitizing muscarinic receptors and the release of guanosine monophosphate (consult a neuropsychiatrist); Williams's Twelve Steps; taking up religion
Excess epinephrine, norepinephrine, or both	Noncompetitive aerobic exercise
Low epinephrine, norepinephrine, or both	Lower your blood sugar by exercise or fasting
Left cerebral hemisphere underactive	Drugs that increase blood flow and glucose metabolism in the left lobe (consult a neuropsychiatrist); talking therapy; Seligman's ABCDE technique
Low immune cell count	Remove stressors
Mental	
Pessimistic explanatory style	Learn Seligman's ABCDE technique; seek a good cognitive therapist
Burnout	Take a long break or leave of absence with the assistance of a therapist; change jobs, or otherwise change the situation that is the source of the burnout; somehow find a new (and better) supervisor
Stress (remember, the higher the stress, the lower the ambition; find your optimun level)	Find one or more strategies in Topic 14.2 that work for you; remove your stressors by changing yourself, changing others, or changing your situation
Excessive reliance on external or extrinsic rewards	Explore how to convert to internal or intrinsic rewards—take an active role in setting your goals and planning action strategies to reach them
People don't pay sufficient attention to you	Try practicing neurolinguistic programming's matching and pacing
Low expectation of self and others	Practice the Pygmalion effect; develop Cousins's sense of "hardiness"

Suggested readings on molar approaches to motivation

Amabile, T. M. (1983). *The Social Psychology of Creativity.* New York: Springer-Verlag.

Caine, R. N., & Caine, G. (1991). *Making Connections: Teaching and the Human Brain.* Alexandria, VA: Association for Supervision and Curriculum Development.

Gazzaniga, M. S. (1985). *The Social Brain.* New York: Basic Books.

Laborde, G. Z. (1983). *Influencing with Integrity.* Palo Alto, CA: Syntony.

Laborde, G. Z. (1988). *Fine Tune Your Brain.* Palo Alto, CA: Syntony.

Rosenthal, R., & Jacobson, L. (1968). *Pygmalion in the Classroom.* New York: Holt, Rinehart & Winston.

Seligman, M.E.P. (1991). *Learned Optimism.* New York: Knopf.

Selye, H. (1952). *The Story of the Adaptation Syndrome.* Montreal: Acta.

16

Brain ergonomics: Workplace design

Ergonomics is the study of how to adapt the workplace to the worker.
It comes from the Greek root *ergon,* or "work," and is also referred to as human-factors engineering. Its efforts are aimed at making the workplace more user-friendly for human workers by minimizing or eliminating harmful stress on their bodies and minds. An ergonomics specialist, for example, would figure out how to make my keyboard bend outward from the middle in a way that would eliminate the stress on my wrist that causes tennis elbow.

This chapter deals with one specific domain of ergonomics: how the brain responds to the workplace. Here we are looking at the elements of workplace design that specifically affect the brain and nervous system. We will not talk about the proper shape of a chair for optimal back support, but about such things as the effect of light on mood and wakefulness. Remember that many of the findings in this chapter are equally applicable to the home, which is a workplace of sorts for all of us.

Temporal considerations

The mind is like a moving picture—you can't stop it. If you stop a moving picture, you have a photograph; if you stop your mind, you have a corpse. Time is inextricably woven into the fabric of mental activity. Some even define intelligence as speed of response. There are several aspects of time that affect the functioning of the brain at work.

for quality and productivity

Topic 16.1 Breaks

We have long known the importance of breaks for minimizing error and fatigue and maximizing productivity, quality, and morale. A recent study (Okogbaa & Shell, 1986) summarizes this research. In addition, the authors offer specific guidelines for minimizing fatigue in computer operators.

As a general rule, workers need five- to ten-minute breaks every one to two hours. The frequency and duration of these breaks will depend on the nature of the work and the worker. To determine the need for breaks, try (1) asking the worker and (2) keeping error logs.

Breaks also support the need in thought processes for "chunking" (see Topic 18.1) and spacing (see Topic 20.2). Work involving higher mental functions such as analysis and synthesis needs to be spaced out to allow new neural connections to solidify. New learning drives out old learning when insufficient time intervenes.

> "God obligeth no man to more than he hath given him ability to perform."
>
> **The Koran**

Applications

1 Allow yourself and your workers to establish optimal periods for breaks. As a simple guideline, when you become aware of more errors or fatigue, take a break.

2 Keep records on error rates over time. Talk with your workers, sharing these records with them. Establish a mutually agreeable policy for taking breaks.

3 Avoid, where possible, rigidly mandating the length of time between breaks. Fatigue may set in earlier or later than your fixed work period, and workers need to recognize it and respond to it promptly. Workers differ: some require longer work periods with longer breaks, while others require shorter periods with shorter breaks. Workers need to feel that they have the authority and responsibility to take a break when they feel the onset of fatigue, particularly where safety issues are involved (driving, operating heavy equipment, lifting loads, etc.).

4 The ideal break involves some level of exercise, such as throwing horseshoes, walking, or playing basketball. This can dissipate the results of overarousal or stimulate people out of boredom or underarousal.

5 During breaks, mind workers should avoid simple carbohydrates and fats (this includes most candy bars and other sweets), which cause sleepiness; proteins and complex carbohydrates such as fruits are fine.

6 Too much caffeine (more than one serving every six hours) causes errors of commission; mind workers are more subject to this phenomenon than muscle workers—the latter burn off excess caffeine more quickly. On the other hand, too little caffeine can cause drowsiness and errors of omission. This could be a serious safety issue for operators of heavy equipment.

7 Display signs like the following ones in break areas to remind workers of the guidelines in Applications 3–6:

"Been sitting all day? Take a stroll outside!"
"Been standing all day? Take a load off your feet!"
"Feeling tense and shaky? Get some exercise."
     (Show pictures of people throwing horseshoes
     or darts or jumping rope.)
"Feeling drowsy? Try exercise, fresh air, light, caffeine."
"Try these foods when you feel nervous—"
     (Show pictures of carbohydrates and fats.)

8 Offer a lunchtime training program to give information on breaks to people.

Topic 16.2 Shifts

For workers who must work a night shift, such as midnight to 8:00 A.M., two issues are important: (1) ensuring good sleep and (2) ensuring alertness at work. Because the body appears to work on a twenty-five-hour cycle (see Topic 7.2), shifts should advance forward, not backward. In other words, day shifts should be followed by afternoon shifts, then by night shifts. Following a day shift with a night shift fights against the natural body clock. For the many other factors that affect quality of sleep, browse through Chapter Seven.

Applications

1   If you are trying to sleep during daylight hours, ensure total darkness. Use blindfolds and black window shades if necessary. Earplugs can also be helpful. The new foam rubber plugs are form-fitting and unnoticeable.

2   Wake up to bright lights to help reset your body clock. (See Topic 7.2 for the recommended light strength and pattern.) Work areas, break areas, and toilets should all be especially well lit for shift workers.

3   An ideal twenty-one-day shift progression built on the twenty-five-hour cycle would look something like the one shown in Table 16.1.

Extraverts adapt more quickly to time-zone and shift changes.

Topic 16.3 Time-zone changes

Extraverts adapt more quickly to time-zone and shift changes, while the physiology of introverts resists time changes. The principal problem is resetting the body's clock; introverts need more help in doing this. The major factors in resetting the body clock are the neurotransmitters serotonin and melatonin. Serotonin can be controlled by diet, and melatonin can be controlled both by diet and by the use of available light. Carbohydrates in general tend to increase serotonin, while dairy products and total darkness tend to increase melatonin.

Applications

1   If you are a more introverted personality, make an extra effort when you must travel through different time zones or change shifts. Light therapy helps (see Topic 17.2); in addition, avoid caffeine, alcohol, artificial sweeteners, and food additives for six hours before you try to sleep after a time-zone change. Consume dairy products, carbohydrates, and fats for maximum facilitation of sleep (milk and cookies, cheese and bread).

Brain ergonomics   **207**

Table 16.1 An ideal sleep-shift progression

Day	Shift starts	Shift ends	Bedtime	Waking time
1	12:00 MIDNIGHT	8:00 A.M.	1:30 P.M.	9:00 P.M.
2	(OFF)		2:30 P.M.	10:00 P.M.
3	(OFF)		3:30 P.M.	11:00 P.M.
4	8:00 A.M.	4:00 P.M.	4:30 P.M.	12:00 MIDNIGHT
5	8:00 A.M.	4:00 P.M.	5:30 P.M.	1:00 A.M.
6	8:00 A.M.	4:00 P.M.	6:30 P.M.	2:00 A.M.
7	8:00 A.M.	4:00 P.M.	7:30 P.M.	2:30 A.M.
8	8:00 A.M.	4:00 P.M.	9:30 P.M.	5:00 A.M.
9	(OFF)		10:30 P.M.	6:00 A.M.
10	(OFF)		11:30 P.M.	7:00 A.M.
11	4:00 P.M.	12:00 MIDNIGHT	1:00 A.M.	8:30 A.M.
12	4:00 P.M.	12:00 MIDNIGHT	2:00 A.M.	9:30 A.M.
13	4:00 P.M.	12:00 MIDNIGHT	3:00 A.M.	10:30 A.M.
14	4:00 P.M.	12:00 MIDNIGHT	4:00 A.M.	11:30 A.M.
15	4:00 P.M.	12:00 MIDNIGHT	5:00 A.M.	12:30 P.M.
16	(OFF)		6:30 A.M.	2:00 P.M.
17	(OFF)		7:30 A.M.	3:00 P.M.
18	12:00 MIDNIGHT	8:00 A.M.	9:00 A.M.	4:30 P.M.
19	12:00 MIDNIGHT	8:00 A.M.	10:00 A.M.	5:30 P.M.
20	12:00 MIDNIGHT	8:00 A.M.	11:00 A.M.	6:30 P.M.
21	12:00 MIDNIGHT	8:00 A.M.	12:00 NOON	7:30 P.M.

2   If you are responsible for managing shift schedules, remember that more extraverted personalities are less disrupted by time-zone or shift changes. This doesn't mean that introverts can't be called on to work night shifts, but you should (a) be sure that they know the precautions to take for minimum disruption and (b) accept their bodily resistance to time changes as normal and not as an attitude problem.

3   Try the following pattern, or something like it, if traveling across time zones gets you down. This pattern assumes a 6:00 P.M. departure in the United States from the East Coast and an 8:00 A.M. (local time) arrival in Europe or Africa, with your body operating as though it were actually 2:00 A.M. You are, in essence, being asked to skip one night's sleep. The solution is to sleep once you arrive or to sleep on the plane. Sleeping once you arrive is best, if you can arrange it. Remember, consume no caffeine or other stimulants for six hours before the flight, and use an eye mask and earplugs. In order to sleep on the plane, however, you must trick your body into thinking it's bedtime shortly after you take off. Following this schedule the week before you leave can help (assume a 6:00 P.M. Saturday departure):

People at work

Day	Rising time	Bedtime
Sunday	7:00 A.M.	11:00 P.M.
Monday	6:30 A.M.	10:30 P.M.
Tuesday	6:00 A.M.	10:00 P.M.
Wednesday	5:30 A.M.	9:30 P.M.
Thursday	5:00 A.M.	9:00 P.M.
Friday	4:30 A.M.	8:30 P.M.
Saturday	4:00 A.M.	8:00 P.M. (AIRBORNE)

If you can manage this schedule, you should get at least a few cycles of sleep and you will feel much better for it. Remember, use an eye mask and earplugs, and take no caffeine, alcohol, or artificial sweeteners after 1:00 P.M. on the day of departure. Your body will then feel as if it's early morning instead of the middle of the night when you land. And when 10:00 P.M. (local time overseas) rolls around on Sunday, your body clock will feel as if it's about 1:30 A.M. (since, if you were following the above pattern at home, you'd go to sleep about 7:30 P.M., or 1:30 A.M. local time). If you hadn't followed the pattern, when it was 10:00 P.M. on Sunday night, your body would feel as if it was 4:00 A.M. Clear? It won't work for everyone, but give it a try if eastward overseas flight really bothers you. Westward flights don't bother most people because they're just like staying up later but being able to sleep a normal night's sleep, in accordance with the body's naturally advancing rhythms.

4   Charles F. Ehret of the Argonne (Illinois) National Laboratory, recommends the anti-jet-lag diet (Yepsen, 1987), an alternating pattern of fasting and feasting, which proceeds as follows:

- Three days before the flight, have high-protein feasts at breakfast and lunch and consume only complex carbohydrates for supper; take caffeine only between 3:00 and 5:00 P.M.
- Two days before the flight, fast on broth soups, salad, and fruit; follow the same caffeine rule.
- One day before the flight, follow the same pattern and same caffeine rule as three days before (feast).
- Flight day is fast day: for east-west flights, fast only half a day, with caffeine in the morning; for west-east flights, fast all day, with caffeine between 6:00 and 11:00 P.M.
- Upon arrival, sleep until breakfast; all three meals on the day of arrival are feasts. Begin and continue on the day of arrival with all the lights turned on and remain active.

5   If you live on the East Coast of the United States and must fly to the West Coast, decide if you will actually be there long enough to justify going through a change of body clock. Jane Howard says, "Often I will go to a two-day meeting in the West, go to bed on Eastern time, and pretend I'm still in the East with respect to meals and caffeine. I go to bed around 9:00 P.M. West Coast time and wake up around 4:30 A.M. Reentry to the East Coast is a breeze; my body clock remains unchanged. I miss out on night life with this plan, but marrieds should feel okay about that."

Studies show that nappers outproduce non-nappers.

Topic 16.4 Naps

Rossi and Nimmons (1991) cite support for two or three twenty-minute naps per day. That is the ideal number for maximum quality, productivity, sense of well-being, and overall health and longevity. Studies show that nappers outproduce non-nappers; however, a goal of three naps a day is out of reach for most people. Perhaps a minimum of one fifteen- to thirty-minute nap per day should be voted a basic human right.

Applications

1   Many companies have official policies that prohibit employees from napping during the workday. These policies serve public relations purposes and are not consistent with research on productivity. Don't associate reasonable napping with laziness; associate it with productivity.

2   There are safety reasons why some people should not be permitted to nap, but even they would be safer workers if they were allowed to nap while off-duty.

3   If you are a citizen and spot a public worker napping, resist calling in to report it as laziness and a waste of the taxpayers' dollars. Appreciate the productivity, quality, safety, and health benefits associated with a nap. Of course, if you see a public worker snoozing the day away, that's another matter!

Topic 16.5 Stress in the workplace

J. Donald Millar, director of the National Institute of Occupational Safety and Health, in a presentation at the 1991 American Psychological Association convention in San Francisco, reported that workers' compensation claims for stress-related problems rose 700 percent in California from 1979 to 1988. Nationally, stress-related claims have recently comprised 12 percent of all workers' compensation claims. During the eighties, roughly one-fourth of all Social Security disability claims were for mental disorders—that's 600,000 people each year.

Millar cites several sources of this increase of stress in the workplace, including an unpredictable economy, conversion from manufacturing jobs to service jobs, and the increasing role of computers (Bales, 1991, p. 32). He also refers to a greater use of contract workers as a way to beat rising medical costs. His recommendations are listed below as Applications. Additional information on the causes and remedies of stress is given elsewhere in this chapter as well as in Chapters Fourteen and Fifteen.

Applications

1 Design healthy jobs. This includes everything from applying principles of ergonomics to asking workers how their jobs could be improved.

2 Monitor jobs to ensure that workers stay healthy. This includes attitude surveys and a variety of participative management techniques.

3 Educate managers and the public on the causes and consequences of stress in the workplace.

4 Improve the availability of mental health services.

5 Notify management of stressors on the job. (contributed by Rick Bradley)

Suggested readings on workplace design and stress
Bales, J. (1991, November). "Work Stress Grows, But Services Decline."
      APA Monitor, p. 32.
"Combatting Stress at Work." (1993, January). *Conditions of Work Digest*
      [Special volume], *12*(1).
Druckman, D., & Swets, J. A. (Eds.). (1988). *Enhancing Human*
      Performance: Issues, Theories, and Techniques. Washington, DC:
      National Academy Press.
Rossi, E. L., & Nimmons, D. (1991). *The 20-Minute Break: Using the New*
      Science of Ultradian Rhythms. Los Angeles: Tarcher.

⚫17

The five senses: Brain messages

The five senses all directly affect our presence of mind. Some tend to have a more disruptive influence than others—for instance, smell generally links up directly with the limbic system and thus has the capacity for quickly becoming a source of stress. You can close your eyes, cover your ears, fold your hands, and quit tasting or eating, but you can't get away from smells except by physically removing yourself from the premises. This chapter explores how the input of our five sensory channels affects our minds. Topics 17.2–17.5 relate to the visual sense, Topics 17.6–17.8 to the auditory sense, Topics 17.9–17.13 to smell, Topic 17.14 to taste, and Topics 17.15–17.18 to the kinesthetic senses. Kinesthetics is the study of touch, space, and motion. You've often heard that you can learn by hearing, by seeing, and by doing. Kinesthetic learning is learning by doing. We will look at four specific aspects of kinesthetics in the workplace: proxemics, room arrangement, touch, and temperature.

Topic 17.1 The five senses in the workplace

Each of us is constantly taking in sensory data as the afferent nerves send visual, auditory, olfactory, tactile, and gustatory messages to the brain. These messages vie for attention with other mental activities, such as creativity, analysis, and inspection, all of which can be interrupted by sensory data. Make sure that sensory input in your workplace is not driving productive mental activity out of your workers.

that influence work

Applications

1 Talk with your workers to find out if there are any sensory distractions that make their work unnecessarily complicated—noises, glares, smells, tastes, or other physical discomforts that can take their minds off the task at hand, however momentarily. Distractions beget errors.

2 Include questions in your annual employee attitude survey about sensory distractions.

3 When you conduct walk-throughs, imagine yourself in the workers' shoes and try to identify sensory distractions that might cause you to make errors.

4 Identify and remove any sensory distractions that hinder your own performance. (contributed by Rick Bradley)

> "It is shameful for a man to rest in ignorance of the structure of his own body, especially when the knowledge of it mainly conduces to his welfare, and directs his application of his own powers."
>
> **Philipp Melanchthon**

Topic 17.2 Light

Light affects mood and alertness by shutting down the production of melatonin, the sleep inducer. Darkness triggers the pineal gland in the base of the brain to secrete melatonin. If alertness is important for safety and productivity, the work environment should be well lighted. If a low degree of alertness, or even drowsiness, is acceptable, then brightness is not as important. Full-spectrum lights are best. Weatherall (1987) points out that most lights are concentrated in the wrong part of the spectrum—orange-violet-red—although blue-green is the most vital part. Absence of this part of the spectrum leads to measurable fatigue and eyestrain.

Light deprivation not only affects performance; it can also lead to a form of depression. So-called winter depression, or seasonal affective disorder, associated with the shorter days and longer periods of darkness of winter, has recently been successfully treated with light therapy.

For travelers passing through several time zones, exposure to bright lights several "mornings" in a row in the new time zone can reset the body clock. In September 1991, our family hosted the matron of the King's College Chapel Choir from Cambridge, England. Charlotte was the choir's first stop in the United States. The group was whisked from the airport to our church, and then straight to our several homes. We arrived at our home around 9:00 P.M. (which was about 2:00 A.M. for Dorothy, the matron). We had a full schedule the following day, so we called Dorothy to tea at 7:30 A.M., turning on every light in the house to help her reset her body clock. We didn't tell her why we were so light-happy, but she reported later that this was one of her best trips ever, and that she had felt unexpectedly refreshed.

Further discussion of light and sleep may be found in Chapters Seven and Sixteen.

Applications

1 Ensure adequate lighting in the workplace. Skimping on lighting can affect morale, quality, and productivity. Weatherall (1987) suggests using the Color Rendering Index (CRI) as a measure of the adequacy of artificial light. In this index, natural light equals 100; the higher the numerical light rating, the lower the need to take a physical sample to a window to determine correct color. Ask at your local lighting-supply company for fluorescent or incandescent bulbs with a CRI of 90 or higher.

2 Provide extra lighting for workers on night shifts. This lighting can be turned off during the day. but on dark, overcast days, use it to help shake off the doldrums.

3 In training sessions, plan carefully when you use transparencies or slides requiring subdued lighting. If it is not possible to lower the lights, plan a break or activity immediately following the presentation to rest the audience's eyes.

Topic 17.3 Night vision

The quality of our night vision decreases with age. At fifty-one, I am already aware of poorer distance vision when driving at night. Also, men tend to have better day vision (note that more women wear sun-protective glasses), and women tend to have better night vision (Moir & Jessel, 1991).

Manley West, a University of West Indies pharmacology professor, researched the rumor that marijuana improved night vision. He found that a nonpsychoactive ingredient in marijuana, Canasil, caused a significant improvement in night vision. At the time of this writing, Canasil, which is the same ingredient in marijuana that relieves glaucoma, is not yet available in the United States.

Applications

1 As you age, take extra precautions when you drive at night, especially if you are a man. Allow extra distance between you and vehicles in front of you, drive more slowly, and take more breaks. Let a younger person or a woman drive when possible.

2 All other things being equal (driving skill, physical condition, road familiarity, etc.), a woman will be a safer driver at night because of generally superior night vision. During the day, men will tend to be safer because they are less subject to fatigue from the sun. Women will generally desire or require more breaks to avoid eye fatigue during the day, with men requiring more during the night.

3 Understand that these differences exist, and don't interpret people who are different from you as weak, malingering, or inferior.

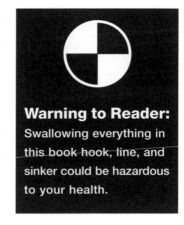

Warning to Reader: Swallowing everything in this book hook, line, and sinker could be hazardous to your health.

Topic 17.4 Color

Faber Birren, in *Color and Human Response* (1978a), reports specific tendencies in people's responses to various colors. I summarize them as follows:

Color	Response
Red	Good for creative thinking, short-term high energy
Green	Good for productivity, long-term energy
Yellow, orange, coral, etc.	Conducive to physical work, exercising; elicits positive moods
Blue	Slows pulse and lowers blood pressure; conducive to studying, deep thinking, concentration; accent with red for keener insights

Color	Response
Purple	Tranquilizing; good for appetite control
Pink	Restful; calming
Light colors	All-purpose; provide minimum disruption across all moods and mental activity
White	Disrupting, like snow-blindness—avoid

Birren recommends light colors for most situations and warns against all-white schemes, which can be disrupting. Here are some other points of general interest:

- Most people like primary colors.
- More discriminating people like purple, blue-green, and pink.
- Brown, white, gray, and black are the least preferred colors; they tend to attract the mentally disturbed.
- Extraverts, brunets, and Latins prefer warmer colors such as red or orange.
- Introverts, blonds, and Nordics prefer cool colors such as blue or green.

I recommend that you approach these findings with caution. Birren does not offer detailed research citations in support of his conclusions, and some of the color research is contradictory. For example, according to some reports yellow walls elicit positive moods, while another report finds that yellow walls in hospital rooms are associated with patients who require more pain-killing medication.

Application

Evaluate the colors used throughout your workplace in terms of the nature of the work performed in each area. Some apparently winning combinations are:

Area	Color
Cafeteria	Purple
Sales room	Yellow, orange, or coral
Conference rooms	Red
Offices	Blue with a tinge of red
Production areas	Green

Topic 17.5 The effect of shapes and designs

Beginning in the crib, all humans benefit from a visually enriched environment: mirrors, artwork, games, posters, colors, shapes. To the degree that your work force will benefit from cortical alertness, provide them with food for the eyes. Consult with them to determine the practicality of your ideas, however. I remember the choral rehearsal room in the Cunningham Fine Arts Building on the Davidson College campus in Davidson, North Carolina. It was beautifully designed, with black wire mesh on the wall behind the conductor, punctuated with thin vertical teak strips, but we singers developed headaches from the dizzying effect created when the conductor moved back and forth in front of the strips.

Applications

1   Dot the walls of your meeting rooms with appropriate posters containing philosophical or other thoughtful or amusing statements. IBM has done a good job of this, with posters reminding workers that "The individual comes first" or "Today is the first day of the rest of your life." These posters are available free from the IBM Gallery of Science and Art, 590 Madison Avenue, New York, NY 10022. (contributed by Jack Wilson)

Don't trust a mechanic who listens to music while working on your car.

2   Provide a budget for artwork and allow employee participation in making selections.

3   Put yourself in the position of your workers and identify overly distracting or boring visual areas in their workplace. Better yet, ask them how to improve the view that meets their eyes at work.

Topic 17.6 The relation of sounds to concentration

The brain responds to organized and unorganized sounds—the first we call music; the second, noise. Furthermore, one person's music can be another's noise. As a general rule, neither music nor noise should be present where careful mental work is required. As Robert Pirsig comments in his *Zen and the Art of Motorcycle Maintenance* (1974), don't trust a mechanic who listens to music while working on your car. If you're listening to music, then you're not listening to the engine. So-called background music does not stay in the background. I write more quickly and effectively when the stereo is off. It is impossible to create a sentence and listen to a passage of Tchaikovsky. If I'm trying to do both, then I'm actually alternating between the two, inevitably adding time and errors to my writing and thinking.

Applications

1   Background music should only accompany routinized tasks and other situations in which the mind is not actively engaged. I've seen it effectively used in

The five senses   **217**

manufacturing assembly operations and in elevators. But don't provide background music for mental work, because it will inevitably occupy the foreground. For example, when I'm placed on telephone hold, I prefer that *no* music be piped into my ear. Why? Because I try to do miscellaneous paperwork while waiting, and the music is distracting.

2 Remember that people have different tastes in music. What is satisfying for one person may be intrusive for another. I've known retail workers who came to hate holiday music when their stores played the same tapes repeatedly for a month.

Topic 17.7 The effect of music on mood

Here are some general guidelines on the human response to various aspects of music:

- The higher the pitch, the more positive the effect generated.
- Slower, minor keys warm the brain, which fosters both cortical and limbic alertness.
- Faster, major keys cool the brain, which fosters better moods.
- Classical composers (e.g., Mozart, Haydn, and Beethoven) and mid- to late Baroque composers except Bach (e.g., Vivaldi, Scarlatti, Handel, and Corelli) are considered universal donors in the musical world—that is, they tend to offend the fewest listeners.

Application

Some appropriate uses of music would appear to be:

Place	Type of music
Retail stores	Faster, higher-pitched music in a major key (e.g., Vivaldi's *The Four Seasons*)
Waiting rooms	No music or TV, please (so people like me can read)
Workplaces where routine work is done	Slower, lower-pitched music in a minor key (e.g., Barber's *Adagio for Strings*)

Topic 17.8 Noise

Noise can be the bane of a mind worker's existence—from conversation to clacking equipment, from dripping water to occasional footsteps. Research indicates that so-called white noise, a low-pitched, sustained noise of low volume, serves to mask all other noises. Such an effect can be created by fluorescent light fixtures!

One day in the Davis Library on the campus of the University of North Carolina at Chapel Hill, I was totally absorbed in reading a series of journal articles back in the bowels of the stacks. Just as I finished an article on the positive effect of white noise in masking out distractions, I became aware of a low, sustained buzz emanating from somewhere above. I wondered—did the designer of this library know about white noise, or was this just a lucky accident?

So-called white noise, a low-pitched, sustained noise of low volume, serves to mask all other noises.

Application

Consult with an acoustical engineer about the proper way to mask noises that represent potential distractions for your mind workers. Machines are available that generate such white noise.

Topic 17.9 The relation of the sense of smell to the limbic system

Smell, according to Charles Wysocki of the Monell Chemical Senses Center in Philadelphia, is the only one of the five senses that has direct link-ups with the limbic system. Accordingly, smell can have a profoundly subtle effect on our level of relaxation or agitation (Kallan, 1991). Remember that some people are allergic to specific odors; be aware of possible allergic reactions.

Application

Be particularly sympathetic to others' complaints about bothersome smells, such as perfume, food, or smoke. Not all people are sensitive to the same odors, and sensitivities can be extremely disruptive.

Topic 17.10 The effect of odors on females

Females are more sensitive to odors than males. It takes a stronger odor to get a typical man's attention than a woman's. This is likely a genetic artifact of natural selection for mothers, who must be alert to olfactory indicators of infants' distress. This gender difference has been definitely established (remembering, of course, that exceptions are common), but its cause is speculative.

Applications

1   Be sensitive to the fact that women regard certain odors as offensive. They do so because the female-differentiated brain has more alert smell receptors than the male-differentiated brain. They are not being stereotypically prissy any more than a man is being stereotypically macho when he is aggressive—this behavior is a result of their different hormonal makeups.

2   There are many tasks that require an acute sense of smell: cooking, chemical analysis, safety inspection (e.g., for gas leaks), quality inspection (e.g., for the right fragrance), even lie detection (e.g., for the odor of perspiration). Consider that females as a group have more sensitivity in olfactory detection.

Topic 17.11 The effect of odors on sleep

Most odors disrupt sleep; the heart rate increases and brain waves quicken.

Peter Badia, of Bowling Green State University in Ohio, reports from his sleep lab research that most odors disrupt sleep; the heart rate increases and brain waves quicken. One odor, heliotropine, which has a vanilla-almond fragrance, does not disrupt sleep, and may help (Kallan, 1991).

Applications

1   Try Amaretto liqueur or almond extract in your hot milk before going to sleep. Or try a few of drops of vanilla extract in your bedtime milk.

2   Eliminate strong odors before going to sleep. Sleeping with an open window can help diffuse odors.

Topic 17.12 The effect of odors on productivity

Fragrances improve performance at about the same rate as a cup of coffee, according to William Dember of the University of Cincinatti and Raja Parasuraman of the Catholic University of America. On a forty-minute test of vigilance (like that needed for air traffic control or distance driving), thirty-second bursts of peppermint or muguet (lily of the valley) scent every five minutes resulted in a 15 to 25 percent improvement in performance. Workers receiving scented bursts showed less decline in performance as the task continued over time.

In the same meeting of the American Association for the Advancement of Science at which Dember and Parasuraman presented their findings, Robert Baron, of the Rensselaer Polytechnic Institute in Troy, New York, reported that pleasant fragrances cause people to be more efficient, increase their risk level, form more challenging goals, negotiate more agreeably, and behave less combatively.

Along the same lines, Shimizu Technology Center America, Inc., reports keypunch operators improving 21 percent with lavender bursts, 33 percent with jasmine, and 54 percent with lemon.

Application

Shimizu Technology Center America, in Boston, sells a process that emits fragrance bursts through existing ventilation ducts. The system, which has been sold to Japanese hotels, banks, nursing homes, and offices, sells for ten thousand dollars.

Topic 17.13 The effect of odors on relaxation

Lavender-chamomile scents reportedly reduce stress; lemon, jasmine, and cypress scents induce a positive mood; and basil, peppermint, pine, eucalyptus, and clove are "refreshing . . . invigorating," according to Junichi Yagi of Shimizu Technology Center America. Gary Schwartz of the University of Arizona in Tucson finds that within one minute, spiced apple scents yield more relaxed brain waves and an average drop in blood pressure of five millimeters per person.

William H. Redd of the Memorial Sloan-Kettering Cancer Center in New York has experimented with bursts of heliotropine to relax patients undergoing magnetic resonance imaging. These patients frequently suffer anxiety, panic, and claustrophobic attacks, which cause average delays of fifteen minutes. This results in the loss of approximately $62.5 million annually in the United States (Kallan, 1991). At the March 1991 meeting of the Society of Behavioral Medicine in Washington, D.C., Redd reported that among eighty-five patients, the heliotropine-receiving group exhibited 63 percent less anxiety than the controls.

Applications

1   Chamomile, spiced apple, lemon, jasmine, eucalyptus, and peppermint are all available in tea-bag form. Consider supplying them in break areas as a hot-drink alternative to decaffeinated coffee.

2   In waiting rooms and other areas where you would like to put people at ease, consider naturally fragrant wood furniture (e.g., cedar or cypress), home-style fragrances (e.g., clove balls or potpourri), natural objects (e.g., pine needles or cones, a potted miniature pine tree, a bowl of apples), and oils (e.g., lavender) for a continuous source of relaxing fragrance. Hospitals in particular should work to rid waiting areas of that unique hospital smell; though I have no research data to back me up, I'm sure it is anxiety-producing.

3   Provide, where possible, work tools that possess a natural texture and odor. There's too much plastic in the world. Picking up a ruler made of wood can add a bit of pleasurable fragrance to an otherwise cold and lackluster act. I've played on an aluminum harpsichord, and it just doesn't offer the same sense of pleasure as performing on a fragrant wooden instrument. I keep a plastic blockflute for use on camping trips, but I never play it at home because it has no pleasing taste or smell that compares to my rosewood version smelling of linseed oil.

Topic 17.14 Gender differences in taste

Female-differentiated brains are more sensitive to sweet tastes, while male-differentiated brains are more sensitive to salty tastes. Hence, the typical female requires more salt to satisfy her and the typical male needs more sugar. A classic example is my wife's tendency to oversalt when she cooks and my tendency to oversweeten hot chocolate when I make it from scratch. Notice how, generally, women tend to shake salt on their meals for a longer period than men, while men tend to add more sugar to their coffee or tea (if they sweeten it at all).

Applications

1   In food preparation, female chefs should try not to oversalt their dishes and male chefs should not oversweeten theirs. Folks can always add salt or sugar to their taste.

2   Do not be offended if you're female and a male adds sugar to your pre-pared dish; do not be offended if you're male and a female adds salt to your prepared dish!

Topic 17.15 Proxemics

Proxemics is the study of how people physically distance themselves from others. Here are several general rules:

- Generally, women are more comfortable at close distances from other women; men are more comfortable at greater distances from other men. This is probably a relic dating from a time when men were genetically selected for their ability to function as isolated hunters outdoors, whereas women were genetically selected for their comfort in more crowded conditions back in the cave and in nursing and caring for their young.
- The smaller the enclosed space, the farther people will want to sit or stand from each other. The larger the enclosed space, the closer they will choose to sit or stand from each other.

- When two people stand face-to-face, they communicate that they like each other. As the imaginary angle between them increases through a right angle to 180 degrees, less liking is communicated.
- The closer two people stand to one another, the more they communicate mutual liking.
- Moderate eye contact communicates liking, while excessive eye contact communicates hostility (as in staring your opponent down); sparse eye contact communicates apathy or aversion.
- Cultural differences exist concerning comfortable distances and gazing patterns. If people from a different culture from yours appear to be standing farther or closer than is comfortable for you, the chances are that it is more comfortable for them. If you adjust the space between you, they will immediately return to the previous distance. I once taught with a man from Jamaica, who would talk to me standing closer than was comfortable for me. At first I interpreted this as a sexual advance. After learning that Jamaicans generally stand closer to others, I felt more comfortable.
- Anthropologist Raymond Birdwhistell has established that, in American culture, masculinity is communicated nonverbally by standing with arms akimbo, feet parallel in the same plane, and pelvis rotated forward (tummy in), while femininity is communicated nonverbally by arms folded together, feet planted asymmetrically, and pelvis rotated backward (tummy out).
- Research in neurolinguistic programming suggests that a group will produce better-quality work if members who reenter a room after a break take different seats. Apparently, this change of perspective yields new insights.

Moderate eye contact communicates liking, while excessive eye contact communicates hostility.

Applications

1 Generally, men require a larger work space than women. If you allow people to self-select how much space they need to perform their work, women will select less space, men more.

2 In small offices, meeting rooms, or waiting areas, place chairs and sofas as far apart as possible to give people more space. Using wider chairs accomplishes a similar purpose.

3 When you desire to communicate explicitly to people that you like them (for instance, in a performance appraisal or sales call), stand or sit face-to-face at

Figure 17.1

a minimal comfortable distance with moderate eye contact. Avoid either staring them down or excessively gazing away (e.g., looking out the window).

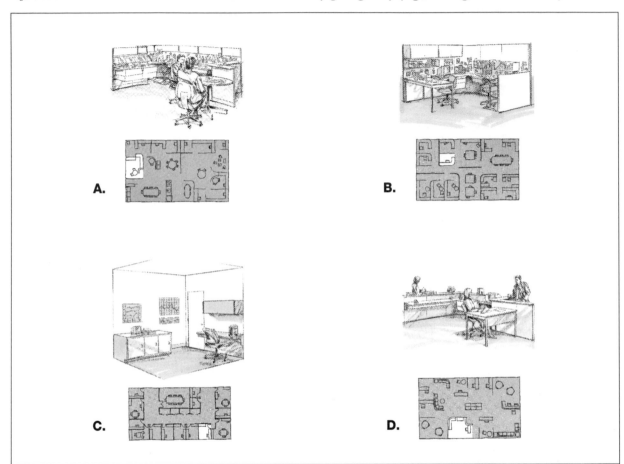

Personality type and office arrangement. A. Preserver; **B.** Explorer; **C.** Challenger; **D.** Adapter. From *The Negotiable Environment: People, White Collar Work, and the Office* by C. L. Williams et al., 1985, Ann Arbor, MI: Miller, Herman. © 1985 by Miller, Herman, Inc. Reprinted by permission.

4 If a person of the opposite sex is coming on to you in an unwanted manner, try using the three nonverbal sexuality communicators of your opposite sex: a woman, for example, to "turn off" a man, would stand with feet planted parallel, arms akimbo, and pelvis rotated forward.

Topic 17.16 Room arrangement

C. L. Williams et al. (1985), in *The Negotiable Environment,* demonstrate that different personality temperaments respond better to different room or office arrangements. Shown in Figure 17.1 are office arrangements for the Preserver, the Explorer, the Challenger, and the Adapter (these personality temperaments are described in Chapter Ten). See if you can identify which is which.

People at work

Application

When you are designing office environments, take into account the preferences of people with differing personality temperaments:

- Explorers generally prefer more books and artwork.
- Preservers generally prefer more action-oriented pictures and objects (cars, airplanes, horses).
- Challengers generally prefer computers and other sources of data.
- Adapters generally prefer to have an area set aside for group meetings (a round table, a corner sofa).
- Flexibles generally prefer lots of surface space for all their piles.
- Focused people generally prefer elaborate storage equipment— staying organized is a must.
- Extraverts generally like lots of eye contact; they prefer windows, open offices, and low walls.
- Introverts generally like to be able to close the door and isolate themselves for extended periods of time.
- Reactives will let you know their wants, and they will probably change from time to time.
- Sedates will probably not care about their office arrangement.

Topic 17.17 Touch

For some people, the sense of touch is an important element of motivation for work. Be aware that artificial touch sensations can demotivate some workers. For some, glass is preferable to plastic, wood or metal to plastic, wood to metal, natural fibers to synthetic fibers, natural plants to artificial plants, china to plastic or paper plates, leather to plastic, and so on.

Application

Consult with workers about what's important to them in their work environment. Specifically ask about what materials they prefer and the importance of tactile sensations to them. If how their materials, equipment, and furniture feel to their touch is not important to them, then there is no need to change them.

Topic 17.18 Temperature

The cooler your brain is, the more relaxed you are. The warmer your brain, the more aroused you are (this arousal can be either limbic or cortical). Hence, the stereotypes of the cool, unflappable British subject and the passionate, hot resident of the equatorial zones. Robert Zajonc of the University of Michigan reports that higher temperatures can affect the level of neurotransmitters in your neurocirculatory system, especially the level of norepinephrine. Interestingly, Zajonc reports that breathing through the nose cools the brain.

Applications

1 One simple way to try relaxing at work is by breathing through your nose.

2 In areas where cortical alertness is necessary, keep temperatures in the upper range of the comfort zone. Too cool a meeting room shuts down cortical functions.

3 In areas where you want people to be relaxed (waiting areas, sales presentation rooms, cafeterias, break areas), keep temperatures in the lower range of the comfort zone.

Suggested readings on the senses

Ackerman, D. (1990). *A Natural History of the Senses*. New York: Random House.

Yepsen, R. B., Jr. (1987). *How to Boost Your Brain Power: Achieving Peak Intelligence, Memory and Creativity*. Emmaus, PA: Rodale.

Part five

Creating new mental paths:

Memory, creativity, and problem solving

Creating new mental paths:

Memory, creativity, and problem solving

Class action: Tools and techniques

The findings from cognitive research presented in this chapter all relate to how we learn. These findings will be applicable to you to the degree that you have an interest in influencing the learning of others (as well as yourself!). Clearly not every finding and every suggested application will find its way into your learning experiences.

This chapter focuses on findings that relate to the design of learning experiences in general. Treat the chapter as a sort of cafeteria line or smorgasbord from which you take what you need today, then return later to take something different as your learning needs change. As a way of helping you to evaluate your learning experiences overall, I have provided a Checklist for the Self-Evaluation of Learning Practices in Appendix G.

Enjoy.

Topic 18.1 Chunking

Make an effort to limit the introduction of new information to groupings of about *seven* of anything. Miller (1956) has demonstrated that seven new and previously unassociated bits of information (like those found in a telephone number) are about as much as most people can work with. Once the seven or so bits of information are mastered, they become a chunk and behave like one bit!

for acquiring knowledge

Applications

1 If you want people to remember a list of ten or more items, either (a) somehow reduce the list to nine or fewer items (preferably seven) or (b) break up the list into two or more units of seven chunks each, then master the first list of seven before moving on to the second, and so on.

2 Where possible, take a longer list of, say, fifteen or twenty items and reduce it to about seven by identifying the biggest categories. Then learn the original list as subcategories of the shorter one. Work on the seven main categories until they have been mastered, then work on each set of subcategories one by one until you have learned the entire list.

3 For verbal passages, start by mastering the first five to nine words or chunks. (Remember, a familiar phrase counts as one chunk.) Then learn the next five to nine words or chunks. Put them all together and continue.

> "What sculpture is to a block of marble, education is to the human soul."
>
> **Joseph Addison**

Topic 18.2 Testing is a learning process

Testing learners helps them to remember, according to Ronald P. Fisher of Florida International University. Some of his findings are summarized as follows:

- Learners who take pretests do better on their finals.
- Learners who take pretests with fill-in-the-blank questions do better on their finals than those who take pretests with multiple-choice questions.
- Learners who take pretests with inferential multiple-choice questions do better on their finals than those who take pretests with factual multiple-choice questions.

Apparently, testing gives the learner an opportunity to practice several effective learning procedures simultaneously. Tests do not have to be punitive, or even graded, to be effective. It is the act of taking the test that is helpful.

Hart (1983) argues that nondirective tests are superior to directive tests, such as multiple-choice and true-false exams, because learners have to identify patterns and select programs.

Applications

1   Use the beginning of a class session to review content from previous sessions. For example, in reviewing a decision-making process, you might throw out a series of questions such as "What is the first step?" "Why does it come first?" "What step is most frequently skipped?" "Why is it hard to remember?" This is a good way to use time while waiting for everyone to get back from a break.

2   Use group competition in tests. For example, divide the learners into small groups and have them make a list of the steps of a process you taught in a previous session. Let the group that finishes first recite the steps to the other groups. If they make an error, let another small group recite from that point, and so on.

3   Let learners in small groups construct a test to give to the other groups. This builds on the principle of "Handle It!" (see Topic 18.5).

4   Use card sorts to see if the steps of a process have been learned. For example, in an organization with an elaborate seventeen-step performance appraisal process, the trainer made decks of seventeen cards each, with each card containing an unnumbered step of the process. The learners had to arrange the cards in the proper sequence, as individuals and as groups. They then were allowed to review each others' work until everyone in the class thought they were right. The "school" solution was then revealed. You should be open to the possibility that in such a case the class may come up with an improvement to the process!

5   If possible, choose tests that require the learner to identify a pattern (e.g., somebody doing a poor job of listening to someone else) and then to identify an appropriate program to apply (e.g., a clarifying question).

6   Start a training session with a pretest that includes some of the more unusual points you will cover in your session. (contributed by Jane Howard)

Topic 18.3 Trust the experts

Research on the effectiveness of various problem-solving techniques suggests that experts are generally better than techniques. In other words, before you take the time to learn a problem-solving technique to solve an electrical engineering problem, first go to an electrical engineer who is familiar with the situation or a worker who is actually doing the work, and see if they can spot the cause and offer a solution.

Experts are generally better than techniques.

Applications
1   If you are teaching problem-solving techniques, caution students that the techniques are a last resort and should be used only when experts are unavailable or have been stumped by the problem.

2   Include a task expert on a problem-solving team or consult someone who is actually doing the job. (contributed by Rick Bradley)

Topic 18.4 Schemas

The British psychologist Fredrick Bartlett (1932) was the first person to propose a theory of abstract cognitive structures called schemas. If schemas are similar to an experience, they render our memories accurate; if they are different, they color our memories accordingly. The biological basis of a schema is a neural pathway that represents the schematic diagram of a specific cognitive process. We have schemas for telling stories or jokes, giving directions, and solving problems. We may even have several different schemas for each task. David Rumelhart (Gardner, 1985, p. 125) describes the standard schema for storytelling; I have summarized his description as follows:

1   State the goal.

2   Enumerate the steps to the goal.

3   Relate the reactions along the way.

4   Describe and comment upon the success or failure in reaching the goal.

Our schemas differ just as our experiences do. Someone who has learned the Chinese language will have different schemas than someone who hasn't. In one sense, the story of our mental life is the story of either (1) forming new schemas or (2) accommodating new experiences to old schemas. Most learning appears to be a process of fitting new information into old schemas. Our existing schemas tend to determine how we evaluate and shape new information, unless we work hard to establish new schemas.

John Bransford of Vanderbilt University has determined that schemas play such a strong role in coloring new learning that learners can't help but modify what they hear and see according to their prior experience. Learners who hear "The doctor's son greeted his father" will typically tend to accommodate this statement to their schema about doctoring and see the son shaking hands with a father who is a doctor, rather than allowing for the possibility that the doctor is actually the mother, standing by and watching her son greet his father, who is not a doctor. Bransford says that this tendency is so strong and so pervasive that the instructor must take responsibility for listening to students discuss their newfound knowledge and clarify incidences of inappropriate accommodation to previous schemas. As Hodgson's law says, we tend to remember a thing the way we want to remember it.

Hart (1983) defines learning as the acquisition of useful schemas, which he calls programs. He defines a program or schema as a sequence used for attaining a preselected goal. Programs are triggered when the learner recognizes a pattern. If the program works (i.e., the learner achieves the goal), fine; otherwise, the learner tries another program or looks for another pattern.

Applications

1   Before teaching someone a new skill or body of knowledge, first find out what the learner already knows that is similar. Then proceed with your instruction, pointing out the ways in which this new learning is similar to or different from the learner's existing schemas. For example, if the learner is to learn arc welding, find out if he or she has had experience with other kinds of welding machines, solderers, and so on. This is a normal part of the technical training model called job instruction training (see Eckles, Carmichael, & Sarchet, 1981, p. 340).

2   As we get older, we have more complex and more numerous schemas to build on. This is particularly helpful in the peg-word technique for memorizing lists. Say that you want to memorize the ten largest cities in the world. You start by making a list of rhyming words for the numbers one to ten. You then think of an association between the rhyming word (the peg word) and the name of the city; the more whimsical or outrageous the association is, the easier it will be to remember. For example:

Number	Rhyme	City	Association
One	Bun	Tokyo	Looks like the bow on the traditional Japanese kimono
Two	Shoe	Mexico City	Mexico as the shoe of the body of the North American continent
Three	Tree	São Paulo	The land of rain forests
Four	Door	New York	The traditional door to the United States for immigrants
Five	Hive	Seoul	A beehive of political activity
Six	Sticks	Osaka	"O sock-a me with the sticks"
Seven	Heaven	Buenos Aires	Heaven is good air
Eight	Gate	Calcutta	"Cut a" gate into the fence
Nine	Line	Bombay	The coastline around the bay
Ten	Pin	Rio de Janeiro	Pin (blame) it on Rio

Once you've memorized the peg words (bun, shoe, etc.), all you have to do is form good visual associations between the peg word and the related item on the list you're trying to memorize. The mind can easily relate the schema of bun, for example, to both sweet rolls and the bow on the back of the kimono. See examples in Lorayne and Lucas (1974) and Buzan (1991).

3 When you think a common schema exists for everyone in a group, you might refer to it in front of the whole class. For example, if you are talking about performance appraisal, you might discuss how it is similar to and different from traditional school report cards.

4 Ask questions and provide examples that relate to the experiences of the learners. Help them see the connection between their experience and what you are teaching.

5 Allow your learners time for exploration. Help them to verbalize both the patterns they recognize and the programs and schemas they choose to apply (Hart, 1983). Here's a model of the process:
1 Recognize the pattern.
2 Implement the program.

3 Evaluate the program. If it fails, reinterpret the pattern, look for a new pattern, try a new program, or try a variation on the failed program.

Topic 18.5 Handle it!

One of the best ways to learn a body of information is to manipulate it in such a way as to make it yours. I have a friend who understood this principle in undergraduate school. After each lecture, he would return to his room with his notes, then sit at his typewriter and rewrite the notes in an outline form that was meaningful to him. Four years later, he had earned his Phi Beta Kappa key! Handle it to get a handle on it.

Applications

1   If you are a teacher and want to hand out an outline of your material, wait until after you've covered it. That forces the learners to write notes of their own and struggle with the wording and outline. This act of having to "handle" the material helps the learners to build on existing schemas.

2   If the material forms some kind of list or chart, put the elements on cards. Then have either individuals or groups arrange the cards in a correct or meaningful order.

3   Have small groups generate their own examples of the point you are making.

4   Use role playing.

5   Have the learners write their own case studies.

6   If the learners are to apply a skill to a job (such as constructive criticism), have them write out a script to use.

7   Examine books on the subject of TRICA (Teaching Reading In the Content Areas). These texts contain hands-on activities and are meant for high school teachers with students who do not read well. The activities work well as an adult learning technique, regardless of reading level.

8   Have the learners prepare a presentation for each other. (Remember, the best way to learn something is to teach it.)

Creating new mental paths

9   Suggest that the learners make a presentation back on the job to others who are unable to attend. Allow time in class to begin work on such a presentation.

10   Give the learners, alone or in groups, an unorganized list of all the elements of your presentation and let them decide how they'd like to organize it.

11   Have individuals or groups rank a list of items according to some criterion. This helps them to grapple with the concepts.

Topic 18.6 Applying classroom ideas to the real world

Whenever you teach a theory or concept, give the learners time to apply it to specific situations. Many learners are unable mentally or unwilling motivationally to apply an idea to an everyday situation.

Practice clarifies and strengthens the neural connections that are formed while learning.

Applications

1   Use printed, video, or audio examples. For example, the excellent course, Interpersonal Management Skills (IMS), developed at Xerox, provides printed worksheets with good and bad examples of the skills applied in different settings (plant, office, home, etc.), an audiotape with examples and practice exercises, and a videotape with both good and bad examples. The IMS program is available from:

> *Learning International, Inc.*
> *225 High Ridge Road*
> *Stamford, CT 06905*

2   Using your schemas, give examples from your personal experience to illustrate a concept, then ask learners to generate other examples in small groups, building on their schemas.

Topic 18.7 Practice

Provide ample time for practice. Supervised practice allows for the feedback necessary to refine the learning, while practice in and of itself is crucial in converting the learning from short- to long-term memory (see Chapter Nineteen). Practice clarifies and strengthens the neural connections that are formed while learning.

Applications

1   Role playing is an effective way to practice, especially for interpersonal skills. Try to make it less intimidating by having several pairs or groups of three do the role play at the same time and then discuss the results together, rather than putting two individuals on the spot in front of the class.

2   Provide case studies, both off-the-shelf and real. They give learners the opportunity to practice applying their learning under your supervision.

Topic 18.8 Focus and attention

The brain cannot focus on more than one stimulus at a time.

In spite of teenagers' claims that they can do homework in front of the television set, the brain cannot focus on more than one stimulus at a time. What may appear to be multitasking, or simultaneous focusing, is in fact a rapid alternation of focus. The more routine a stimulus is, the less it interferes with rival stimuli. So if you're listening to the news while driving on the interstate with moderate traffic, you will miss far less of the news than when you are driving around the Place de l'Étoile in Paris trying to maneuver across eight lanes of circular traffic.

Applications

1   Avoid playing music if you want the learner to concentrate. My wife and I once attended a workshop together. The leader asked us to complete a worksheet individually and silently. As we began our seatwork, the leader started to play some background music. I believe it was a fifties' tune. Well, my wife knew every word to that and each succeeding tune, silently sang along with them, and found it impossible to concentrate on the worksheet. The background music became foreground for her.

2   Don't introduce a new skill on top of a prior one until the prior skill has become routinized. Practice the skills separately until one is mastered; then you may build upon it. My daughter understood this well when, at the age of eight, she took Suzuki violin lessons. One day, as I was supervising her practice, she lost patience with my approach and glared at me, saying, "I'll keep my wrist right or I'll keep my feet right. Take your pick. But don't make me do them both at the same time."

Topic 18.9 Visualization

Remember the importance and effectiveness of visual and mental rehearsal in combination with physical rehearsal and practice in preparation for an event. See Druckman and Bjork (1991) and Gawain (1978).

Creating new mental paths

Application

If you are an athlete, executive, actor—anyone wanting to present a smooth, masterful performance—close your eyes and internally simulate the performance in your mind. Allow yourself to accompany this visualization with approximate physical movements or pantomime.

Topic 18.10 Subliminal hooey

While subliminal self-help tapes are a fifty-million-dollar industry, claims that they help you to quit smoking, learn languages, and so on don't bear out. You can't just sit back and learn with no conscious awareness that learning is taking place. In fact, many of these tapes with so-called subliminal images have, under close examination, been found to have no such images (Druckman & Bjork, 1991).

Application

Don't waste your money on subliminal tapes. Spend it on tapes with actual content that you want to learn consciously.

Suggested readings on learning

Buzan, T. (1991). *Use Your Perfect Memory.* (3rd ed.). New York: Penguin.

Caine, R. N., & Caine, G. (1991). *Making Connections: Teaching and the Human Brain.* Alexandria, VA: Association for Supervision and Curriculum Development.

Druckman, D., & Bjork, R. A. (Eds.). (1991). *In the Mind's Eye: Enhancing Human Performance.* Washington, DC: National Academy Press.

Druckman, D., & Swets, J. A. (Eds.). (1988). *Enhancing Human Performance: Issues, Theories, and Techniques.* Washington, DC: National Academy Press.

Hart, L. A. (1983). *Human Brain and Human Learning.* New York: Longman.

Lorayne, H., & Lucas, J. (1974). *The Memory Book.* New York: Stein & Day.

19

Learning that sticks: Insights for

Research on memory has taken a significant turn in the last ten years. Memory used to be regarded as a structure; now it is seen as a process. A memory was thought of as a single unit with an identifiable place of residence somewhere in the brain, which was recalled when necessary. Now a memory is regarded as a reconstruction from many different chunks stored redundantly through the brain.

Bartlett (1932, p. 213) foresaw this development when he wrote: "Remembering is not the re-excitation of innumerable fixed, lifeless, and fragmentary traces. It is an imaginative reconstruction, or construction, built out of the relation of our attitude towards a whole active mass of organized past reactions or experience, and to a little outstanding detail which commonly appears in image or in language form. It is thus hardly ever really exact, even in the most rudimentary cases of rote recapitulation, and it is not at all important that it should be so."

This new view of memory was brought dramatically to the public's awareness after John Dean's testimony at the Watergate hearings. Viewers were initially impressed with Dean's avowed excellent memory for detail. But when his testimony was later compared to accurate records of conversations, viewers (and Dean himself) were flabbergasted to learn that most of his testimony was at best flawed and at worst made up.

Creating new mental paths

enhancing memory

Topic 19.1 Defining memory

Memory is learning that sticks. When learning occurs, new synapses form, old synapses are strengthened, or both. These new or strengthened connections *are* the new learning. The synaptic connections are the molecular equivalent of a chunk of newly learned material, such as a telephone number. Initially, as we learn, a protein called C-kinase is deposited among certain hippocampal neurons, according to Daniel Alkon of the Marine Biological Laboratory, Woods Hole, Massachusetts. Apparently, C-kinase causes the branches of the brain cells to narrow. When they have narrowed and formed new synapses, learning has occurred. Unless the learning is converted into long-term memory, however, it will disappear, just as new muscle fiber will break down if it is not used. Again, we must use it or lose it.

With continued use, the hippocampal cells extend the storage of the new learning to the cerebral cortex, which then becomes the primary location of long-term storage and retrieval. When a new learning chunk reaches the cerebral cortex, it apparently is stored for the long term. Larry Squire of the University of California, San Diego, describes the hippocampus as a kind of broker that binds memory until the cortex takes over and becomes its handler. And Gazzaniga (1988) reports that memory occurs not just in the brain, but throughout the

> "My memory is the thing I forget with."
>
> **A schoolchild**

nervous system. In animal research, animals with no hippocampus can remember remote items but not recent items, while those with intact hippocampi remember recent items better than remote items, which is the normal condition. Anders Bjorklund, of the University of Lund in Sweden, has demonstrated that aging rats with deteriorated hippocampi are unable to learn new skills, yet are able to learn and remember after receiving transplants of good hippocampal cells from young rats.

Memory appears to be fully developed by eight years of age. At that point, we remember an average of one bit of information out of every 100 we receive. There is some debate about the relation of memory to IQ, but I come down on the side of those who hold that they are apparently unrelated. As I read the research, I am convinced that if memory and IQ appear to be directly related, it is because those with higher IQs usually attempt to acquire more learning than those with lower IQs. In a competition of humans versus five-year-old rhesus monkeys, the University of Texas Health Science Center in Houston reported that, after viewing a series of slides, humans *and* monkeys got 86 percent right on a ten-item test in which they were shown the slides with new slides mixed in and were asked to press a lever upon recognizing a familiar slide! One of the reasons that people who score high on conventional IQ tests also have excellent memories is that conventional IQ tests include so many questions whose correct answers rely on good memory. A purer IQ test would separate memory as just one variable.

Applications

1 Remember that it is not sufficient to learn a new concept, skill, or body of information. You must convert it into long-term memory. In other words, if you take the time to read a book or article, say, on how to be a better listener, you probably will not remember the skills or concepts unless you practice one or more of the three strategies described in Topic 19.5.

2 Additional techniques for establishing new learning in long-term memory are suggested in Chapters Eighteen and Twenty, and later in this chapter.

Topic 19.2 The three stages of memory formation

Forming a chunk of memory is like making a photograph. Regard photography as a three-stage process: capturing the image on light-sensitive film, developing the film with chemicals, and fixing the image permanently with chemicals. A similar process happens in memory-chunk formation: capturing the chunk (immediate memory), developing the chunk (short-term memory), and fixing the chunk (long-term

Creating new mental paths

memory). Bolles (1988) makes the case that the concept of short- and long-term memory is an outdated one, based on computer structure; the debate continues.

Immediate memory is a kind of buffer area that can hold thousands of pieces of data for two seconds or less. For example, when you look up a telephone number that you've never seen before, you'll forget it a few seconds later unless you keep repeating it. New information will push out old unless the old is paid attention to.

Short-term memory appears to function in the hippocampus as a kind of broker that selects chunks of data to remember. A chunk is defined as an unfamiliar array of seven (plus or minus two) pieces, or bits, of information—for example, a seven-digit telephone number, a new word such as *phlyxma* (I made this up!), or a new definition composed of familiar words. George Miller (1956), in a classic article in *Psychological Review*, first identified that people learn most efficiently in units of seven plus or minus two. Groups of seven occur throughout literature and history (the Seven Wonders of the World, the seven mortal sins, the seven virtues, . . .). Interestingly, the Australian aborigines have only seven words for numbers, equivalent to one, two, three, four, five, six, and seven. Another word means simply many, or more than seven. It is perhaps because the aborigines have little or no need for long-term memory that they recall only what is reinforced daily. The word for three surely would occur every day, or at least every other day, whereas a word for sixty-three wouldn't get a chance to be reinforced every two days. Therefore, three would remain in short-term memory, but sixty-three would disappear and have to be reinvented.

Decision theorist Herbert Simon says that it takes about eight seconds of attention to add one new chunk to short-term memory. Once a chunk has been completely mastered, it becomes a bit and can then be combined with other bits to become a new chunk. In other words, a new chunk loses its identity as a chunk after it becomes second nature to us. Chunks become bits, just as images on film become printable negatives after developing.

Long-term memory appears to be located in the cerebral cortex. Apparently, hippocampal short-term memory communicates with the cortex through what we call simple human will or effort; over time, it establishes chunks in long-term storage. A key to the formation of long-term memory is the level of the neurotransmitters epinephrine and norepinephrine. James McGaugh, a psychobiologist at the University of California, Irvine, showed that rats with low epinephrine levels had poorer recall ability, but that booster shots of epinephrine after they had learned something improved their retention. He further found that injecting older rats after they had learned a maze improved their memory. Larry Stein, also at Irvine, shocked rats when they stepped off a platform that was

New information will push out old unless the old is paid attention to.

surrounded by water. Weeks later, when the rats were put back on the platform, they remembered and didn't step off. However, when he blocked their norepinephrine, he found that, while they could *learn* not to step off, they couldn't *remember* and stepped off into repeated shocks. When we have strong experiences, norepinephrine tells the brain to print it, and we hang on to such memories. Apparently, trivial experiences, about which we don't get juiced up, are lost. Blocking norepinephrine prevents us from remembering new information. This is why some people with amnesia can remember distant events but not recent ones.

Epinephrine and norepinephrine are released by the adrenal medulla when the body is subjected to physical or emotional stress. In addition to causing increased blood flow, this release causes extra glucose production. The rate of glucose breakdown is a measure of cortical activity. So although you can relax when you are reading, you need to put in a little sweat equity (known as grunting and groaning) in order to convert what you learn into long-term memory.

We acquire one or two bits of information per second during concentrated study; by midlife we have acquired roughly 10^9 bits. Our average brain capacity is 2.8×10^{20}, or approximately ten million volumes (books) of a thousand pages each.

Karl Pribram of Stanford University writes of the holographic structure of long-term memory. Each memory seems to be stored throughout the brain, rather than in a single confined location. Apparently, memories hook on to related networks of other memories, so that, for example, redheads are all somehow loosely tied together in your storage, and you can dump out a long list of redheads upon request. These networks become diffuse and interdependent. Neal Cohen of Johns Hopkins University trained rats to learn a maze, then operated on them. If less than one-fifth of the cortex was removed, *regardless of where it came from,* the rats exhibited no memory loss. If more than one-fifth of the cortex was removed, a proportional loss of memory occurred. So there appears to be no one location within the cortex for memory storage; instead, each memory seems to have an extensive set of backups.

Applications

1 After a learning episode of an hour or so, take a break and do something to pump up your epinephrine levels: walk about, do isometrics, climb some stairs, do laundry, move some boxes—anything that will generate epinephrine and norepinephrine to help fix the memory. Then go back and review the old material before going on to something new.

2 Making the effort to reorganize new material you've read or heard about is, in itself, a form of stress that will help you convert the material to long-term memory.

> Our average brain capacity is 2.8×10^{20}, or approximately ten million volumes of a thousand pages each.

Creating new mental paths

Topic 19.3 Maintenance requirements

Once a long-term memory is formed, there appear to be three major obstacles to retrieving it: *clogging at the synapse, deterioration of the neuronal pathways involved,* and *stress.* Clogging at the synapse occurs over time as protein particles accumulate on both sides of the synaptic gap; it consists of pregap or dendritic clogging and postgap or axonic clogging. This clogging is similar to the protein accumulation on contact lenses. Just as this protein accumulation can be removed by soaking and baking, synaptic clogging is removed by the neurotransmitter *calpain,* found in calcium. Calpain acts like an internal PacPerson that scurries around the synapse gobbling up protein particles. Another finding, by Richard Wurtman of Massachusetts Institute of Technology, is that Alzheimer's patients have buildups of rock-hard amyloid protein and a deficiency of acetylcholine, which is necessary to break down amyloid protein.

Deterioration of the neuronal pathways occurs naturally through aging (see Topic 4.1 for a list of factors that contribute to the deterioration of neurons), but there is one source of deterioration over which we have control. That is lack of production of the neurotransmitter acetylcholine, whose presence is crucial to the maintenance of neuronal membranes. With insufficient acetylcholine, these cell membranes become brittle and fall away. The dietary source of acetylcholine is fat. Diets with levels of fat below the recommended daily allowance represent a threat to acetylcholine levels. Normal or even high fat content in your diet, however, does not ensure sufficient acetylcholine. Other factors, such as genetics, disease, medication, or stress, can influence acetylcholine levels downward.

Stress causes the limbic system to work in the foreground, thus drastically reducing the availability of the cortical system. As a result memory retrieval is highly ineffective and unreliable. For example, when I make a presentation, I experience stress. If I am prepared and speak from well-organized notes, the presentation goes well. On the other hand, if I have not organized the presentation, have no notes or outline, and am winging it, I do less well. The difference is not how well I know the material—I know it equally well in both cases. The difference is that, under stress, I cannot access or retrieve the material as effectively. The notes help guide the retrieval. This has the added effect of reducing the stress.

Electroshock can improve memory by approximately 300 percent, with effects that last for about three weeks. Apparently electroshock shakes some of the protein off the synapse. Some improvement of memory is possible with the drug physostigmine, which inhibits the formation of cholinesterase, an enzyme that breaks down neurotransmitters such as acetylcholine. Improvements have also been seen in studies at Northwestern University Medical School with a drug called nimodipine, which appears to inhibit calcium buildup in people who consume too much calcium. In experiments with rabbits, older rabbits learned more quickly after taking nimodipine. More recently, researchers at Northwestern University Medical School have found that cycloserine and monoclonal antibodies appear to have profoundly positive effects, improving and speeding up memory as well as improving memory disorders such as Alzheimer's disease. These two chemicals act on the nimodipine receptors in the hippocampus to allow calcium to enter and help in forming new synapses.

Applications

1   Maintain the recommended daily allowances for fat and calcium. See Appendix B.

2   Remove or minimize as much as possible the stress in your life. See Topic 14.2.

3   Consult your neurologist for possible experimental drug treatment of memory problems.

4   If someone you know, especially an older adult, seems confused or is having memory problems, check for an excess or deficiency of dietary calcium.

Topic 19.4   The two kinds of memory chunks

Richard Hirsh of McGill University describes two kinds of memory chunks: facts and skills; fellow Canadian Endel Tulving calls them semantic and episodic units. *Facts* are more discrete chunks of memory, such as word definitions, symbol meanings, and associations with dates, places, and faces, hence Tulving's reference to them as semantic. *Skills* are more continuous chunks of memory, such as stories and kinesthetic sequences (tying shoes, riding a bicycle). Skill learning is primarily associated with the limbic (animal) brain, whereas fact learning is primarily associated with the cerebral cortex, which develops after the limbic area. Perhaps this is why we can't remember much from the first several years of life. Hirsh reports that damage to the hippocampus prevents learning of new facts, but allows new skills to be learned.

Fact and skill learning abilities may be associated with hemispheric specialization. The area devoted to fact learning may be a kind of articulation apparatus located in the verbal area of the cortex (see Topic 3.1), while the area devoted

Creating new mental paths

to skill learning may be a kind of visual-spatial notepad located in the visual-spatial area of the cortex (the right hemisphere for males and both hemispheres for females). I know of no research to back this up, but it would seem to be a logical inference from existing studies.

Application

It is possible that you have more strength in one kind of memory unit than in another. If so, emphasize your strength rather than regretting your weakness. I am sure that my skill (visual-spatial) memory is superior to my fact (language) memory. So I should abandon the frustrating pastime of trying to keep my foreign language ability up, and enjoy my ability to learn new musical instruments.

Topic 19.5 The three strategies for remembering

Minninger (1984) has categorized all the many memorization gimmicks into three categories: *intend, file,* and *rehearse.* This approach has been around for some time. Erasmus wrote in 1512, "Though I do not deny that memory can be helped by places and images, yet the best memory is based on three important things: namely study [rehearse], order [file], and care [intend]." *Intend* to remember something; that is, don't assume that it'll just stick after exposure—you need to make a point of wanting to remember it. *File* it by organizing it and playing with it in your own special way. And *rehearse* it, or practice it, as a way of showing that you intend to remember it. Do it and say it repeatedly.

Intend, file, and rehearse.

These three generic strategy types are the means by which we convert short-term memory to long-term memory.

Applications

1   Here are some ways to apply the intend strategy:

- Before reading an article or book, preread it by reviewing the section headings, pictures, charts, graphs, figures, appendixes, and bibliography to get a feeling for how it is laid out and what it covers. This will serve as a kind of advance organizer that will make the reading more meaningful.
- Before taking a course or workshop, do all you can to be ready to receive the material: review the course syllabus if it is available; familiarize yourself with the course outline, agenda, handouts, or bibliography if you can; and read relevant material suggested by a librarian, the instructor, the bibliography, graduates of the course, or common sense. Contact other prior participants to discuss what they learned.

- Consciously decide to remember something, then select a way to file it (see Application 2 below). D. J. Herrmann (1991) provides many good suggestions in his *Supermemory: A Quick-Action Program for Memory Improvement*. His approach is not as technical as those of Buzan (1991) and Lorayne and Lucas (1974).
- Once you've decided to memorize information, one way to show your intention is to *chunk* it (see Topic 18.1) and learn the chunks. Divide and conquer.
- Understand and practice the concept of state dependence described in Topic 19.6.

Our memory for images is better than our memory for words.

2 Following are some ways to apply the file strategy:

- Make a flowchart, Pareto chart (see Topic 23.3), or any other kind of organizational chart that structures what you've learned in a way that's meaningful to you.
- Using self-sticking notes or a material like flannel board, write out a single chunk of what you've learned on its own separate sheet. Then arrange the chunks on a wall in a way that makes sense to you. Restudy the arrangement from time to time and rearrange the notes as needed. When you've fixed the organization the way you like it, make a flowchart or some other kind of chart or outline and put it away for easy review or retrieval. Keep it in your portable notebook for frequent rehearsal.
- Describe the person or object you want to remember in such a way that it evokes the name of the object. For example, you might associate the name Ann Woodward with this description: "She who keeps the extra timber for repairs to Green Gables."
- Substitute words (perhaps with rhymes) as an aid to remembering a name. Try to make it graphically visual. For example, if Harvey Darrow has bad acne, associate the name with the substitutes "larvae barrow," while visualizing a wheelbarrow containing dirt filled with larvae (acne). At a party, if you want to remember the name Ted Miller, and Ted is extremely lacking in personality, remember him as the Dead Miller. I invite folks who reverse my first and last names to remember my name as rhyming with the "fierce coward" (Pierce Howard). See *The Memory Book* (Lorayne & Lucas, 1974) and *Use Your Perfect Memory* (Buzan, 1991) for many ideas on visualization techniques for memory. These authors remind us that our memory for images is better than our memory for words, and our memory for concrete words is better than our memory for abstract words.

- Lorayne and Lucas (1974) recommend another technique called linking, which is a way to remember a list of things. If you need to stop by the grocery store to pick up milk, bread, hose, and shrimp, link each word to the next one on the list by some exaggerated visual connection. For example, a huge carton of milk has a loaf of bread for a stopper, with a pair of hose connected to the loaf to pull it out in order to pour the milk in a saucepan to boil the shrimp. Once you've made these linking associations, all you have to remember is the first image—the big bottle of milk—and the rest follows.
- Use the peg-word technique, described in Topic 18.4, Application 2. The peg-word technique is actually a variation on the loci technique of Simonides, the ancient Greek orator. Simonides associated parts of a speech with parts of familiar places (loci); for example, each spot in a familiar walkway or building would be associated with a paragraph or subtopic of the speech.
- To remember a number, such as a telephone number, substitute the phonetic consonant equivalents for the numbers and fill in with vowels to make up words. To substitute consonants, try:

1 = *d* or *t* or *th* (one vertical stroke)
2 = *n* (two vertical strokes)
3 = *m* (three vertical strokes)
4 = *r* (last letter of the sound of four)
5 = *L* (Roman numeral for 500; five fingers spread out look like an *L*)
6 = *j*, soft *g*, *sh*, or *ch* (*J* and 6 are mirror images; the others sound like the *s* or *x*)
7 = *k*, hard *g*, or hard *c* (angular, like a 7; *g* and *c* sound like *k*)
8 = *f, v,* or *ph* (cursive *f* looks like an 8; *v* and *ph* sound like *f*)
9 = *b* or *p* (*b* looks like an upside-down 9, *p* like a backward 9; *b* and *p* sound alike; they are labial consonants)
0 = *z, s,* or soft *c* (first letter in zero)

So, to remember the telephone number for our favorite Indian restaurant, I came up with Lub Duk Tiki-Ba, or 591-7179 (LBD-KTKB). Leave out the vowels and substitute numbers for consonants according to the above list (or think up your own). See Lorayne and Lucas (1974), Buzan (1991), and Minninger (1984) for more examples. Try to create outrageous, gruesome, or bawdy images—they're easier to recall and can be your private joke on the world.

3 Here are some ways to apply the rehearse strategy:

- Obtain or create the material on audiotape and review it while driving, jogging, walking, or busing.
- Create a tickle file. Assign a file folder for each month, week, or day and insert notes you want to review in the appropriate folder.
- Use a highlighter or pen while reading to note sections for review, then periodically review the highlighted sections.
- When you are idle (stopped at a red light, walking, etc.), recall recently memorized material and rehearse it. Review this material with a walking or jogging partner.
- Make a set of flash cards of the steps in a process or some other sequential list of items you want to remember, with the correct sequence of each card indicated on the back side. Shuffle the cards and sort them.
- For many additional suggestions, information, and training opportunities, get on the mailing list of the Buzan Centre:

The Buzan Centre of Palm Beach, Inc.
415 Federal Highway
Lake Park, FL 33403
800-964-6362 or 800-Y-MINDMAP

Topic 19.6 State dependence

People recall information more readily when they can remember the state in which they learned that information. This is the basis of the old advice to play back in your mind everywhere you've been in the last thirty minutes when you want to find an object you've lost in that time period. In one research study, subjects memorized a list in the basement of a building and were tested. They then moved to one of the upper floors of the building and were given the same test, but scored poorly. When they were asked to visualize the basement in which the memory task occurred, their scores improved, and when they were returned to the actual basement room where they had memorized the list and were tested again, their scores improved even more. This phenomenon is called state dependence, the theory that recall of learning can depend on the state or other situation that existed when the learning took place.

State dependence is reported to hold true for *place* (as in the basement example), *mood* (if you were angry when you learned, remember the anger), *odors* (remember that the olfactory sense is located in the limbic system), and *physical condition* (if you were drinking coffee while you were learning, you will remember better if you drink coffee). Why? Apparently, the synapses formed to create a specific memory are connected to neural networks that form the basis of conditions associated with the time and place of learning. Recalling the place (e.g., a specific room in a house) in which you learned a person's name will help access the name, because the two are connected by neural networks. This is similar to taking a photo of a person standing against a background.

> If you were drinking coffee while you were learning, you will remember better if you drink coffee.

Applications

1   When you are with someone who is having a hard time remembering something you both want to remember, get that person to focus on the place, the mood, and his or her physical condition when the information was learned. The same goes for you if you're trying to remember something.

2   Be careful to learn things under conditions that are easy to replicate when you need to remember them.

3   When you are trying to teach job-related skills, create a learning environment that approximates the conditions on the job. (contributed by Rick Bradley)

Topic 19.7   Helping others remember

Research into witness management has led to some interesting techniques for eliciting latent memories from a witness. For example, build on a witness's schemas (see Topic 18.4), then identify something in the witness's background that he or she can relate to the scene of the crime. Another witness management technique is to minimize questions, asking only a few open-ended questions from which the witness can reveal his or her schemas. The interviewer then builds on the information the witness has volunteered.

Applications

1   Use the witness's interests to elicit memories. For example, if the witness is a soap opera addict, ask first, "Was there a television set in the room? Describe it. What was on top of it? Beside it? On the wall above it?" You use the TV set to retrieve images of the rest of the room. If you start with an impersonal question that the witness cannot immediately relate to his or her experience, you are less likely to get the desired level of detail. If your witness likes woodwork, try starting with items made of wood. Ask someone who's bookish about printed matter, an artist about artwork, a musician about a piano, and so on.

2   Ask open-ended questions beginning with words like *when, where, how many, how long,* and *what*. These types of question starters are more likely to get someone talking and exploit their memory than closed-ended questions that typically elicit yes-or-no responses, such as "Did you arrive before 8:00 P.M.?"

Topic 19.8 The difference in short- and long-term memory

The real difference between short-term and long-term memory is the difference between learning a telephone number long enough to dial it immediately and learning it long enough to dial it a week later. That distinction is often confused in people who seem to remember remote events (e.g., elderly people may recall episodes from their childhood) but can't remember something they were told yesterday. Bolles (1988, p. 234) writes: "Memories for recent and for long-ago events depend on the same constructive abilities and the same emotional, factual, and interpretive levels of memory. If a person can still remember past events well and still tell interesting stories about the long ago, he has the equipment to do the same for more recent events. Failure to remember the present in such cases suggests a failure to pay attention to the present, not an inability to learn new details." This suggests that, for many, what may appear to be poor short-term memory may in fact be a symptom of depression. Depressed people may not pay sufficient attention to events or care enough about them to remember them.

What may appear to be poor short-term memory may in fact be a symptom of depression.

Applications

1   If you want another person to think you have their attention, then focus on what they are telling you, including their name. To say, "I have to hear a name three times before I remember it" just doesn't wash—it simply leaves you sounding like someone who doesn't pay attention. If you don't want to forget the name, keep saying it to yourself, associate it with other images, and ask questions about it, such as "Is it a popular name in your family?" "What part of the world does it come from?" "Is it a nickname?"

2   If someone, particularly an older person, appears forgetful, remember that it could be something as simple as his or her mind having wandered momentarily, or something as major as depression.

Summary

Bolles (1988, p. 23) describes the process of memory like this: "We remember what we understand; we understand only what we pay attention to; we pay attention to what we want." In other words, *experience* arouses *emotion*, which fixes *attention* and leads to *understanding and insight*, which results in *memory*. Bolles continues: "Attention is like digestion. We do not store the food we eat; we break it down so that it becomes part of our body. Attention selects parts of experience and uses it to nourish our memories. We do not store this experience, we use it. Of course, we eat many things that we do not digest and we also experience many things without paying them any attention" (p. 183).

Suggested readings on memory

Bolles, E. B. (1988). *Remembering and Forgetting: An Inquiry into the Nature of Memory.* New York: Walker.

Buzan, T. (1991). *Use Your Perfect Memory.* (3rd ed.). New York: Penguin.

Edelman, G. M. (1987). *Neural Darwinism: The Theory of Neuronal Group Selection.* New York: Basic Books.

Lorayne, H., & Lucas, J. (1974). *The Memory Book.* New York: Stein & Day.

Minninger, J. (1984). *Total Recall: How to Boost Your Memory Power.* Emmaus, PA: Rodale.

Rosenfield, I. (1988). *The Invention of Memory: A New View of the Brain.* New York: Basic Books.

20

We are all teachers and students:

Not only have we all experienced classroom learning, but many of us will have the opportunity in the near or distant future to teach something to a group. Sales representatives teach their prospects as a part of their sales presentations. Other people may conduct a training class for employees, teach an elementary or secondary school class, teach at the university, conduct an evening class at the community college, give religious instruction, orient new employees, train employees on the job in new skills and technologies, or teach (i.e., persuade) power brokers to pursue a certain path. This chapter is intended for the teacher in all of us.

The best lesson plan in the world is less effective than it could be if the teacher using it fails to bring to that plan what only good teachers can bring. That is the role of the teacher: to present content for learning in such a way that students are most likely to learn. This chapter looks at what brain research says about the teacher's role as a facilitator of learning.

Hart (1983) suggests that any educational environment be characterized by the following four general features:

1   High expectations

2   A nonthreatening ambiance

3   A goal of 100 percent mastery

4   An air of reality (i.e., it consists of more than just books)

Creating new mental paths

Helping learning happen

Topic 20.1 Advance organizers

Students tend to learn more when they are given some warning about what they are to learn. Perhaps this brings relevant schemas into the foreground or at least prepares them to put forth appropriate effort in forming new ones. Techniques used to alert learners about the nature of an upcoming learning episode are called advance organizers because they assist the learners in calling up relevant schemas in preparation for learning.

Applications

1   Send out preliminary reading materials.

2   Provide an outline or agenda of the learning experience both in advance of the session and at the beginning of the session.

3   Review the objectives at the beginning of the session.

4   Tell people what you are getting ready to do. Abruptly moving into an activity is disturbing to many people.

5   Have attendees meet with their supervisor or team members before the class to agree on expectations.

> "Those who educate children well are more to be honored than even their parents, for these only give them life, those the art of living well."
>
> **Aristotle**

6   At the beginning of the session, give participants some kind of big-picture overview of the material to be covered; this provides a map for the terrain.

7   Ask participants what their expectations are. (contributed by Jane Howard)

Topic 20.2 Spacing

In a 1978 experiment, British postal workers learned to use a new machine. Those who studied one hour a day learned twice as fast as those who studied four hours a day in two two-hour sessions. The two-hour group learned in half as many days, but spent twice as many hours learning. In other words, the more hours per day they spent in instruction, the more total time they required. Clearly this would be desirable only under a deadline. Prefer spaced to massed learning where possible. Learning is "spaced" if it is composed of multiple modules with a significant time lapse between modules. Shorter modules for a given quantity of learning mean that it is more spaced.

Harry Bahrick, a psychologist at Ohio Wesleyan University, believes that you should institutionalize spacing concepts. His research establishes the superior effect of cumulative learning. The more you study and review, the more you remember. He found that high school Spanish students who took five courses remembered about 60 percent of the vocabulary twenty-five years after high school, while students taking only one course remembered almost none, in spite of the fact that neither group had used their Spanish to a significant degree after high school. Again controlling for usage, he compared 1,726 adults who had finished high school fifty years previously and found that those who had gone on from high school algebra and geometry to take college-level math at or above the level of calculus scored 80 percent correct on an algebra test. Those who took only high school algebra and geometry and did as well as the college math group in their high school math courses managed to score only slightly better than a control group who had taken no algebra or geometry at all in high school or anywhere else! Bahrick laments that we spend millions helping people learn, then let them forget what they learned.

Applications

1   Try to schedule learning modules of no more than two to four hours per day; allow time and space for practice between sessions. Build in frequent breaks when this isn't possible.

2   If you must have an all-day seminar, take extra care to allow participants time to read in advance and to practice and review afterward.

3 Schools should change from the quarter system to the semester system, and from longer class periods to shorter class periods (and to more of them).

4 Schools and other learning organizations should require review of prior material both during the course and in subsequent courses.

5 Schools should have cumulative courses that review and integrate prior courses and should give cumulative final examinations.

6 Schools should offer courses that meet, for example, once a week for two or three years, rather than three times a week for four months. The general rule should be to spread out learning as much as possible to maximize retention.

7 Plan training carefully for new employees, so as not to overwhelm them during their first days on the job. (contributed by Rick Bradley)

8 Schedule more frequent, shorter staff meetings.

Topic 20.3 Breaks

Research indicates at least two good reasons to take breaks after each learning module. First, the new neural connections formed by the learning need time to fix and strengthen themselves without competition from additional novel stimuli. A simple walk around the block can serve to provide such jelling time. This is like the need in darkroom photography for a "fixing" chemical to stabilize the photographic image. Second, because of fatigue factors, errors increase as break time decreases.

Some form of exercise is an excellent follow-up to a learning episode.

Applications

1 Some form of exercise is an excellent follow-up to a learning episode, because of the impact of the extra epinephrine on the formation of neuronal connections. Perhaps you could lead your students in stretching, bending, and breathing exercises after a learning episode.

2 The best time of day to take in new material is just before going to sleep. Research indicates that material studied then tends to be remembered better. Sleep, in one sense, is another way to take a break. Encourage learners to do memory work before going to sleep.

3 In classes of adults, announce that students can leave the room whenever they wish, but also have periodic, scheduled breaks. (contributed by Jack Wilson)

Topic 20.4 Incubation

To come up with creative responses to problems, time is needed for the information to incubate. As Louis Pasteur remarked, "Chance favors the prepared mind." Do your homework, then let intuition work on it. When I was a first-year student at Davidson College, I had a tennis class under Coach Lefty Driesell. One day, after Lefty hit a ball past me, I shouted out, playfully, "LUCK!" Driesell stopped dead in his tracks, glared at me, and said, "There's no such thing as luck, Howard. It's preparation meeting the opportunity."

Applications

1   Allow for a substantial break, when possible, after problem-definition activity and before idea-generation activity.

2   Many of us participate in team-building retreats. The best use of these overnight problem-solving sessions is to present the information (attitude survey results, etc.) before bedtime, then, in the morning, after it has incubated, to come up with creative responses in a planning session.

3   Teams and departments often push through meeting agendas, grasping at the first suggestion that develops in order to get to the next item. Make it a group norm to allow for more incubation time when a matter is not urgent. Better planning often results.

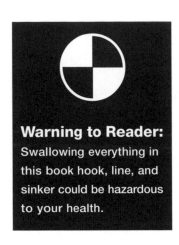

Warning to Reader:
Swallowing everything in this book hook, line, and sinker could be hazardous to your health.

Topic 20.5 Follow-up

The best way to ensure that classroom learning is forgotten is to fail to provide opportunities for follow-up and follow-through. Studies show that a larger portion of the material learned in a classroom setting is retained when the learner or the teacher make provisions for follow-up.

Applications

1   Have learners write goal letters to themselves and mail them out several months later. They all will receive letters from their conscience about what they intended to work on after the training session.

2   Make sure that after returning to the job, the learners schedule a conference with their supervisor or team to review accomplishments and possibilities for applying the learnings on the job.

Creating new mental paths

3   Develop refresher modules of short duration for students to take periodically.

4   Have class reunions.

5   When using a series of spaced modules, provide homework assignments (practice or reading) between sessions. Review the homework, sharing successes and failures, at the beginning of each session.

6   Plan during class how each participant will apply new learnings to the job—for example, by writing scripts, developing implementation schedules, identifying obstacles to success, or writing personal development plans.

7   Send out audio- or videotapes that recap the major points of the training session.

Topic 20.6 Control

The teacher is the one person most able to influence the learner's sense of control over the learning process. If the learner feels in control, a wider range of learning, both rote and meaningful, can occur. If the learner feels highly controlled, only rote learning can occur. Caine and Caine (1991) call this taxon (list) and locale (map) learning. Locale learning encourages creativity, analysis, synthesis, planning, problem solving, and complex decisions. When the learner feels relaxed and in control, the cortex is fully functional and this higher-level, more meaningful learning is possible. When the learner feels out of control of the learning process, he or she "downshifts" (Caine & Caine, 1991) from cortical locale learning to the limbic system's taxon, or rote, learning.

In this condition, the cortex essentially shuts down. The only learning possible involves rote memorization or learning of simple skills, and the only creativity or problem solving possible is that which is based on habits, instincts, or other already learned routinized behavior.

Sometimes persons of lower ability appear to be able to learn only simple, routine skills, when in fact they can only learn routines because they are under stress. Away from sources of stress, they can be more creative and complex in their learning behavior.

By being stressful or perceived to be stressful, the learning environment, or classroom, can itself prevent cortical learning. Make sure your classroom does not force downshifting. (For a more extended treatment of stress and control issues, refer to Chapter Fourteen.)

Applications

1   At the beginning of a class, clearly establish learner control by reviewing class norms; for example, you might say, "Feel free to take a break when you need to," "Please let me know if you're physically uncomfortable and I'll see what can be done about it," or "Please feel free to ask any question whenever the need arises—the only dumb question is the unasked question."

2   Help learners set their own goals for learning.

3   Use effective listening techniques, such as active and reflective listening, paraphrasing, and clarifying, that have the effect of focusing on the learners and underscoring their control.

4   Ask open-ended questions; they invite the learner to be more involved in the process. Avoid questions with yes-or-no responses; they discourage involvement. And avoid questions starting with "Why . . . ?" This type of question tends to create stress in learners and make them defensive (see Flanders, 1970).

5   Use some of the Applications suggested in Topics 18.3 through 18.6. Each of these four learning strategies places the learner in the driver's seat.

6   Respect differences in learning styles. Pete Stone, an innovative elementary school principal in Charlotte, North Carolina, accommodates students' stylistic differences to the maximum: their need for cool or warm temperatures, preference for dim or full light, desire for snacks, and need for physical activity.

7   Build in opportunities for participant involvement—role plays, case studies, small-group work, and so on. (contributed by Rick Bradley)

8   Allow participants to select their own seats without assigning them. If you want to mix them up after a break, ask them to select new seats with new people on either side. Each participant will still maintain the same sense of control.

Topic 20.7 Relaxation

As discussed in Topic 20.6, encouraging the learner to feel in control is a major strategy in preventing downshifting, or moving from cortical alertness to limbic arousal, or stress. Another strategy would be to help learners who are already under stress (e.g., those coming into your class after a bad encounter) to upshift, or move from

    Creating new mental paths

limbic fight-or-flight arousal into cortical arousal and alertness. When a person comes to your learning experience full of stress, it must be relieved before meaningful learning can occur. The primary strategy to use in the classroom is relaxation.

Applications

1 Play tapes with sounds of nature—rainstorms, desert winds, the beach, birds—before class, during breaks, or during silent individual work like reading or filling out worksheets. Nature sounds have a way of refocusing a person away from absent stress into the here and now.

2 Play tapes with simple classical music (Mozart is a good common denominator)—again, before class or during breaks—as a way of helping people refocus. Don't play music during individual work, however.

3 If you are the teacher, lighten up from time to time in a way that is appropriate for you. This keeps students alert and prevents them from downshifting.

4 If you are the student, practice some of the relaxation techniques described in the Applications to Topic 14.2.

Topic 20.8 Rapport

Researchers, particularly in the field of neurolinguistic programming (NLP), have tried to identify why some therapists seem to work magic on clients. They have found that effective therapists tend to establish rapport with clients by matching and pacing—in other words, by mirroring the clients' posture and following their tempo. The research suggests that matching and pacing another person has the effect of establishing rapport and increasing trust and openness. Matching and pacing are discussed further in Topic 15.4.

> Matching and pacing another person has the effect of establishing rapport and increasing trust and openness.

Applications

1 Using Figure 15.1, find authentic ways of establishing rapport by matching and pacing your learners.

2 When you have a student who seems to be resisting your help, identify the biggest differences between the two of you and see if you can eliminate some of these differences or at least minimize their effect.

3 Move toward a learner who is asking a question or making a comment; establish rapport by getting closer and using eye contact. (contributed by Jane Howard)

We are all teachers and students

Topic 20.9 Positive expectations

Rosenthal and Jacobson (1968) established that positive expectations tend to yield positive results and negative expectations yield negative results. See Topic 15.3 for more on this subject.

Applications

1 Communicate clearly to all learners that you are confident in their ability to excel.

Positive expectations tend to yield positive results and negative expectations yield negative results.

2 Communicate to all learners your confidence in your own ability to teach effectively.

3 Communicate to all learners your confidence in previous learners' successful application of classroom learning to the real world.

4 Resist the temptation to give up on some students; maintain clearly high expectations for all of them. Remember, you may have some students who've been told all their life that they're failures, so don't be discouraged if you don't make much of a dent in their self-concept. If enough of us treat them with positive expectations, we increase the chances of their success.

5 If it is appropriate, mention other groups, classes, or organizations that have successfully completed the program.

Topic 20.10 Enuf's enuf (habituation)

Habituation is the psychological term for "enough is enough." Our sensory receptors become aroused when a new stimulus begins, but if the new stimulus continues without variation in quality or quantity, our sensory receptors shut down from their aroused state, having become habituated, or accustomed, to the monotonous stimulus. A change in the quality or quantity of the stimulus will arouse the receptors again. This is why, for example, it is hard to pay attention to someone who speaks in a monotone. It is also why people often add salt, pepper, or other seasoning after several bites. Druckman and Bjork (1991) emphasize the importance of varying training conditions to prevent habituation and its attendant inefficiency in learning.

Applications

1 Have someone videotape you while you are teaching (or simply set up a videotape camera, aim it in your general direction, and let it run). Review the tape and critique yourself for signs of repetitive behaviors that might tend to lessen the alertness of your students: talking at the same pitch, the same volume, or the same speed (never even slowing down to make a dramatic point); using the same vocabulary (complex Greek- or Latin-derived words rather than simple Anglo-Saxon ones); standing or sitting in the same place; walking in the same pattern (desk to window, window to desk, desk to window, etc.); limiting eye contact (always looking at the same three or four students, or from the window to the ceiling and back); or waving your arm the same way for emphasis.

2 Seek out authentic ways to vary your behavior to maximize students' alertness. Remember when the teacher played by Robin Williams in *Dead Poets Society* jumped up on his desk or walked the class into the hall to view a picture? He knew how to avoid habituation. Fight it like the **pLaGuE**!

3 Minimize learning tasks that exceed five to ten minutes, and search for ways to vary the tasks to maximize the students' arousal: contrast lecture with discussion; whole-group or small-group learning with individual seatwork; reading with writing; standing with sitting; remembering and mastering with creating; practicing with critiquing.

4 After each break, encourage learners to take a seat in a different part of the room.

5 Jump, clap, shout, throw, wave, stomp, roll, whisper.

6 Offer graphs to trainers for feedback on how well they do with this habituation paradigm. Once I was asked to observe a superintendent of schools as he conducted a staff meeting. He had a reputation for horrible meetings. The first thing I noticed was his monotone. I charted his variation in pitch, volume, tempo, vocabulary, posture, and gesture over time. The resulting graph showed nothing but a group of flat lines. It made the point and he understood why and how to improve.

Topic 20.11 Developing prestige

In their research, Caine and Caine (1991) found that students perform better when they perceive the teacher as prestigious. They further found that this prestige comes primarily from two perceptions: that the teacher has expertise and that he or she is caring. Expertise is assumed from the appearance that the teacher has mastered the subject, is not dependent on notes (except to help in sticking to the subject!), and has practiced what is being preached. Caring is assumed from the appearance that the teacher accepts and values each student as a human being.

Applications

1 Practice the Applications in Topics 20.8 and 20.9.

2 Try visualizing the class process in much the same way that a skier visualizes the downhill sequence before jumping off. Keep notes on potential problems you spot while visualizing, then solve them after you finish.

3 Try a dry run in which you move through the class process rapidly, again keeping notes on potential problems.

4 Try putting notes on the borders of your transparencies to avoid the distraction of looking down at notes in your hand.

5 Try the lesson plan out first on a test group (officemates, your family, a group of employees, or even paid guinea pigs). Have them critique you or simply serve as a live test audience.

6 Arrive early and greet people by name; don't rush away as soon as the lesson is over.

7 During breaks, mix and mingle.

8 Lightly pencil your notes onto blank flip-chart pages prior to class. The notes will go unnoticed by participants and you'll be perceived as being well versed in your subject. (contributed by Rick Bradley)

9 When seeking input from a group, capture their responses on a flip chart or transparency. (contributed by Rick Bradley)

10 Acknowledge input from the group. (contributed by Rick Bradley)

11 Work hard to understand your audience and their issues and concerns. Use this understanding to build class outlines. Use real-life examples they can relate to.

> Caring is assumed from the appearance that the teacher accepts and values each student as a human being.

Creating new mental paths

12   If you have been brought into an organization as an outside expert or guest, have someone from the organization introduce you to the group. (contributed by Jane Howard)

13   Display or mention licenses, certificates, apprenticeships, degrees, and awards.

Topic 20.12 Atmosphere

Research has identified a long list of learning-atmosphere variables, each of which suggests its own applications. See more on workplace design in Chapters Sixteen and Seventeen.

Applications

1   Faber Birren, in *Color and Human Response* (1978a), has suggested the many effects of color on people. See Topic 17.4 for a listing of these effects.

2   Ensure abundant light, especially at the beginning of a session, for those who may not be fully awake.

3   Remember that a moderate amount of background noise (so-called white noise) is helpful for concentration. In a room that is too quiet when participants are working silently at their seats, one can run the fan of an overhead projector. (contributed by Jane Howard)

4   You can take advantage of the knowledge that arousal (both limbic and cortical) is associated with a warmer brain, pleasant moods with a cooler brain. R. Zajonc, of the University of Michigan, has found that slow, minor-key music warms the brain, and breathing through the nose cools the brain (Izard, Kagan, & Zajonc, 1984).

5   Provide sufficient telephones nearby to reduce students' stress at being unable to keep in touch with their offices. I've been in many workshop situations in which fifteen to twenty people had only one telephone in the building available to use during breaks—not a good situation.

6   Avoid serving high-carbohydrate foods for snacks; they produce a pleasant mood and sleepiness. Choose proteins and low-carbohydrate foods—fruit, vegetables, low-fat crackers, non-fat dips—which are better for mental activity. Supply juices and diet sodas rather than full-strength sugared colas.

We are all teachers and students

7   Make sure that ample caffeine-free beverages are available to prevent overarousal, which makes concentration difficult.

8   Encourage participants to sit in a different place after each break—NLP research indicates that this improves participation and freshens the participants' perspective.

9   Have a no-smoking policy during class, unless an excellent exhaust system is available.

10   Allow fifty square feet per person in the classroom; less is stressful.

11   Plan the lighting in the room carefully when you are using slides or an over-head projector. Develop alternatives if the room must be darkened too much.

Synaptic structures show growth from enriched environments throughout the life span, including old age.

Topic 20.13 Richness

Mark Rosenzweig of the University of California, Berkeley, conducted a classic experiment in which two groups of rats were compared for the impact of environmental richness on brain development. One group was placed in a dull cage, the other in an enriched Disneyland-type cage. The brains of the highly stimulated rats grew larger and developed denser concentrations of synapses. Other research, including research on humans, has confirmed these findings. See particularly the work of Marian Diamond (1988), also of the University of California, Berkeley, who concludes that synaptic structures show growth from enriched environments throughout the life span, including old age.

Applications

1   Have a variety of posters, corporate and otherwise (e.g., "Today is the first day of the rest of your life"), on the walls of the classroom.

2   As you complete flip-chart diagrams, lists, and so on, tear them off and tape them to the wall for visual reinforcement.

3   Place games and puzzles around the border of the room and on the students' tables for manipulation during idle minutes.

4   Have a computer around for experimentation with relevant software, or for playing games during breaks.

Creating new mental paths

5   Hang appropriate photographs on the walls.

6   Place artwork on the walls of the classroom and in nearby hallways.

7   Have books for browsing in the classroom.

8   Supply several daily newspapers in the classroom, such as the *Wall Street Journal* and *USA Today*.

9   Place mirrors in appropriate locations for self-stimulation. Mirrors enhance self-concept among infants and relieve boredom among adults. In one amusing incident, tenants of an office tower complained of long elevator waits. The owners installed mirrors in the elevator waiting area and the complaints disappeared. Preening makes the wait grow shorter!

10   Post information about local resources such as restaurants and shopping centers—include maps.

11   If it is appropriate, have participants bring in and display samples of their own work. As an example, for NationsBank Quality Team meetings, which bring facilitators from across the company together for two- or three-day seminars, participants are asked to show how quality is being visibly promoted in their area. The walls and tables are filled with posters, buttons, banners, T-shirts, memos, job aids, and team pictures. It creates real excitement. (contributed by Rick Bradley)

12   Use graphics and color on overhead projections, slides, participant guides, and so on. (contributed by Rick Bradley)

13   Ditch the black flip-chart marker. Use a variety of colors. (contributed by Rick Bradley)

14   When headed for a particularly boring meeting, make sure to carry along at least three colors of ink pens and colored paper to take notes with. (contributed by Rick Bradley)

15   Include extra, relevant reading materials such as articles for participants to read if they finish individual tasks before other people are done. (contributed by Jane Howard)

Topic 20.14 Peer feedback

Peer feedback is more influential than teacher feedback in obtaining lasting performance results; too much teacher feedback can be harmful (Druckman & Swets, 1988). Apparently the approval or disapproval of one's peers is the best reinforcer. Excess feedback from the teacher can be perceived as insincere if it is too effusive or demotivating if it is too discouraging.

Applications

1   Emphasize peer feedback for student performance in small groups or one-on-one interaction.

2   One effective technique is to have graduates of a seminar meet in pairs over breakfast or lunch six months later for a follow-up session in which they discuss their successes and failures in implementing class concepts and skills.

3   When doing a role play, have all the participants do the exercise at the same time in groups of three—two to actually play the roles and one to help by making suggestions to a participant who is stuck and by providing feedback. (contributed by Jane Howard)

Suggested readings on the role of the teacher or trainer

Caine, R. N., & Caine, G. (1991). *Making Connections: Teaching and the Human Brain*. Alexandria, VA: Association for Supervision and Curriculum Development.

Diamond, M. (1988). *Enriching Heredity: The Impact of the Environment on the Anatomy of the Brain*. New York: Free Press.

Druckman, D., & Bjork, R. A. (Eds.). (1991). *In the Mind's Eye: Understanding Human Performance*. Washington, DC: National Academy Press.

Druckman, D., & Swets, J. A. (Eds.). (1988). *Enhancing Human Performance: Issues, Theories, and Techniques*. Washington, DC: National Academy Press.

Hart, L. A. (1983). *Human Brain and Human Learning*. New York: Longman.

Rosenthal, R., & Jacobson, L. (1968). *Pygmalion in the Classroom*. New York: Holt, Rinehart & Winston.

21

The psychobiology of creativity:

The call for creativity strikes fear in some while arousing enthusiasm in others. Why? This chapter addresses that question, based on the current state of research on creativity.

Topic 21.1 The creative act

Teresa Amabile (1983, p. 33), a leading researcher in creativity, has defined creativity conceptually as follows: "A product or response will be judged as creative to the extent that (a) it is both a novel and appropriate, useful, correct or valuable response to the task at hand, and (b) the task is heuristic rather than algorithmic." She then identifies three criteria for distinguishing more creative contributions from less creative ones: (1) *novelty* (we haven't seen or heard this before), (2) *relevance* (it relates to satisfying the need that originally prompted the contribution), and (3) *spontaneity* (the contributor didn't use a formula to "mechanically" come up with the contribution).

Margaret Boden (1990), thinking in parallel with Amabile, distinguishes between psychological creativity and historical creativity. The first is merely something new for the individual doing the creating, while the second is something new for humanity. To quote Boden: "A merely novel idea is one which can be described and/or produced by the same set of generative rules as are

Creating new mental paths

Cultivating a precious resource

other, familiar ideas. A genuinely original, or creative, idea is one which cannot" (p. 40).

How do we know whether or not a contribution possesses these three
features? Amabile (1983, p. 31) proposes a consensual definition: "A product or
response is creative to the extent that appropriate observers independently agree
it is creative. Appropriate observers are those familiar with the domain in which the
product was created or the response articulated." Her definition reflects
Aristotle's comment in the *Rhetoric* that he can't tell how to make good art; he can
only describe the art that observers over the ages have agreed was good.

> "'Tis wise to learn;
> 'tis godlike to create!"
>
> **John Godfrey Saxe**

Application

The merely novel is often represented to us as being creative. Novelty by itself,
however, is an insufficient basis on which to judge something to be creative.
Novelty without relevance falls somewhere between whimsy and the psychotic.
Novelty without spontaneity is tiresomely formulaic—it leads viewers to
respond, "I could have done that myself," for example, after seeing a painting
with a repeating pattern of colors and squares or hearing a twelve-tone-row
composition. The classic example of nonspontaneous art is "painting by the numbers." Stress the necessity for all three elements, either in your own creative
processes or in those of your students, co-workers, and children.

Topic 21.2 The psychology of the creative personality

Amabile (1983) identifies three components of creativity in individuals: *domain-relevant skills, creativity-relevant skills,* and *task motivation.* These three components must all be present for an individual to be fully creative.

To have *domain-relevant skills,* the individual must possess the knowledge, technical skills, and special talents peculiar to the domain in which he or she wishes to be creative. Without this, it may be easy to create novel and spontaneous contributions, but relevance will be, at best, random. The presence of these skills is dependent on innate logical ability and perceptual-motor skills, as well as on formal and informal education. Amabile defines a talent as a skill in which an individual has an apparently natural ability. Thus, someone can play the piano technically well but have no talent for it, leaving listeners less than impressed. Or a person can master the technical side of a welding process, but, not having talent for it, be frustratingly error-prone. This definition of talent fits well with Gardner's definition of the six domains of intelligence summarized in Topic 12.2.

Amabile identifies *creativity-relevant skills* in three different areas:

1 *Cognitive style:* This includes the ability and willingness to break perceptual sets (as opposed to functional fixedness), be comfortable with complexity, hold options open and not push for closure, suspend judgment rather than reacting to things as good or bad, be comfortable with wider categories, develop an accurate memory, abandon or suspend performance scripts, and see things differently from others.

2 *Knowledge of heuristics:* Heuristics are insightful tips for coming up with new ideas (for a more complete treatment of heuristics, see Topic 23.4). Probably the most famous heuristic comes out of the NLP literature (see Topic 15.4): "If what you're doing is not working, try something different." This is based on the axiom, "If you always do what you've always done, you'll always get what you've always gotten." A dated but highly effective introduction to heuristics is Zuce Kogan's *Essentials in Problem Solving* (1956). Also full of insightful tips are Adams (1980), Bandler and Grinder (1982), de Bono (1967), Fisher (1981), P. Goldberg (1983), and von Oech (1983).

3 *Work style:* A positive work style consists of the ability to sustain long periods of concentration, the ability to abandon nonproductive approaches, persistence during difficulty, a high energy level, and a willingness to work hard.

Creating new mental paths

Amabile finds that two prerequisites determine our level of performance in these three areas of creativity-relevant skills: experience and personality traits. Experience in generating ideas in and out of the classroom contributes heavily to a person's creativity. You can't do it unless you've done it! Among the personality traits critical to creativity-relevant skills are:

- Self-discipline
- Delay of gratification
- Perseverance
- Independent judgment
- Tolerance for ambiguity
- Autonomy
- Absence of sex-role stereotyping
- Internal locus of control
- Willingness to take risks
- Ability to be a self-starter
- Absence of conformity to social pressure

Amabile has found that the creative personality must also have *task motivation,* or a positive attitude toward the task—that is, he or she must want to do it. Unwillingness to do a task results in measurably lower creativity, using the parameters of novelty, relevance, and spontaneity. In addition, research has conclusively demonstrated that *internal motivation* (see Topic 15.1) is a prerequisite for creative behavior. Internal motivation (doing something because we want to) produces greater novelty, domain relevance, and spontaneity than external motivation (doing something because a boss, spouse, or teacher wants us to). If we perceive that we are doing something because we want to, even if another person wants it too, then creativity is enhanced. The highest creativity occurs when we discover the need for a creative response ourselves and choose to contribute independently of any possible external constraints. When external constraints (e.g., deadlines, rewards, or punishers) are imposed on a personally desirable task, creativity can still flourish if we are able to cognitively minimize those constraints. When we are unable to forget about them, creativity suffers.

The one exception to this negative effect of external motivation is a situation in which the guidelines for success are carefully spelled out. For example, a school art contest or a sales-force contest with specific rules and guidelines can generate creative behavior. The guidelines can free us to be spontaneous and novel within a clearly defined playing field. Apparently, the rules have the effect of increasing both the perceived fairness of the contest and our perceived chances of winning.

Internal motivation is a prerequisite for creative behavior.

The psychobiology of creativity

Applications

1   When you expect others to be creative, take the time to develop their buy-in. Negotiate with them until you perceive that they want to do the task and feel in control of the process. Avoid setting goals and methods *for* others if you expect creative behavior—set them *with* others, in joint discussions and mutual agreements. Setting goals unilaterally for others typically breeds fears and resentments that stifle creativity.

2   In looking for creative talent, value technical expertise (domain-relevant skills) as much as the more creative behaviors.

3   In looking for creative talent, look for indications that the individual is a self-starter who can work without close supervision.

4   Reward creativity *after* the fact rather than *before*. Working for a reward generally stifles creativity, whereas unexpected rewards encourage further creativity. On the other hand, always rewarding creativity after the fact will stifle creativity in the long run, because the reward becomes expected. Usually, it is best to just be comfortable accepting creative people's own satisfaction with their contribution. Many creative people report discomfort, even resentment, when a to-do is made over their contribution. It is the creative process itself that is rewarding, and they are eager to return to it.

> Many creative people report discomfort, even resentment, when a to-do is made over their contribution.

5   When commissioning a problem-solving team, ensure that they understand their goal and have management support to implement their solution. If their solution has limits (e.g., the project can't cost over ten thousand dollars), state them up front. (contributed by Rick Bradley)

Topic 21.3 The biology of the creative personality

Whatever finally comes to be established as the biological basis of creativity, it will certainly be a composite of three of the Big Five personality factors (see Chapter Ten): the Explorer, Challenger, and Flexible. Although the precise biological foundation has not been finally defined, many elements of that foundation have been tentatively identified. Exploring (high in the Openness trait) is probably related to higher acetylcholine, calpain, and C-kinase levels, with the key biological difference between Exploring and Preserving lying in the degree of complexity of the synaptic connections. Inasmuch as the corpus callosum is thicker in right-brain-dominant people, we will probably find it thicker in creative minds. The Challenger trait will

Creating new mental paths

probably be found to have as its basis high serotonin and low endorphin levels. In fact, many creative personalities (see Amabile, 1983) report the need to do something special to calm down for work, such as meditation or music. This suggests less active opioid receptors than the norm. Finally, the Flexible trait is related to lower testosterone and higher dopamine levels (Geen, Beatty, & Arkin, 1984).

On a somewhat different molecular plane, creativity can be described as a function of theta waves, which occur somewhere between sleep and alertness (Goleman, Kaufman, & Ray, 1992). Thomas Edison built this fact into his Menlo Park invention setting in the following manner: he would sit in a comfortable chair, holding heavy metal balls draped over the side of the chair in each hand and poised directly above two pans positioned on either side of the chair. He would attempt to doze, until he was startled into waking by the sound of the balls landing in the pans. At this moment, he reports, he had his best creative insights. In this brain state, we relinquish control of our mental processes. On the continuum from tight mental self-control to the loss of control we experience in sleep, creativity occurs toward the sleep end of the continuum.

Applications

1   The diet to increase creativity is no different from the diet recommended for overall good health (see Appendix B). A word of warning, however: consumption of simple carbohydrates and fats tends to interfere with creative activity by reducing arousal, while consumption of proteins and complex carbohydrates, unless it is excessive, has no apparent negative impact on arousal.

2   Creative episodes are most productive when they are preceded by some form of meditation or aerobic exertion (see Topic 14.2). Richard Restak (1991) calls this attentional—as opposed to intentional—mental space.

3   Plan a physical group activity (team building, an icebreaker, an Outward Bound type of initiative) prior to a brainstorming session; see Fluegelman (1976) for ideas. (contributed by Rick Bradley)

4   More introverted people will probably be at their creative best in the mornings, while more extraverted people will probably be at their creative best in the evenings (see the discussion of extraversion, arousal, and caffeine in Topic 6.2).

5   When you are trying hard to come up with a new idea and are feeling frustrated by it, try letting go of your control by walking, dozing, or relaxing in other ways.

6 Look for reports of research by Candace Pert of Johns Hopkins University in Baltimore, who reportedly is developing a "creativity pill."

Topic 21.4 The four stages of the creative process

Graham Wallas (1926) identified four phases of the creative process, which have lasted to the present day. Using the common language of more recent writers, I would summarize them as follows:

1 *Preparation:* Doing research, gathering facts, assembling people or materials—whatever is needed to have all domain-specific information at our disposal before the creative act. Chick Thompson (1992) reports that Yoshiro NakaMats, professional Japanese inventor and holder of 2,300 patents, sees memory work as the basis of the freedom necessary for creativity.

2 *Incubation:* Allowing the collected materials to gestate, to be assimilated into our preexisting schemas, and to interplay unconsciously or consciously in our minds without the stress of having to produce. Incubation can be as short as a fifteen-minute break or as long as a lifetime. It asks us to let go of the data long enough to gain some perspective. A commonly reported form of incubation is dreaming. Elias Howe dreamed of primitives with spears that had eyes at the end, which led to the invention of the sewing machine; Friedrich August Kekulé's dream of snakes biting their own tails led to the discovery of the ring structure of the benzene molecule.

3 *Inspiration:* The actual "Aha!" or "Eureka!" moment when preparation and incubation produce inspiration. This stage has also been called illumination and discovery. It can take the form of focusing our attention on coming up with a solution, through the sheer force of our will, or it can consist of merely participating in a structured idea-generating session such as brainstorming.

4 *Evaluation:* The attempt to verify that the proposed solution is domain-relevant and logically fits the requirement of the original need or stimulus. It is also called confirmation. The question asked is "Will it work?"

Amabile integrates these four stages of the creative process into a flowchart that includes the three components of creativity: task motivation (incubation), domain relevance (preparation and evaluation), and creativity skills (inspiration). That flowchart is shown in Figure 21.1.

Creating new mental paths

Chick Thompson (1992, pp. xi–xviii) tells the story of Yoshiro NakaMats and his three-phase philosophy of creativity:

1   *Suji* (knowledge), similar to Wallas's preparation step

2   *Pika* (inspiration), similar to the incubation and illumination steps combined

3   *Iki* (practicality), similar to the evaluation step

Figure 21.1

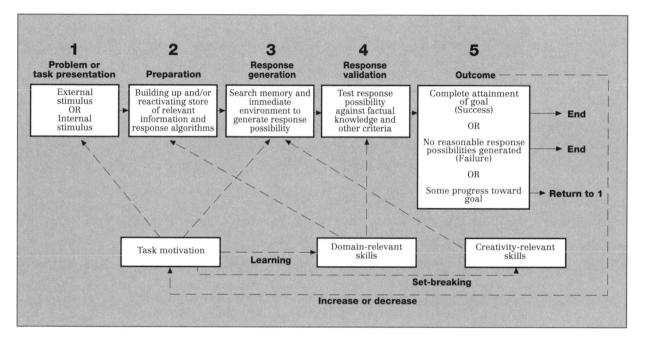

Thompson describes this process as "Ready, Fire, Aim." NakaMats has a static room consisting only of natural materials (plants, natural fibers, and wood, but no plastic) and a dynamic room with music, video, and other media for stimulation. After spending *pika* time in these two rooms, he goes for a swim, during which he expects to have his inspiration, much like Thomas Edison's ball-in-the-pan method (see Topic 21.3).

Applications

1   When you expect yourself or someone else to come up with a creative contribution, be sure to allow adequate time for preparation and incubation. Ask "What information or material is needed before action can be taken?"

2   Always take a break between preparing for your creative act and actually trying to execute it. There's good scientific evidence for sleeping on it!

The componential framework of creativity. The solid lines indicate the sequence of events of the creative process, while the dotted lines indicate where each of the three components of creativity have their greatest impact on the process. From *The Social Psychology of Creativity* by T. M. Amabile, 1983, New York: Springer-Verlag. Reprinted by permission of Springer-Verlag.

3   Many structured exercises are available to assist in the process of idea generation. One element they have in common is that they find a way to hold judgment in abeyance until all contributions are on the table for consideration. These exercises are based on research that shows evaluative activity to be stressful, thus activating the limbic system (see Chapter Two). When the limbic system is activated, the cerebral cortex is significantly shut down, inhibiting creative production. Two of the more common exercises are brainstorming (excellent for extraverts) and brainwriting (excellent for introverts), both of which are included as Appendixes H and I.

4   Identify your places of greatest inspirational moments and keep paper and pencil in each location ready for quick recording. For me, these locations are the bathroom, car, and bedroom.

Topic 21.5 Creativity and madness

Throughout history, writers have linked creativity and mental derangement. Consider:

> "[Persons] outstanding in philosophy, poetry,
> and the arts are melancholic."
> **Aristotle**

> "Great wits are sure to madness near allied,
> And thin partitions do their bounds divide."
> **John Dryden**

> "The lunatic, the lover, and the poet,
> Are of imagination all compact."
> **William Shakespeare**

Ruth Richards, in the April 1992 *Harvard Health Letter,* reviews studies that show a high incidence of mood disorders among more creative personalities. There is growing evidence that creative outlets in and of themselves have a therapeutic benefit for those with mood disorders.

Applications
1   Encourage creative responsibilities for those with bothersome mood swings.

2   Do not insist that creative personalities have perfect mood control.

Suggested readings on creativity

Amabile, T. M. (1983). *The Social Psychology of Creativity.* New York:
  Springer-Verlag.

Boden, M. A. (1990). *The Creative Mind: Myths and Mechanisms.* New York:
  Basic Books.

Csikszentmihalyi, M. (1990). *Flow: The Psychology of Optimal Experience.*
  New York: HarperCollins.

Goleman, D., Kaufman, P., & Ray, M. (1992). *The Creative Spirit.*
  New York: Dutton.

Koestler, A. (1964). *The Act of Creation.* New York: Macmillan.

Thompson, C. (1992). *What a Great Idea! The Key Steps Creative
  People Take.* New York: HarperCollins.

22

Getting the creative juices to flow:

The previous chapter was concerned with the definition of creativity. This chapter will attend to how it may be measured and developed.

Topic 22.1 Assessing for creativity

Amabile (1983) reviews the various personality, biographical, and behavioral inventories that have purported to measure aspects of creativity. Most, in effect, measure aspects of only one component, creativity-relevant skills; for the most part, they do not measure either domain-relevant skills or task motivation (see Chapter Twenty-One for definitions).

Applications

1   The *NEO Five Factor Inventory* and *NEO-PI-R,* described in Topics 10.1 and 10.2, can give as good a profile of the personality traits relevant to creativity as any other inventory. Most multifactor personality tests today have "creativity" scores that are derived from scores on the individual scales related to creativity.

2   Global Creativity Corporation (P.O. Box 294, Mill Valley, CA 94942, 415-331-4823) has developed the *Innovation Styles Profile,* a brief, twenty-eight-question questionnaire that yields a descriptive profile of how the respondent

Removing obstacles to creativity

might typically approach the creative act. The same information could be derived from a multifactor inventory, but if all you want to do is measure creativity styles, this is an effective instrument. Other brief instruments are included in many of the books written about creativity, such as Fisher's "Test Your Intuitive Quotient" in his book, *Intuition* (1981).

3 If you want to measure creative behaviors (the tests in Applications 1 and 2 only measure traits), then you must turn to the *Torrance Tests of Creative Thinking* (also called the *Minnesota Tests of Creative Thinking*), developed by E. Paul Torrance (1974).

4 Martin Seligman (see the discussion of his learned-optimism theory of motivation in Topic 13.1) has developed the *Seligman Attributional Style Questionnaire* (1984), which, in my judgment, is the best instrument available for measuring extrinsic and intrinsic motivation. Another version of the test is available in his book, *Learned Optimism* (1991).

5 I know of no one test that purports to measure completely all three components of creativity as Amabile has described them. I suggest that you review the specific facets of the three components listed in Topic 21.2 (or in Amabile,

> "One must *be* something to be able to *do* something."
>
> **Johann Wolfgang von Goethe**

1983) in order to identify which of them are most relevant to your measurement problem. Then piece together a testing protocol to measure those facets.

Topic 22.2 General principles for developing creativity

The presence of creativity in individuals will, of course, be founded on the development of their *domain-relevant skills, creativity-relevant skills,* and *task motivation.* The methods for developing domain-relevant skills are well known: schoolwork, reading, professional associations, mentoring, training classes, and coaching and counseling. The material in Chapters Eighteen through Twenty describes how these methods can be most effective. The methods for developing intrinsic motivation are also covered in some detail in Topics 15.1 and 15.2.

Amabile (1983, pp. 161–164) reports several principles concerning the development of creativity in young children, which I summarize below:

- Ability grouping benefits higher-ability students only.
- Parents' and teachers' expectations significantly determine creativity (see Topic 15.3 for Rosenthal's work on the self-fulfilling prophecy).
- Teachers tend to wrongly perceive boys as having the greatest variability in creativity—that is, they see them as having both the most and the least creativity, with girls seen as average. If you are a teacher, beware of this tendency!
- More informal classrooms generate more creativity.

At the university level, Amabile (p. 164) identifies the differences between professors who are successful in facilitating creativity and those who inhibit it. I summarize her discussion as follows:

Facilitating professors	Inhibiting professors
See students as individuals	Discourage students' ideas
Encourage independence	Are insecure
Model creative behavior	Have low energy
Spend time with students outside class	Emphasize rote learning
Expect excellence of students	Are dogmatic
Maintain enthusiasm for the subject and learning	Are not up-to-date
	Have narrow interests
Accept students as equals	Are unavailable outside the classroom
Recognize student competence	
Are interesting lecturers	
Are good one-on-one	

Creating new mental paths

Amabile also identifies several guidelines (pp. 166–167) for establishing an environment in the workplace that results in increased creativity. I summarize them as follows:

■ Give employees the responsibility for initiating new activities.

■ Empower employees to hire assistants (allow a budget for doing the less creative work, such as number crunching or assembly).

■ Provide freedom from administrative interference.

■ Provide job security.

Combine the following Applications with the suggestions in Chapters Eighteen through Twenty to develop creative behavior.

Applications

1 Train individuals and teams in techniques for suspending judgment, such as brainstorming (see Appendix H) and brainwriting (see Appendix I).

2 Encourage people to use heuristic techniques, such as those in Adams (1980), Bandler and Grinder (1982), de Bono (1967), Fisher (1981), P. Goldberg (1983), Kogan (1956), Senge (1990), and von Oech (1983).

3 Introduce the works of writers who deal in paradox and perceptual flexibility, such as Escher (1983), Falletta (1983), M. Gardner (1979), Hofstadter (1979), Korzybski (1948), Polya (1971), Poundstone (1988), and Zdenek (1985). These are only a few of many such works, but they represent an excellent start. Digesting these volumes will result in an impatience with conventional assumptions and a greater tolerance for ambiguity.

Constant disruption is the enemy of creativity.

4 Allow yourself and others long periods of uninterrupted concentration. Constant disruption is the enemy of creativity. Quality circles are an attempt to provide workers with periods of concentration so that they can creatively solve nagging problems in the workplace.

5 Develop the habit of bringing your assumptions to the surface and questioning them. Three excellent readings in this area are Kuhn (1970); Senge (1990); and Watzlawick, Weakland, and Fisch (1974).

6 Develop the practice of exploring how two or more ideas or objects can be combined to produce new ideas or objects. Koestler (1964) calls this bisociation. Some examples of bisociation from the history of invention are listed in Table 22.1.

Table 22.1 Examples of bisociation

Person	Idea A	Idea B	Result of bisociation
Archimedes	How to measure gold content of Tyro's crown	Overflowing bathtub	Displacement theory
Pythagoras	Musical pitches	Blacksmith forging iron rod	Discovery of relation of length to pitch in music
Alexander Fleming	Mucus from nose falls into culture	Spore flies in window and lands in culture dish	Penicillin
Blaise Pascal	Mathematics	Gambling	Probability theory
Friedrich August Kekulé	Chemistry	Dream of snakes swallowing each others' tails	Benzene ring
Johannes Gutenberg	Grape press	Coin stamp	Printing press

7   Build the habit of playing creative games such as charades, Facts 'n' Five, or Pictionary—ask at your library, bookstore, or game store for help in identifying more such games and learning how to play them. There are many books filled with creative games and exercises for kids.

8   Many books provide specific methods for lessening dependence on so-called left-brain activity. Chick Thompson (1992) describes techniques that are helpful for developing creativity in a wide range of business and personal settings. Betty Edwards (1989) provides hints on right-brained approaches to learning to draw.

9   Get on the mailing list of The Global Intuition Network. Write:

> *Dr. Weston H. Agor*
> *Global Intuition Network*
> *P.O. Box 614*
> *University of Texas at El Paso*
> *El Paso, TX 79968-0614*

Topic 22.3   Obstacles to creativity

Over the years, I have maintained a list of what I call obstacles to creative behavior, which I have used with various workshop populations. Each obstacle can be evaluated in many ways. For example, *fear* is a known obstacle to creativity. But fear can emanate from any one of many sources: ourselves, our co-workers, our spouse, our boss, the corporate culture, the neighborhood, and more. To deal with fear as an obstacle, we must first be clear as to its source. Following are specific obstacles to creativity:

- *A critical nature:* An overly critical nature serves as an inhibitor of creativity. Goleman, Kaufman, and Ray (1992) call this psychosclerosis, or hardening of the attitudes. It is especially active during the preparation phase and is often referred to as the voice of judgment or functional fixedness.

- *Personality type:* Creativity is minimized among the Preserver ("Stick with what works"), Adapter ("Don't rock the boat"), and Focused ("We need it yesterday") personality types. See Chapter Ten for information on these personality types.

- *Poor diet:* A normal healthy diet is imperative (see Topic 5.1 and Appendix B), with special caution against excessive simple carbohydrates and fats and insufficient protein and complex carbohydrates.

- *Poor physical condition:* While you don't have to be a marathoner to be creative, you must be sufficiently active and healthy to maintain the alertness necessary for creativity.

- *Fear:* Fear activates the limbic system and proportionally shuts down the cerebral cortex, the center of creative activity. It is often accompanied by lack of faith in one's ability.

- *Unproductive conflict style:* Negotiators who look for win-win situations breed more creativity than Adapters, Challengers, or Preservers (see Chapter Ten).

- *Poor group health:* If the team with which you are involved (a work group, your family, etc.) is functioning poorly, your creativity and that of the team will be inhibited.

- *A highly developed superego:* An overly active conscience (full of don't's) inhibits creativity.

- *Left-hemisphere dominance:* All logic and no play makes Jo a dull person.

- *A conservative culture:* If your organization's culture is characterized by celebrating the status quo, creativity is inhibited.

- *Inappropriate questioning skills:* Closed-ended (yes-no) questions inhibit creativity, while open-ended questions encourage creativity.

- *Perceptual fixedness:* If you continue to see what you've always seen, you'll continue to get what you've always gotten. Perceptual fixedness can only be helped by extraordinarily close and precise observation—by seeing what is there, not what you expect to be there.

Getting the creative juices to flow

- *Unchanging perspective:* If you continue to look at the mountain from the same side, you'll always see the same mountain.
- *Need for power and control:* Control freaks, those who always must be right ("My way or the highway"), are the ultimate obstacle to creativity, both for others and for themselves.
- *Pessimism:* Seligman (see Topic 13.1) has demonstrated conclusively that personal, pervasive, and permanent pessimism results in less productivity, including creative productivity.
- *Time pressures:* Amabile warns that unnecessary time constraints are one of the biggest killers of creativity. This is a special problem when you're trying to encourage creativity during a brief period of time during a school day.
- *Over- or underachievement:* Mihalyi Csikszentmihalyi (1990), a psychologist at the University of Chicago, defines flow as that magical quality of total absorption in the task at hand that occurs when our skill level matches the task. When our skills are deficient for the task, we become frustrated by our attempt to overachieve. When our skills are excessive for the task, we become bored by our attempt to underachieve.

Application

Identify the obstacles to creativity in your life. Develop a plan to eliminate or minimize these obstacles in areas where you wish to be more creative.

Suggested readings on developing creativity

Amabile, T. M. (1983). *The Social Psychology of Creativity.* New York: Springer-Verlag.

Csikszentmihalyi, M. (1990). *Flow: The Psychology of Optimal Experience.* New York: HarperCollins.

de Bono, E. (1967). *New Think.* New York: Basic Books.

Goleman, D., Kaufman, P., & Ray, M. (1992). *The Creative Spirit.* New York: Dutton.

Koestler, A. (1964). *The Act of Creation.* New York: Macmillan.

Seligman, M.E.P. (1991). *Learned Optimism.* New York: Knopf.

Thompson, C. (1992). *What a Great Idea! The Key Steps Creative People Take.* New York: HarperCollins.

Torrance, E. P. (1974). *Torrance Tests of Creative Thinking.* Bensenville, IL: Scholastic Testing Service.

23

Creative leverage: A guide to prob

The word problem *comes from the Greek* pro-, *or "forward," and* ballein, *"to throw or drive,"* and means something thrown forward, as when we put something on the table for inspection. A question asked, a diseased animal being inspected, and an unidentified fingerprint at a crime scene all have been "thrown forward," or singled out from the ordinary for our inspection and consideration. *Webster's New World Dictionary* defines a problem as "anything requiring the doing of something." In other words, when you have a problem, you can't just keep doing business as usual. You must do something that is not normally a part of your routine—special attention is required.

Before plunging into the details of problem-solving styles, definitions, and techniques, I want to make one point perfectly clear: *the best problem solver is an expert in the subject involved.* An expert might be an engineer, a consultant, a professor, a competitor, or even someone who knows the task intimately—the worker. No technique is as good as an expert. So, depending upon the seriousness of the problem, *consult an expert before trying one of these techniques.* For example, if you've got a cold, treat yourself, but if the symptoms are more complex, consult an expert—your doctor. The techniques mentioned in this chapter are intended to serve either (1) when relevant expertise is unavailable or (2) when the experts have been stumped. I was once called in to help solve a problem that had stumped the experts for about nine months. A $500,000 machine had been failing

Creating new mental paths

lem-solving breakthroughs

in the field 50 percent of the time. By applying the right technique (root-cause analysis, described by Plunkett & Hale, 1982), I led a group of ten experts to find the cause of the problem in six hours.

Topic 23.1 Styles for approaching problems

In the last ten years, attempts to define problem-solving styles have flourished. These styles are all based on various combinations of personality traits (see the Big Five traits discussed in Chapter Ten). The literature on problem-solving styles is extensive, and I will not treat it here. Suffice it to say that all the attempts at defining styles are based on extreme scores on the Big Five. Four of the ten possible Big Five extreme scores appear to be most commonly associated with problem-solving style:

- *Preserver:* The Preserver aims at a quick solution based on tried-and-true principles.
- *Explorer:* The Explorer aims at an innovative solution based on a new insight.
- *Challenger:* The Challenger aims at the truth based on unrelenting logic.
- *Adapter:* The Adapter aims at harmony and buy-in through building consensus.

Applications

1 When faced with a problem of some magnitude, consider which style is most relevant to understanding and solving it. For many complex problems, a combination of all styles is particularly powerful.

2 To assess your own style and the styles of those around you, use the worksheet in Appendix D to find the Big-Five trait descriptors most typical of you and yours, or you might contact the publisher of the tests and models identified in Table 23.1.

Table 23.1 Appropriate techniques for different types of problems

Kind of problem	Appropriate technique	Where to learn technique
Problem with unknown cause	Root-cause analysis	Education Research (1987) Kepner & Tregoe (1981) Plunkett & Hale (1982)
Problem with known cause or cause irrelevant	Creative problem solving (assorted varieties)	Bransford & Stein (1984) Hayes (1989) Nadler & Hibino (1990) Nierenberg (1985) Prince (1970) Rickards (1974)
Decision among solutions with certain outcomes	Matrix-decision analysis	Education Research (1988) Hayes (1989) Kepner & Tregoe (1981) Moody (1983) Plunkett & Hale (1982)
Decision among solutions with uncertain outcomes	The decision tree (based on probability theory)	Behn & Vaupel (1982) Hayes (1989) McGuire & Radner (1972) McNamee & Celona (1987) Moody (1983)
A jumbled list	The analytic-hierarchy process (also called scaled comparison)	Moody (1983) Saaty (1982)
Adversarial problem solving	Explanatory coherence	Thagard (1992)

Creating new mental paths

3   When you are assembling teams to solve problems, encourage diversity—in personality, styles, expertise, departmental experience, and so on. (contributed by Rick Bradley)

4   The diversity recommended in Application 3 may also help with general acceptance of the team's solution to the problem afterward. (contributed by Jane Howard)

Topic 23.2 Types of problems

Problems lead, hopefully, to solutions. In light of that, I think in terms of two types of problems:

1   Problems for which the possible solutions are unknown
2   Problems for which the solutions are known, but the best solution
      is not obvious.

The goal in solving the first type of problem is to generate ideas, whereas the goal in solving the second type is to make a decision.

Problems where the solution is unknown can be further subdivided into two categories:

1   The cause of the problem is unknown and must be discovered.
2   The cause of the problem is known, or is unknown and irrelevant.

An example of the first would be a blown fuse (or tripped circuit breaker). If you do not discover the cause of the electrical overload, you risk fire (at most) or the unavailability of that electrical circuit (at least). An example of the second would be having a flat tire in the desert with no jack available. The cause of the flat is most likely irrelevant; you just need some good ideas.

Problems where the best solution is not obvious can be subdivided into three categories. Although these situations are frequently referred to (erroneously, I think) as problems, they are more aptly called decisions. The verb *decide* comes from the Latin *de-* ("off") and *caedere* ("to cut"), or "to cut off." In other words, decision time is the time to cut off debate and affirm the solution to the problem at hand. In its purest form, then, a problem is a mess without a solution, and a decision situation is a mess with two or more possible solutions. The three classes of solution are:

1   Solutions with certain outcomes
2   Solutions with uncertain outcomes
3   Solutions in need of being prioritized

An example of the first is deciding which home to buy—the outcomes are certain, in the sense that their features are plain to the eye. An example of the second is whether or not to risk major surgery—the outcomes are unknown, although to some degree they are predictable. An example of the third is having a list of twenty projects that need to be undertaken, yet having a budget for only a few of them.

Applications

1   When you commit to trying to solve a problem, first determine what kind of problem it is. Once you know that, you will know what your objective is. This information is summarized in Table 23.2.

Table 23.2 Kinds of problems and the nature of their solutions

Kind of problem	Nature of appropriate problem-solving activity
Problem with unknown cause	Finding the cause
Problem with known cause or cause irrelevant	Generating ideas that could fix the problem
Decision among solutions with certain outcomes	Deciding on one best solution
Decision among solutions with uncertain outcomes	Deciding which solution has highest probability of success
A jumbled list	Determining priority order

2   Often, it is not enough to figure out what kind of problem you are facing—you must also determine an appropriate technique to use in solving that problem. Refer to Table 23.1 for the names of possible techniques to use in solving each kind of problem and resources for learning these techniques.

Topic 23.3 Describing a problem

The first step in any problem-solving process is taking time to describe the problem as presented. All too often, in the American "pioneer" spirit, we concentrate on the quick fix and take pride in coming up with solutions immediately upon discovering a problem. But research continues to support the thesis that time taken to plan at the front end is inversely proportional to the time required for execution.

In other words, the effectiveness of problem solving is enhanced by the time taken to understand and gain consensus about the problem at the front end.

The following Applications present five of the more popular and effective techniques for describing problems.

Applications

1 *Mind mapping* (see Figure 23.1) is a technique attributed to Tony Buzan (1991). You start by writing down the main problem you're trying to describe in the middle of the page. Circle that problem, then think of everything that might be related to the problem, jotting down words and phrases around the page, linking smaller concepts to bigger concepts. This is a free-form method of outlining that is modeled on the image we have of neural networks in the brain.

2 The *Ishikawa* or *fishbone diagram*, also known as the cause-and-effect diagram, has become popular in world business as part of the Total Quality Revolution. A simple treatment of it is available in Walton (1986); see also Gitlow, Gitlow, Oppenheim, and Oppenheim (1989). The fishbone chart is a cross between traditional outlining and mind mapping—it is not as logically restrictive as outlining and not as free-form as mind mapping. The chart assumes that any given problem will have about four major areas (commonly, but not always, identified as people, methods, machinery, and materials). These four areas become the fins of a fishbone. Ideas related to the big ideas become bones on the fins (see Figure 23.2).

3 The *Pareto chart* is also known as the Eighty-Twenty Rule, or the law of the mighty few. Simply put, it is a frequency distribution of problems that enables you to identify the mighty few (usually about 20 percent of your problems) that, if fixed, could give you the maximum payoff (i.e., reduce your problems by about 80 percent). Other common phrasings of the Pareto principle are: Which 20 percent of your sales prospects could get you 80 percent of your sales goals? Which 20 percent of your quality problems account for 80 percent of your cost variances?

4 The *actual versus ideal* comparison, also referred to as *current state versus desired state*, *is versus should*, and *performance versus standard*, has become the most common way of beginning a problem-solving process. Simply put, first list all the details associated with the current problem (the *actual* problem situation). Second, describe what the situation would look like (sound like, smell like, etc.) if the problem were fixed (the *ideal*). This contrast between actual and ideal

Figures 23.1 (left)
and 23.2 (right)

provides the focus for generating ideas that might solve the problem, allowing you to move from the actual to the ideal state.

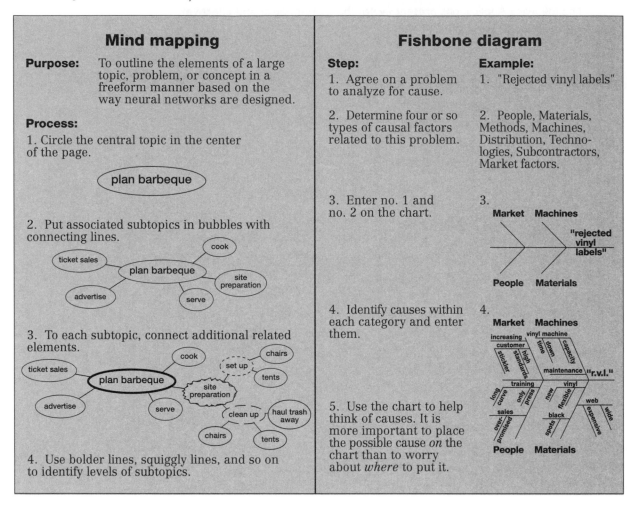

Mind mapping

Purpose: To outline the elements of a large topic, problem, or concept in a freeform manner based on the way neural networks are designed.

Process:

1. Circle the central topic in the center of the page.

2. Put associated subtopics in bubbles with connecting lines.

3. To each subtopic, connect additional related elements.

4. Use bolder lines, squiggly lines, and so on to identify levels of subtopics.

Fishbone diagram

Step:

1. Agree on a problem to analyze for cause.

2. Determine four or so types of causal factors related to this problem.

3. Enter no. 1 and no. 2 on the chart.

4. Identify causes within each category and enter them.

5. Use the chart to help think of causes. It is more important to place the possible cause *on* the chart than to worry about *where* to put it.

Example:

1. "Rejected vinyl labels"

2. People, Materials, Methods, Machines, Distribution, Technologies, Subcontractors, Market factors.

5 *CEDAC* was developed by Productivity Design, Inc., in Boston. It is a variation on the Ishikawa diagram (see Application 2 above) in which cards or self-sticking notes are used for greater ease of movement.

For information, contact:

Nate Apkon, President
Productivity Design, Inc.
648 Beacon Street, Sixth Floor
Boston, MA 02215
617-262-1717

Creating new mental paths

Topic 23.4 Solutions: Algorithms and heuristics

Research on human attention throughout the years has demonstrated strongly that we cannot concentrate on more than one focal point at a time. This truth can be built into our approach to problem solving if we focus on one aspect of the problem at a time. Algorithmic problem-solving methods naturally do this by dividing problem solving into steps.

Many will argue that the practice of proceeding one step at a time kills creativity. For these people, heuristic problem-solving methods approach a problem more globally. For example, "If pushing doesn't work, try pulling" is a classic heuristic approach to problem solving. It encourages a big-picture approach in which we think about all aspects of the problem at once. This works best for experts who are intimately familiar with the technical details of the problem and can draw on extensive mental networks.

The word *heuristic* comes from the Greek *heuriskein,* meaning "to find or discover"; Archimedes supposedly said "Eureka!" or "I found it!" when he discovered the specific-gravity method for determining the purity of gold. When heuristic methods fail to yield a solution, an algorithmic (stepwise) approach should be tried.

Applications

1   Of the many problem-solving methods identified in Table 23.1, four are particularly noteworthy for their concentration on breaking the problem-solving process down into discrete parts: root-cause analysis, matrix-decision analysis, the decision tree, and the analytic-hierarchy process.

2   The more familiar you are with the details of the problem, the more likely you are to have success with heuristic approaches. Heuristics are really just rules of thumb for approaching problems. Here is an assortment of these rules of thumb:

- To detach something, attach it to something else.
- If you can't remove it, counteract it.
- Find a similar problem. Is its solution applicable?
- Reframe the problem. A different definition can yield new possible solutions.
- Simulate the problem to understand it better.
- Work backward from the actual state to the former ideal state.
- Remove the unnecessary.
- Dream—fantasize a solution assuming that all restrictions have been removed.

Creative leverage

- Simplify by removing some variables.
- Establish subgoals; break the problem into smaller ones.
- List your assumptions and challenge them.
- Study, then incubate.
- Expand, reduce, reverse, substitute, rearrange, regroup, alternate.
- Make overt the covert.
- Try less of the same.
- Try advertising instead of concealing.
- When one way fails, try the opposite.

3 For more heuristic techniques, see Adams (1980, 1986), Bandler and Grinder (1982), de Bono (1967), Fisher (1981), P. Goldberg (1983), Kogan (1956), and Nierenberg (1985). Also, get yourself on the mailing lists of these excellent resources for problem solving:

Mindware (catalog)
1803 Mission Street, Suite 414
Santa Cruz, CA 95060
800-447-0477

Shamrock Press (catalog)
1277 Garnet Avenue
San Diego, CA 92109
619-272-3880

4 When heuristics don't work, try a more algorithmic approach.

Topic 23.5 Games and problem-solving ability

Games are helpful in maintaining flexibility in solving problems.

A wide variety of games, puzzles, and toys come under the heading of brain-teasers, including such items as Rubik's Cube, the tangram, the Tower of Hanoi, Jim Fixx's word-game books, and Martin Gardner's mathematical and logical puzzle books. These games are helpful in maintaining flexibility in approaching problems. People who report that they enjoy and play these games also score higher on problem-solving tests.

Applications

1 Make a habit of giving games and puzzles to your children starting at an early age, with the games becoming gradually more sophisticated.

Creating new mental paths

2   Do not tease adults for being attracted to brainteasers; they are avoiding perceptual fixedness and developing their mental flexibility.

3   If you work in a facility with a waiting area, consider putting out games and puzzles as well as magazines.

4   Encourage the appropriate use of games and puzzles in the workplace.

Topic 23.6 Sleep, relaxation, and problem solving

Often, a problem on your mind interferes with sleep and relaxation. One way to eliminate this bother is to do a mental dump: write down everything in your mind related to the problem or concern. By writing it down, you will rest knowing that the elements will not be forgotten.

Sleep also serves as a good break between the data-collection and solution aspects of problem solving. By collecting all relevant data and then sleeping on it, you allow unconscious forces to develop a pattern, insight, or inspiration relative to the data.

If sleep time is not available, simply engage in a relaxing activity after finishing the preliminary problem solving and before trying to come up with a solution. Patterns will emerge in this gestation period.

Applications

1   Keep writing materials by your bed in case you need to do a mental dump.

2   When you are trying to solve a problem, take a break (sleep, nap, walk, have lunch) before trying to come up with a final solution.

Summary

Problem solving is many things. If I were forced to recommend an overall approach—one that would fit most situations—it would be the following one:

1   *Ask an expert.* Consider carefully who the possible experts are (a worker on the job, a consultant). If no one is available or helpful, then . . .

2   *Decide what kind of problem it is* (see Table 23.2).

3   *Select a method* to use for that kind of problem (see Table 23.1). If you are an expert in the problem's area of expertise, first try a more holistic approach (see the list of heuristic tips in Topic 23.4, Application 2). If heuristics don't work, or if you're not an expert, then try an algorithmic approach.

4   *Evaluate your recommended solution* in light of Sternberg's flexible domain of intelligence (see Topic 12.1). Remember that you can change yourself, the other person, or the situation. If one doesn't work, shift to another venue!

Suggested readings on problem solving

Adams, J. L. (1980). *Conceptual Blockbusting: A Guide to Better Ideas.* (2nd ed.). New York: W. W. Norton.

Adams, J. L. (1986). *The Care and Feeding of Ideas: A Guide to Encouraging Creativity.* Reading, MA: Addison-Wesley.

Anderson, J. R. (1993, January). "Problem Solving and Learning." *American Psychologist, 48*(1), 35–44.

Bandler, R., & Grinder, J. (1982). *ReFraming: Neuro-Linguistic Programming and the Transformation of Meaning.* Moab, UT: Real People Press.

Gitlow, H., Gitlow, S., Oppenheim, A., & Oppenheim, R. (1989). *Tools and Methods for the Improvement of Quality.* Homewood, IL: Irwin.

Hayes, J. R. (1989). *The Complete Problem Solver.* (2nd ed.). Hillsdale, NJ: Lawrence Erlbaum.

Moody, P. E. (1983). *Decision Making: Proven Methods for Better Decisions.* New York: McGraw-Hill.

Plunkett, L. C., & Hale, G. A. (1982). *The Proactive Manager: The Complete Book of Problem Solving and Decision Making.* New York: Wiley.

Part six

The quest for knowledge:

The brain-philosophy connection

The quest for knowledge:

The brain-philosophy connection

How we view the world: Epistem

> "If believers could come to realize there isn't ten cents' worth of difference in their substantive plans, perhaps they might then begin to see the magical part for what it is."
>
> **Michael Gazzaniga,**
> *The Social Brain*

The word epistemology *comes from the Greek* epi- + histanai, *meaning "to stand under."* This strong image suggests the essence of empiricism, which maintains that if the majority of people can agree during their waking hours that something exists, then it does. The more modern derivation of *epistemology,* "to understand," seems weaker to me. The phrase "to stand under" rings of rugged empiricism, a more radical practicality. It suggests the structure that lies at the core of a thing. There it is—therefore we know it.

Epistemology is defined as the study of the origin, nature, methods, and limits of knowledge. The word *knowledge* derives from the Middle English *knowen,* meaning "to know as a fact." It is interesting to note the similarity of "to know" (Old English *cnāwan*) and "to gnaw" (Middle English *gnawen*). We gnaw something until we get to the bone, the core. To gnaw something is to know it. We know by gnawing. We pry until the bare bones stand there before us, and then we accept what we see as knowledge—we *acknowledge* it.

Of all the branches of philosophy, epistemology is the most closely linked to cognitive science, the study of the mind-brain. But how do we come to accept something as knowledge? What are the methods by which we determine what is knowledge? How is knowledge recognized? And how do we distinguish what is knowledge from what is not?

These are some of the questions we will explore in this chapter.

ology and the search for peace

Topic 24.1 Northrop: Health as morality

At one time, all first-year students at Yale were exposed to F.S.C. Northrop's *Logic of the Sciences and the Humanities* (1947). This classic twentieth-century formulation of the structure of knowledge set a high standard for talking about commonality among everything from mathematics to dreams. For a peek into Northrop's structure, look at my summary of his model in Table 24.1.

Table 24.1 Northrop's structure of knowledge

The real world can be known by:

Concepts by postulation (by talking about it) OR	Concepts by intuition (by receiving information through the five senses)
Intellection (imageless and senseless)	Differentiated aesthetic continuum (sensing and aware of contrasts)
Imagination (images without sensing)	Undifferentiated aesthetic continuum (sensing without patterns; mysticism)
Perception (images with sensing)	Concepts of the differentiations (color alone, shape alone, etc.)
Logical intuition (sensations made global)	Field concepts by inspection (differentiation—e.g., clouds —considered inseparable from the context—e.g., the sky)

How does an epistemologist propose to engage in ethical reasoning? I find Northrop's approach intriguing. Essentially, he proposes that our ethical behavior should be an extension of our physical existence. If we can take our own physical existence as a given, and as being good in and of itself, then ethical reasoning depends on the status of our physical existence. Hence, any action or thought that preserves or restores life in its purest form is good, while any action or thought that alters or diminishes life from its purest form is evil. Such an approach emphasizes the human being as a neighbor, with equal responsibility for maximizing the health of self and neighbor, of people and animals, of ambulatory creatures and the Earth itself.

Applications

1   Be a good neighbor.

2   Consider the impact of your actions on the physical and psychological health of whoever or whatever receives the effect of your actions. If you can imagine a groan resulting from an action, consider abandoning it. If you can imagine some form of contentment resulting, proceed. This is very similar to Tolstoy's ethic of love, in which he defined love as any act that enhanced life in its natural form and hate as any act that detracted from it. This led him to vegetarianism and an avoidance of drugs.

3   Try to determine what your senses are telling you (Northrop's concepts by intuition) before deciding on an interpretation (concepts by postulation).

Topic 24.2   Bartlett: Schema as reality

Fredrick Bartlett (1932; see Topic 18.4) sees the schema as the ultimate basis of our personal reality. Hence, our individual knowledge is a collection of schemas. I am aware, as I review my French-language ability in preparation for a trip to Paris, that as an American-born English speaker I have no built-in schema for the French medial consonant construction (*va t'il, y a t'il*); thus it is extremely difficult for me to recognize it in spoken form. In a less technical vein, I was reared with a strong schema for reciprocity, so I feel unsettled until I have returned a good deed and, yes, until someone else has returned my original good deed! My schema "Eat to show mama you love her" has led to a pesky tendency to overeat as an adult.

We tend to see reality through the filtering effect of our schemas.

Applications

1   Know your schemas. Be aware that we tend to see reality through the filtering effect of our schemas. We screen out what doesn't fit. Forming new schemas takes conscious effort.

The quest for knowledge

2   Be aware of others' schemas. Know that their disagreements with you are probably due to conflicting schemas. Peter Senge (1990) calls these schemas "mental models"; he asks us to take the time to identify our assumptions with our significant others at work or home, then use them to make decisions, solve problems, and make plans. By getting these assumptions out into the open, we may be able to pursue the mature approach of selecting the assumptions that seem most effective for the occasion at hand. Maybe your assumption is more appropriate than mine. Maybe we'll find a schema we both possess that allows a win-win situation.

3   Practice Senge's left-hand-column method (Senge, 1990). After a significant interchange with one or more people, try writing out the key statements you made in the right-hand column, labeled "What I Said." In the left-hand column, labeled "What I Was Thinking," enter the thought that lay behind your words. This is a helpful process for checking out your assumptions and paradigms and getting them on the table. Here are a couple of examples:

What I was thinking	What I said
"The bottom may fall out any day."	"Yes, I think we're right on target."
"Courtesy will soften the blow."	"May I take your coat?"

Topic 24.3   Healy: Reality as schema

Jane Healy (1990) reports that excessive television watching by children produces adults who have failed to develop schemas for active engagement with their environment. By viewing a world (television) in which no time or need for reflection (or internal talking) exists, children build only minimal skills for listening and responding. Their responses become formulas based on favorite programs. So if you have a child who often watches soap operas, he or she stands a strong chance of developing the schema of "disappointment leads to crying, which leads to restoration," as opposed to "disappointment leads to thinking through the cause and working toward restoration." Obviously the first schema is part of a fantasy world and will normally lead to frustration in the "real" world.

Applications

1   Withhold all television watching until reading, mathematical, learning, and interpersonal habits are firmly established.

2   Find a way to get children (or, increasingly, adults) who've succumbed to the

Watch television with
your children to
compare your version
of reality with what
television programming
is offering.

"entertain me" syndrome of the TV addict into a long-term, intensive, small-group experience. This could be anything from a volleyball team to a support group.

3 Watch television with your children to compare your version of reality with what television programming is offering. Discuss how you, your children, and the television characters see the world differently and similarly.

Topic 24.4 E-Prime: Language as scapegoat

David Bourland, Jr. (reported in Bois, 1966), argues that the verb *to be* has misled us into the harmful habits of (1) unequivocally absolute statements ("Russia *is* the evil empire") and (2) inflammatorily ambiguous statements ("My way *is* better than yours"). Bourland argues that we should banish the verb *to be* from the language, forcing ourselves to use more descriptive, less judgmental statements. Compare "Thou art a hot number" to "Shall I compare thee to a summer day?" or "He is lazy" to "His breaks average thirty minutes, and he produces 80 percent of his quota." Bourland refers to English without *to be* as E-Prime. He has developed a formula to describe it: $E^I = E - e$, where E is the traditional, intact English language, and e is the verb *to be* with its many inflections.

Applications

1 On official documents such as performance appraisals, contracts, or memos of record, prefer action verbs to the verb *to be*. By eliminating words like *is* and *are* (and, hence, the passive voice and subjunctive mood), your writing will be more descriptive and informative and less blameful and judgmental.

2 When you catch yourself in an argument with someone, try talking in E-Prime. First, it slows you down and leads to more thoughtful language. Second, it eliminates many phrases that tend to alienate and offend people, such as "That's a stupid thing to say" or "You're just plain wrong."

3 Use E-Prime when you are developing course outlines, scripts, speeches, and presentations.

Suggested readings on epistemology

Korzybski, A. (1948). *Science and Sanity: An Introduction to Non-Aristotelian Systems and General Semantics*. (3rd ed.). Lakeville, CT: International Non-Aristotelian Library.

The quest for knowledge

Northrop, F.S.C. (1947). *The Logic of the Sciences and the Humanities.*
    Cleveland, OH: World.
Senge, P. (1990). *The Fifth Discipline.* New York: Doubleday/Currency.

25

Sacred systems and shifting para

This chapter presents several molar approaches to understanding the structure of knowledge. Perhaps one or more of these commonsense approaches will provide you with a comfortable tool for being a nonprovincial citizen of the world!

Topic 25.1 Pirsig: The Twenty-Third Psalm

Robert Pirsig (1974) introduced epistemology to the less academic public in his autobiographical novel, *Zen and the Art of Motorcycle Maintenance*. The motorcycle, and his intimate knowledge of it, served as his primary metaphor for what epistemology is all about—a way to focus on the structure of what is out there, how it works, and what happens when you tinker with it. At one point he moves from the highway to the classroom and peeks at the epistemology of religion. What results is, I think, a profoundly simple formula for helping us see the universal truths that are embedded in the particularity of a specific religion.

The formula is as follows: take a passage from one of the world's religions, identify the unique term it uses for a godhead or messianic figure, and then consistently substitute a value that is important for you personally wherever that religious term appears. As an example, for the Twenty-Third Psalm of the Old Testament, the key religious term is *Lord,* with all its many pronoun and synonym

The quest for knowledge

digms: Everyday epistemology

forms. Learning is an important value for me. If I substitute *learning* for *Lord* (the way a computer does a search-and-replace operation), the Twenty-Third Psalm then reads: "*Learning* is my shepherd; I shall not want. *Learning* maketh me to lie down in green pastures; *learning* leadeth me beside the still waters. *Learning* restoreth my soul. . . . *Learning* preparest a table before me in the presence of mine enemies; *learning* anointest my head with oil; my cup runneth over . . ." This search-and-replace exercise provides personal meaning for me in an otherwise impersonal, general statement. It also provides a meditative moment to explore just how much my value does mean to me. The next time I may substitute the name of my wife: "Jane is my shepherd . . ." Thus we see how, over the years, the formulas of religion have emerged from the collective experience of its practitioners.

> "International government does not mean the end of nations, any more than an orchestra means the end of violins."
>
> **Golda Meir**

Applications

1   Try the search-and-replace exercise yourself. Identify a personal value that you try to follow in your life (loyalty, love, forgiveness, etc.). Pick a passage from each of the world's great religious texts, then read it to yourself while substituting your value words. You will gain a sense of how other religions can be personal for you—how you might, in fact, be able to relate to people who follow those religions. You will also enjoy momentarily enlivening what otherwise tends to read like imageless jargon.

2   Take a favorite religious passage and do the search-and-replace exercise. Then try rewriting the passage based on this new and personal reading of it.

3   When a conversation with someone else becomes difficult, hostile, adversarial, or otherwise bogged down, become aware of the key words you both are using. Then try substituting words or concepts that have more potential mutual acceptance.

Topic 25.2 Stevens: The pineapple

Among poets, perhaps Wallace Stevens is known as having the most epistemological approach. In both his poetry and his essays, he celebrates the mind as the maker of meaning. His most extended treatment of this subject is "The Man with the Blue Guitar" (1967), in which a complex metaphor finds the man playing the role of the mind, the guitar playing the role of the outside world, and the music made by the man with the guitar playing the role of knowledge. Knowledge is the result of the mind acting on the world, just as music is the result of the person acting on the guitar. A briefer treatment of epistemology than "Blue Guitar" is his "Someone Puts a Pineapple Together," in which he draws out a series of verses, each of which describes a scene that exhibits the structure of a pineapple (Stevens, 1951, p. 86). Here are a few selected lines:

The hut stands by itself beneath the palms.

Out of their bottle the green genii come.

A vine has climbed the other side of the wall.

The sea is spouting upward out of rocks.

The symbol of feasts and of oblivion . . .

White sky, pink sun, trees on a distant peak.

These lozenges are nailed-up lattices.

The owl sits humped. It has a hundred eyes.

Each of these statements represents a different way of looking at the same reality (a pineapple), just as the world's religions are different ways of looking at the world. That is the essence of epistemology—developing an appreciation and understanding of the structure that underlies our language and perceptions.

Applications

1 Develop the habit of mind that looks for similarities of structure among the elements of your environment—the cloud that looks like a boat, the worker's arm movement that resembles the act of wringing a towel dry (this could be a helpful analogy to use in training a new worker), or the patterns implicit in numerical data, such as cyclical dips and rises. Seeing patterns is the first step in learning, just as the child must understand the common structure in all the things that parents and teachers are calling an "R" before being able to use it as an "R."

2 Cut out pictures from magazines that draw attention to the structural similarity among otherwise different objects. Schott Glass Technology, Inc., Duryea, Pennsylvania, placed a wonderful advertisement in the March 21, 1988, issue of *Business Week* (pp. 76–77) in which several crystal glasses are paired with their real-world flower shapes, like tulips and roses. The caption: "Great design does not happen by chance." Pictures like this serve as a reminder to appreciate the underlying sameness throughout nature.

3 Read *Mathematics in Western Culture* (Kline, 1953) for a careful historical treatment of the structures that pervade the natural world.

Topic 25.3 Kuhn: The shifting paradigm

It has become the vogue to talk about paradigm shifts. Thomas Kuhn (1970) started it all in *The Structure of Scientific Revolutions*. In this insightful study of the history of science, he gave the world a new verbal toy to play with. The word *paradigm* comes from the Greek *para*, or "beside," and *deigma*, or "shown." A paradigm is something shown beside the real thing; it is a pattern or model, like a set of drawings that explains the structure underlying specific phenomena. Kuhn gets more specific when he defines paradigms as "universally recognized scientific achievements that for a time provide model problems and solutions to a community of practitioners" (p. viii). New paradigms emerge because of their capacity to solve more problems, especially problems that the old paradigm couldn't solve. As Kuhn writes: "The failure of existing rules . . . is the prelude to the search for new ones" (p. 68). A paradigm shift is generally preceded by a

New paradigms emerge because of their capacity to solve more problems.

proliferation of theories that try to explain what the old paradigm can't. Kuhn traces in some detail the shift from Priestley's phlogiston theory to Lavoisier's oxygen theory, from Newton's ether to Einstein's relativity, from corpuscular theory to wave theory.

Because paradigm shifts generally require major "retooling," the people affected by the potential shift tend to resist strongly. They wish to forestall the expense and learning curve associated with accepting a new paradigm. Retooling is an extravagance, so when it happens, it suggests that a new paradigm has emerged. This perfectly explains the transition from the assembly-line production paradigm, which held strongly around the world through the 1950s, to what now appears to be the Total Quality Management paradigm of the 1990s. Over the last forty years, gurus have proposed a variety of theories to explain what the old production paradigm couldn't. Theories such as Theory X-Y, Theory Z, Statistical Process Control, and DIRTFOOT (Do It Right The First Time) have all vied to replace the time-and-motion studies of the production paradigm in the business world.

Kuhn points out that new paradigms tend to be defined by (1) younger people and/or (2) people who are new to the field. In both cases, the pushers of the new paradigm are not wedded to the conventional ways of doing things. Hence, the Japanese, with a past record of poor quality in manufacturing, have pushed the quality paradigm.

Lance Morrow wrote a feature essay in *Time* magazine entitled "Old Paradigm, New Paradigm" (January 14, 1991, pp. 65–66), in which he listed examples of old and new paradigms. Here are several of his plus several of mine:

Old paradigms	New paradigms
Fidel Castro	Vaclav Havel
Apartheid	F. W. De Klerk and Nelson Mandela
The American Century	The Pacific Rim
Cigarette smoking	Smoke-free spaces
Labor unions	Self-directed work teams
CBS News	Cable News Network
Charisma	Teamwork
Knowledge	Information
Northern Ireland	The new Germany
Letter writing	Faxing
Nationalism	Pluralism
Communism	Democracy

The quest for knowledge

Applications

1   Paradigms are useful frameworks for solving problems. Be open to the possibility that a new paradigm may emerge in your lifetime that will increase your effectiveness. It doesn't matter whether you invent or discover the new paradigm yourself or follow another person's lead—just don't get caught holding on to an old paradigm for loyalty's sake. If a new set of guidelines appears able to answer more questions than the current set, go for it.

2   Paradigms will shift more frequently now and in the future than in the history that Kuhn described. W. Edwards Deming's dictum of continuing improvement is a paradigm in and of itself and calls for constant attention to opportunities for modifying paradigms.

3   In problem-solving situations, allow your paradigms to surface and be examined. (contributed by Rick Bradley)

4   View the series of three videos narrated by Joel Barker—*Discovering the Future* (published by Charthouse International, Burnsville, MN 55337). This is a helpful series to show and discuss with a group that needs to change. It stresses the importance of questioning our assumptions by taking a fresh look at things.

> Don't get caught holding on to an old paradigm for loyalty's sake.

Topic 25.4 Pemberton: Sanity for survival

William Pemberton, a retired management and clinical psychologist residing in Mill Valley, California, presents the approach of general semantics as the key to peace, both local and global. In his recent *Sanity for Survival* (1989), Pemberton lays out his version of semantic theory, which is an evolution of an earlier theory presented by Korzybski (1948) and Bois (1966). The semantic approach is the study of human evaluative processes, or how people come to like or dislike, embrace or reject, love or hate, approve or disapprove. All we have is what we think. If you love me, you'll love what I think. Love me, love my thinking. Reject my thinking and you reject me. The semantic approach urges us to consider the difference between what we say and what we are talking *about*. We confuse the two, thinking that they are the same. But what our nerve endings receive is different from what is out there. What we receive is *about* what is out there. What we receive is not real—it is *about* what is real. And we all have different "abouts," or schemas (see Topic 18.4).

The way we assess what is out there becomes what we think and say about it. Our assessment, our "about," becomes our sacred system: love me, love my thinking. Love me, love what I'm about. Identification with other people occurs when our assessment fits their assessment. Stress occurs when identification doesn't occur—that is, when our interpretation doesn't match theirs. Yet we are both interpreting or assessing what is out there. The semantic approach is to converse about our separate sacred systems. Ultimately, the semanticist expects us to individually acknowledge our inability to perfectly know what is out there and therefore to be more humble about our "abouts," our sacred systems. Perhaps only by sharing our "abouts" with others can we sense where we are incomplete and come closer to what is actually out there, to what we are all talking about.

Pemberton sees five stages of semantic development. In Table 25.1, I summarize them based on his book and on a presentation he led in Lake Geneva, Wisconsin, in 1990. According to Pemberton, the responsibility of people at more advanced stages is to consistently model their stage around those who are stuck at earlier stages, hoping to draw them forward. If we are to avoid killing each other, we must learn how to talk with others whose sacred systems are shockingly different from ours. Pemberton urges us to follow the Law of Noninvalidation: rather than invalidating others' sacred systems by responding with sullen silence, an outright attack, or joking, a three-step response should be used:

1   *React genuinely.* Acknowledge that they got to you: "Wow, you zinged me that time!"

2   *Paraphrase them.* Aim to understand their interpretation—what they are saying *about* the subject: "Let me see if I understand you . . ." Pemberton calls this a PACT, or positive adult creative translation.

3   *Question them.* Ask open-ended questions to draw out additional detail, background, and examples. Ask questions that begin with *who, what, when, where,* or *how many.* Avoid *why* questions, which tend to elicit stress.

Applications

1   When people knowingly or unknowingly attack your sacred systems, remember to react genuinely, paraphrase them, and continue asking open-ended questions. The goal is to share what each of you sees similarly and differently about what is out there.

2   Remember the Law of Noninvalidation. Do not practice the destructive habit of invalidating other people's interpretations or assessments of what is out

Table 25.1 Stages of scientific thinking

Stage	Age	Concern	Philosophy	Deviant	Definition
1. Sensing	Infant	Me	Hedonist	Demon	Egocentric
2. Pre-science	Child	Those like me	Absolutist	Sin	My version's right
3. Early science	Youth	Those like us (gang)	Relativist	Sick	Your terrorist, my freedom fighter
4. Modern science	Adult-1	Those who touch my life in a relevant way	Transactionalist	Effective	We talk about the way we talk
5. Advancing science	Adult-2	Everybody	Epistemologist	Unknown potential	E.g., F.S.C. Northrop—highly advanced stuff

there. Acknowledge that their assessments are different from yours, seek to understand theirs better, and offer to help them understand yours better. It is very frustrating when someone's assessment doesn't match yours. But remember, *both* of you are interpreting, *both* of you are talking about what is out there. Create an atmosphere in which you can learn from each other.

Note: Based on ideas in *Sanity for Survival: A Semantic Approach to Conflict Resolution* by W. H. Pemberton, 1989, San Francisco: Graphic Guides.

Topic 25.5 Comparing models of development

In Topic 25.4, I presented Pemberton's five stages of development in semantic science. There are many other similar models of development. I thought it would be helpful to place a few of them side by side (see Table 25.2) to compare their interpretations of the process of growing up.

Table 25.2 A comparison of several models of maturational thinking

Pemberton 1989	Kohlberg 1984	Piaget 1977	Covey 1990	Peck 1987
Sensing	Pleasure/pain	Sensorimotor	Dependent	Egocentrism
	Pragmatic	Preoperational		
Pre-science	Reciprocation	Concrete operations	Dependent	Formalism
Early science	Law and order	Concrete operations	Independent	Skepticism
Modern science	Rational/legal	Formal operations	Interdependent	Mysticism
Advancing science	Brotherly love	Formal operations	Interdependent	Mysticism

Pemberton refers to his first stage, sensing, as an insane stage, characterized by the chaos of selfishness. This insane stage represents the Child ego state of transactional analysis. Roughly 10 percent of the population are in this stage. It is the adults stuck in this stage who cause much of the havoc, misery, embarrassment, and war in the world. Hence, Saddam Hussein and the Reverends Jimmy Swaggart and James Bakker. Pemberton calls stages 2 and 3 unsane; they are similar to the Parent ego state, full of righteousness but without the freedom from accountability of stage 1. He believes that about 40 percent are in stage 2, and 30 percent in stage 3. He calls stages 4 and 5 the sane stages, with about 15 percent in stage 4 and 5 percent in stage 5. These are the healthiest stages (the word *sane* comes from the Latin *sanus,* one of whose meanings was "healthy"). It is these 20 percent who are willing to abide by the Law of Noninvalidation (see Topic 25.4), who talk about what is out there without confusing their own assessments with the real world. I believe that T. H. Huxley was comparing stages 2 and 3 with stages 4 and 5 when he wrote, "Irrationally held truths may be more harmful than reasoned errors."

Applications

1   Establish the goal for yourself of feeling at home in stages 4 or 5. Read from the authors referred to in this chapter. Practice conversing with those whose sacred systems differ from yours with the goal of understanding rather than winning; participate in what Senge (1990) calls dialogue rather than discussion.

2   Expect your leadership to demonstrate at least stage-4 behavior. Cast your vote for leadership that is willing to communicate.

Suggested readings on molar approaches to epistemology
Kuhn, T. S. (1970). *The Structure of Scientific Revolutions.* (2nd ed.). Chicago: University of Chicago Press.
Pemberton, W. H. (1989). *Sanity for Survival: A Semantic Approach to Conflict Resolution.* San Francisco: Graphic Guides.
Pirsig, R. M. (1974). *Zen and the Art of Motorcycle Maintenance: An Inquiry into Values.* New York: Morrow.
Stevens, W. (1967). *The Collected Poems of Wallace Stevens.* New York: Knopf.

26

The mind in relationships:

There is only one universe, yet there are many ways of understanding it: religious (Christianity, Islam, Judaism, Buddhism), political (monarchy, democracy, dictatorship), economic (capitalism, communism, socialism), scientific (acupuncture, chiropractic, traditional Western medicine), and countless more. Epistemology is the study of how we may get beyond these many ways of knowing to the one universe itself.

Often the best way to make a point is through telling a story. Let me share with you a tale from *Il Novellino,* a thirteenth-century Italian collection of stories drawn from Oriental, Greek, and Trojan traditions and translated by Bob Lundry, a fellow consultant in Bronxville, New York.

The Sultan and the Jew

Once upon a time it happened that the Sultan was urgently in need of money. He thought of all the possible ways of getting it, he searched in every corner of the room of the treasury, he asked counsel from all his loyal advisers with a voice and a countenance that, to tell the truth, were not very appropriate for a man who ruled over so many people in so large a part of the world. But the fact is, there was no way to come up with any money.

Communication that connects

He was very preoccupied and even a bit put out, when his thoughts ran to a rich Jew who traded all over the far corners of the world, and a smile lit up his face. His plan was made: to trap the rich Jew with a question about religion.

His ambassadors found the Jew in his shop, surrounded by rich and rare merchandise. . . .

When the Jew was in the presence of the Sultan, the Sultan asked him which was the best religion, awaiting an answer with an impenetrable face. He was sure he would find him guilty. If the Jew were to say that the Jewish religion was the best, he could be accused of sinning against the Sultan's faith. And if the poor Jew were to answer that the Muhammadan religion was the most perfect, the Sultan, with a triumphant look, would cry: "Then why do you follow the Jewish faith?"

The poor Jew saw what his master was thinking, but he did not lose his calm. He turned his penetrating eyes to the Sultan and, with a benevolent voice that did not betray his inner turmoil, he responded in this way:

"Master, there once was a father who had three sons

> "No truth so sublime but it may be seen to be trivial to-morrow in the light of new thoughts."
>
> **Ralph Waldo Emerson**

*and a ring with a precious stone, the best in the world.
Each of the sons begged the father to leave him the ring.
The father, seeing that each of them wanted it, summoned
a fine goldsmith and said to him: 'Maestro, make me two
rings precisely like this one, and put in a stone that exact-
ly resembles this one.' The goldsmith, who was extremely
able in his art, made the two rings so perfectly similar to
the original that no one except the father was able to know
which was the true one. When he felt death drawing near,
the father sent for his three sons and gave each a ring in
secret, and so each believed he possessed the true one.*

*"And so, Sir," the Jew concluded, "I say to you of the
faiths, that there are three. The Father who is in heaven
knows the best one. And the sons, who are we, each
believe we have the good one."*

*The Sultan was so struck by the wise and profound
answer that he did not know what to say to accuse the
Jew, and he let him go. Thus, the rich Jew escaped the
clutches of the desperate Sultan, who surely would have
confiscated all of the Jew's goods upon hearing either of
the expected answers.*

(Reprinted from personal correspondence with permission of the translator.)

Epistemology shows us how to come up with such good answers to such
good questions. The Sultan's question was based on a narrow point of view, while
the Jew answered from the global perspective of an epistemologist, more interested in the structural interrelatedness of things than in their uniqueness. The
epistemologist, in a sense, is trying to know God, not from the point of view of a
particular religion, but from that of a universal citizen of spaceship Earth. This
chapter identifies the basic communication skills that are the building blocks of
sanity and survival, of global as well as interpersonal understanding.

Topic 26.1 The skills of interpersonal communication

*Effective communication
is the ultimate expres-
sion of the human brain.*

The building blocks of sanity are the skills of interpersonal communication.
Effective communication is the ultimate expression of the human brain (Black,
1991). At the molecular level, communication takes place through the intermin-
gling of salts, proteins, and neurons. At the molar level, it is accomplished through
a basic set of nine fundamental tools:

The quest for knowledge

1   *Asking questions:* Preferring open-ended questions beginning with words like *what, when,* or *where* to closed-ended yes-or-no questions

2   *Listening:* Paraphrasing your partner's comments and asking questions to be certain you understand their meaning

3   *Giving constructive criticism:* Offering criticism in a descriptive, nonblameful manner while accompanying it with some appropriate form of recognition—using a "good news, bad news" format

4   *Giving recognition:* Telling someone concretely and specifically what he or she has done that you appreciate and what its specific consequences are for you or the organization or both

5   *Building on others' ideas:* Referring to your partner's previous idea as you add to it, rather than competitively proposing your own

6   *Giving instructions:* Allowing your partner to repeat your instructions back to you so that together you may ensure correctness

7   *Being assertive:* Expressing your opinions and feelings objectively, without aggression

8   *Managing conflict:* Learning the underlying needs of conflicting parties and finding a single strategy that satisfies both sets of needs; using the win-win approach

9   *Giving nonverbal signals:* Using the body's ability to communicate liking, acceptance, and attentiveness through immediacy, relaxation, and activity

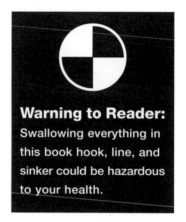

Warning to Reader: Swallowing everything in this book hook, line, and sinker could be hazardous to your health.

     Books, articles, tapes, films, and workshops abound on each of these topics. One of the better ones is a book by Michael and Tempe Thomas, *Getting Commitment at Work* (1990). I don't know of a single resource that provides instruction in all nine skills. Currently, I'm trying to convince my wife and partner, Jane, to write such a book.

Applications

1   Evaluate your effectiveness in each of the nine skills by asking significant people around you for feedback. Get them to grade you on each skill, then identify your priorities for development and systematically learn an effective model for your priority skills. Practice daily.

2   Practice communication skills with children; they enjoy the attention. Volunteer as a tutor. It's a good practice opportunity as well as a way to make a contribution. (contributed by Rick Bradley)

3   Many resources can be identified by talking with your public library's reference librarian. In addition, you might try asking a member of the American Society of Training and Development to help you identify local resources for specific skill development. If you call their national headquarters in Alexandria, Virginia (703-683-8100), they will be happy to give you the name of a member who lives near you.

Topic 26.2 The process of communication

The skills of interpersonal communication should be understood as part of a larger epistemological process. Several varieties of this developmental skill are discussed in Topics 25.4 and 25.5. The simplest version of the process is the one described by Stephen Covey (1990). He sees the task of the individual as moving from dependence to independence to interdependence. Consistent practice of all the communication skills helps us to accomplish this move.

Applications

1   Don't just practice communication skills as single tools in your interpersonal toolbox—be clear what you are building with them. Know your goal, whether it is interdependence, wisdom, sanity, peace, or love. Covey's *The Seven Habits of Highly Effective People* (1990) does the best job I've seen of providing a context and process for such skill development.

2   Other effective approaches to defining a context for the development of communication skills are available in Pemberton (1989) and Peck (1987).

Mental, physical, and relational health in individuals and organizations

Without learning there is no growth.

The organization is an extension of the individual. The health of the organization, whether it is a marriage, a business, a team, or a bridge club, is directly related to the health of the individuals comprising it. Peter Senge (1990, p. 139) writes, "Organizations learn only through individuals who learn. Individual learning does not guarantee organizational learning. But without it no organizational learning occurs."

Without learning there is no growth. Kazuo Inamori asserts: "If employees themselves are not sufficiently motivated to challenge . . . there will simply be no growth" (Senge, 1990, pp. 139–140). To decide that we have arrived at the right answers for all time is to decide that growth is no longer important. In fact, our pronouncements are at best approximations of the truth. Every day we do what we can to get one micron closer. The quest is eternal. Personal mastery is one of Senge's five disciplines necessary to the learning organization. He writes, "People with a high level of personal mastery live in a continual learning mode. They never 'arrive'" (p. 142).

Of course, there is a sense in which we will never know the secret truths of the universe. Cautions against the scientist's arrogant presumption of omniscience are spelled out by Capra (1984), Gleick (1987), and Heisenberg (1962). We can never know with certainty. At best we can estimate probabilities. We can continually improve our estimates, but when we tamper with a system to improve it, our intervention can cause an unforeseen, unpredictable turbulence in the system. We must learn to be comfortable with chaos. Control is an illusion. In Michael Crichton's apocalyptic novel *Jurassic Park* (1990, p. 313), the scientist Malcolm says:

> *And now chaos theory proves that unpredictability is built into our daily lives. It is as mundane as the rainstorm we cannot predict. And so the grand vision of science, hundreds of years old—the dream of total control— has died, in our century. And with it much of the justification, the rationale for science to do what it does. And for us to listen to it. Science has always said that it may not know everything now but it will know, eventually. But now we see that isn't true. It is an idle boast. As foolish, and as misguided, as the child who jumps off a building because he believes he can fly.*

I do not mean to sound the death knell of science—only an end to the illusion of omniscience. Between the extremes of Aristotle and Plato there is the voice of W. Edwards Deming. Aristotle would confine us to the realities of the way things are, while Plato would propel us toward the clouds of the unknowable. In between, Deming urges us to ask daily, "What can I do to improve, today?" Indeed, life is a banquet, and each of us bears individual responsibility for the wisest possible behavior at the banquet table. We cannot blame the farmer, the cook, the server, or the diner, for we are all of them in one. Life is a banquet, and each of us is to blame for its quality. Enjoy.

Suggested readings on everyday epistemology

Capra, F. (1984). *The Tao of Physics.* (2nd ed.). Toronto: Bantam.

Covey, S. R. (1990). *The Seven Habits of Highly Effective People.* New York: Simon & Schuster.

Peck, M. S. (1987). *The Different Drum: Community-Making and Peace.* New York: Simon & Schuster.

Pemberton, W. H. (1989). *Sanity for Survival: A Semantic Approach to Conflict Resolution.* San Francisco: Graphic Guides.

Senge, P. (1990). *The Fifth Discipline.* New York: Doubleday/Currency.

Thomas, M. C., & Thomas, T. S. (1990). *Getting Commitment at Work: A Guide for Managers and Employees.* Chapel Hill, NC: Commitment Press.

27

Updating your owner's manual:

From the gaping head wounds of World War II to the drug-sizzled brains caused by poison-trafficking cartels, we try to learn from our misery. A recent television program described how doctors, noticing that symptoms of crack cocaine addicts resemble those of patients with Parkinson's disease, have made advances in the treatment of Parkinson's disease. But we do not have to wait for tragedy in order to make progress. Scientific exploration and discovery today makes the nineties an exciting time to be alive. And the more we are open to learning the work of others, the more exciting our nineties will be.

Recently we overheard our daughter, Allegra, talking with a girlfriend, who was lamenting her steady boyfriend's unwillingness to talk seriously about their relationship. Allegra told her friend that she had learned in her dad's book about females being wired to talk and males being wired to do, and that she had tried the suggestion of getting a boy to do something so that talking would become an accompaniment to the activity rather than an activity in and of itself. "And you know?" she added to her friend, "It really worked! He talked while we were walking and didn't seem to mind it at all. Give it a try."

What I like about this story is that (1) it shows an experimental, evaluative approach in responding to research and (2) it builds on differences rather than using differences to blame and justify resentments. I hope that this book will become something of a cafeteria for you. By that I mean that you can come to it for nourishment

The quest for knowledge

Continuing the search

and ideas and take what appears to be helpful to you. Return to it when you are baffled by a concern that is covered by one of these chapters—for example, problems related to aging parents or friends; concerns about an unmotivated child, friend, or worker; or a gnawing dissatisfaction with your ability to memorize. This book should yield up to you a specific practical idea or at least suggest relevant resources.

In a sense, I have been sowing seeds, and I'm inviting you to reap from one or more of the many I have thrown out. My observation is that the Age of Research is alive and well. From the health and fitness enthusiasts to the corporate quality gurus, people are spreading the gospel of continuing improvement. But you can't continually improve without doing, following, and evaluating research, and then implementing the findings appropriately in your own life. I emphasize, however, the need to be critical. Just as I have included the Caveat Box throughout this book, I urge you to keep your nonsense detector turned on whenever you encounter suggestions for improvement. Recently, perusing an issue of a futuring magazine, I saw an advertisement for a pill "to make you more intelligent." Amused and alarmed, I called the telephone number provided and asked the woman who answered to send me a copy of the research results of the product testing. They had none! She said that all they could send me was a somewhat more lengthy version of the advertisement I had read. I'm still waiting. I declined, incidentally, to accept their offer of a free thirty-day supply.

> "We should live for the future, and yet should find our life in the fidelities of the present; the last is the only method of the first."
>
> **Henry Ward Beecher**

This kind of irresponsible advertising will face us with more frequency, more force, and more marketing savvy. We must all do what we can to be as informed as possible about what works, what's dangerous, and what's simply inert. In that spirit, I have included in the back of the book a Reader Participation Card, which I hope you will use to let me know what works, what doesn't, and what new ideas you'd like me to add (citing you as the source) in subsequent editions of this book.

In Chapter One, I identified five core principles of cognitive science and suggested that we revisit them in the final chapter. Well, here we are. Perhaps, in fact, it would be helpful to restate these core principles and identify examples of them that appear throughout this owner's manual:

Nativism. The importance of seeing the widespread role of genetics and inheritance can be seen in the discussions of gender, intelligence, personality, and diet, among others.

Unity. The mind-body continuum is especially apparent in the discussions of disease, aging, motivation, and emotion.

Connectivity. The importance of the synaptic gap—and especially of maintaining its healthy state—is clear in the discussions of memory, learning, exercise, and drugs.

Interconnectivity. Recognizing the relatedness of the thousands of systems within the brain is crucial to understanding the material on memory, creativity, workplace design, and epistemology.

Control. The vital factor of the individual's control over his or her life situation is basic to the discussions of motivation, epistemology, intelligence, learning, and aging.

The advances in brain research are breathtakingly rapid. As I write and you read, some piece of information in this book is being challenged or enhanced. Who knows where the next major advance will be and what difference it will make in our lives? Just last month I learned that toenails are now used to extract certain forensic evidence that formerly had to be taken from blood samples.

As research expands our sense of what is true and what is real, paradigms begin to shift, sometimes imperceptibly, sometimes earthshakingly. In looking over the ways in which cognitive science affects our lives, ten paradigms seem to me to be in the middle of major shifts:

The quest for knowledge

Traditional paradigm	Emerging paradigm
1. Motivators are external.	1. Motivators are internal.
2. There are four personality traits.	2. The Five-Factor Model emerges.
3. Aging lowers ability.	3. Use it or lose it!
4. IQ is a single-faceted, academic concept.	4. IQ is a multifaceted, street-smart concept.
5. There are no sex differences.	5. The sexes are wired differently.
6. Nurture is the main factor.	6. Nature is the main factor.
7. Germs cause disease.	7. The mind controls disease.
8. Diet is unrelated to the brain.	8. Diet influences mental function.
9. The brain is seen as a computer.	9. The brain is seen as a pharmacy.
10. Memory is retrieval of complete episodes.	10. Memory is construction of episodes from pieces of information.

Perhaps these ten perceived shifts will form the basis of another book! Until then . . .

The owner's manual for the brain:

Everyday applications from mind-brain research

Appendix A

A listing of sex differences

Male-differentiated brains	Female-differentiated brains
Have better general math ability	Have better general verbal ability
Are better at spatial (three-dimensional) reasoning	Are better in grammar and vocabulary
Are better at chess	Are better at foreign languages
Are better at map reading	Have better fine-motor (hand-eye) coordination within personal space
Are better at blueprint reading	Have better sensory awareness
Have better vision in bright light (see less well in darkness)	Have better night vision (are more sensitive to bright light)
Have better perception in blue end of spectrum	Have better perception in red end of spectrum
Have more narrow vision (tunnel vision), but better depth perception	Have wide peripheral vision for "big picture"— have more receptor rods and cones
Have more stuttering and speech defects	Perceive sounds better
Enroll more in remedial reading (4:1)	Sing in tune more (6:1)
Take more interest in objects	Are more interested in people and faces
Talk and play more with inanimate objects	Read character and social cues better
Identify salty tastes better	Identify subtle tastes better
Require more space	Require less space
Have a better aural memory	Have a better visual memory
Are more easily angered	Are slower to anger
Talk later (usually by four years of age)	Talk earlier (99% are understandable by three years of age)
Are more sensitive to salty tastes	Are more sensitive to bitter tastes, prefer sweets
Have relatively insensitive skin	Have extremely sensitive skin
Have right hemisphere larger than left	Have left hemisphere larger than right
Favor right ear	Listen equally with both ears
Solve math problems nonverbally	Tend to talk while solving math problems
Handle multitasking more easily	Are less at ease with multitasking

Male-differentiated brains	Female-differentiated brains
Have better memory for relevant or organized information	Have better memory for names and faces, and for random and irrelevant information
Use less eye contact	Use more eye contact
Have a shorter attention span	Have a longer attention span
Don't notice the smell of Exaltolide (a musklike odor)	Are especially sensitive to the smell of Exaltolide, especially before ovulation
Are more sensation-seeking	Are less sensation-seeking (but American females are more sensation-seeking than English females)
Are more frequently left-handed	Equal numbers are right- and left-handed
Use left hemisphere in spelling	Use both hemispheres in spelling
Have differentiated hemispheres: right for math and spatial skills, left for language	Have undifferentiated hemispheres
Have corpus callosum that shrinks about 20% by the age of fifty and is thinner relative to brain size	Have corpus callosum that is thicker relative to brain size and doesn't shrink over time
Left hemisphere shrinks with age	Left hemisphere shrinks symmetrically, minimally
Prefer greater distance from same-sex others	Are more comfortable than men are when they are physically close to same-sex others
Are three times more likely to be dyslexic or myopic	Are less likely to be dyslexic or myopic
React to pain slowly	React to pain more quickly; can tolerate long-term pain or discomfort better
When left alone, tend to form organizations with hierarchical, dominant structures	When left alone, tend to form informal organizations with shifting power sources
Male preschoolers:	Female preschoolers:
■ Average 36 seconds for goodbyes	■ Average 93 seconds for goodbyes
■ Occupy more play space	■ Occupy less play space
■ Prefer blocks and building	■ Prefer playing with living things
■ Build high structures	■ Build long and low structures
■ Are indifferent to newcomers	■ Greet newcomers
■ Accept others if they are useful	■ Accept others if they are nice
■ Prefer stories of adventure	■ Prefer stories of romance
■ Identify more with robbers	■ Identify more with victims
■ Play more competitive games (e.g., tag)	■ Play less competitive games (e.g., hopscotch)
■ Use dolls for "dive bombers"	■ Use dolls for family scenes
■ Are better visual-spatial learners	■ Are better auditory learners

Note: Based on *Brain Sex* by Anne Moir and David Jessel, 1991, New York: Carol Publishing/Lyle Stuart.

Appendix B

Eating right

Limit
Egg yolks

Organ meats

Fried foods

Fatty foods (pastries, spreads, dressings)

Animal protein (has no known benefits and may cause cancer)

Alcohol

Certain shellfish (there is some debate over which; scallops are apparently okay)

Emphasize
Fish

Skinless poultry

Lean meats

Low or nonfat dairy products

Complex carbohydrates (fruits, vegetables, starches)

Eliminate
Dietary supplements (megadoses have no known benefits and may be toxic)

Calcium, fish oil, or fiber supplements (they have no known
    benefits and must be taken in food)

Specific limits
Fat

    No more than 30% of daily calories

    (1 tablespoon of peanut butter = 8 grams = 90 calories)

Saturated fats

    Less than 10% of the fat allowance (includes coconut oil and animal fat)

Complex carbohydrates

    At least 55% of daily calories

Vegetables

    Five or more servings, especially of green and yellow

    vegetables (1 serving = $\frac{1}{2}$ cup)

Fruits

Five or more servings, especially of citrus fruits

(1 serving = 1 medium-sized fruit or $1/2$ banana)

Starches

Six or more servings; includes rice, potatoes, pasta, legumes,

and whole-grain bread and cereal (1 serving = 1 slice of bread)

Protein

Eight grams per kilogram of body weight (for a 180-pound man,

an 8.4-ounce hamburger patty; for a 120-pound woman,

a 5.6-ounce hamburger patty)

Alcohol

Less than 1 ounce daily (2 cans of beer or two small glasses of wine;

none for women who are pregnant or trying to conceive)

Salt

Six grams a day (about 1 teaspoon)

Note that in general, Americans eat too much fat, cholesterol, and protein, and too few complex carbohydrates.

Note: Based on *Diet and Health: Implications for Reducing Chronic Disease Risk* by National Research Council, Committee on Diet and Health, 1989, Washington, DC: National Academy Press.

Appendix C

Aerobic versus nonaerobic exercise

Aerobic exercises:
Minimum required times for health effects

Twelve minutes	Fifteen minutes	Twenty minutes
Jumping rope	Jogging	Walking
Running in place	Running	Outdoor bicycling
Jumping jacks	Dancing	Stationary bicycling
Chair stepping	Mini-trampoline	Ice skating
Rowing	Treadmill	Roller skating
Cross-country skiing		Swimming

For the above, add several minutes for warming up.

Nonaerobic exercises:
Why they are nonaerobic

Stop and go	Short duration	Low intensity
Tennis	Weight lifting	Golf
Softball	Sprinting	Canasta
Football	Isometrics	Frisbee
Calisthenics	Square dancing	
Handball	Downhill skiing	
Racquetball		
Basketball		

Note: Adapted from *The New Fit or Fat* by Covert Bailey, 1991, Boston: Houghton Mifflin. © 1977, 1978, 1991 by Covert Bailey. Reprinted by permission of Houghton Mifflin Co. All rights reserved.

Appendix D

Name: **Big-Five feedback form**   **Date:**

Resilience scale

Reactive						Responsive			Sedate			Resilience scale
20	25	30	35	40		45	50	55	60	65	70	75	80

Positive descriptors: alert, aware, empathetic, expressive, energetic

Negative descriptors: tense, high-strung, depressed, neurotic, restless

Positive descriptors: secure, calm, Rock of Gibraltar, concentrating, steady, unflappable, stress-free

Negative descriptors: lethergic, laid-back, unresponsive, unaware, insensitive, tunnel-visioned

Extraversion scale

Introvert						Ambivert			Extravert			Extraversion scale
20	25	30	35	40		45	50	55	60	65	70	75	80

Positive descriptors: private, reserved, serious, works alone, self-minimizing, prefers writing

Negative descriptors: seclusive, fearful, submissive, retreating, eccentric, loner

Positive descriptors: conversational, energetic, assertive, confident, happy, optimistic, sociable

Negative descriptors: outspoken, talkative, overbearing, aggressive, exhibitionistic, heedless, shallow

Openness scale

Preserver						Moderate			Explorer			Openness scale
20	25	30	35	40		45	50	55	60	65	70	75	80

Positive descriptors: seeks depth, practical, expert knowledge, down-to-earth, efficient, traditional, practice until perfect, conservative

Negative descriptors: narrowness, no big picture, misses new opportunities, lacks perspective, set in ways, closed to new experiences, rigid

Positive descriptors: broad interests, curious, likes novelty/variety, chases ideas/theory, imaginative, liberal, understands big picture

Negative descriptors: dabbler, amateur, easily bored, impractical, head in clouds, lacks detail, lives in fantasy

Agreeableness scale

Challenger						Negotiator			Adapter			Agreeableness scale
20	25	30	35	40		45	50	55	60	65	70	75	80

Positive descriptors: independent, skeptical, direct, self-interested, competitive, questioning

Negative descriptors: rejecting, hostile, rude, self-centered, combative, argumentative

Positive descriptors: friendly, tolerant, trusting, team player, considerate, accepting

Negative descriptors: syrupy, spineless, gullible, dependent, doormat, unprincipled, conflict averse

Conscientiousness scale

Flexible						Balanced			Focused			Conscientiousness scale
20	25	30	35	40		45	50	55	60	65	70	75	80

Positive descriptors: relaxed, spontaneous, open-ended, multitask, experimental, roles not goals, accepts uncertainty

Negative descriptors: lackadaisical, quitter, indecisive, chaotic, irresponsible, nonproductive, permissive, procrastinator

Positive descriptors: industrious, dependable, will to achieve, productive, organized, decisive, persevering, driven

Negative descriptors: overbearing, compulsive, workaholic, suppressed, meticulous, stubborn

Big-Five feedback form

Appendix E

Guide for evaluating the intelligence (mental self-management) of someone you are recruiting or interviewing

1 Does this person have the ability to administer a project from beginning to end in compliance with project requirements (cost, time, quality, etc.)?

    a. Interview evidence:

    b. Reference evidence:

2 Does this person have the ability to scan relevant resources and obtain accurate, current, relevant, and effective information to use in solving problems? Include habits and attitudes toward reading (using the library, periodicals, books, etc.) and asking questions (particularly the habit of asking open-ended questions).

    a. Interview evidence:

    b. Reference evidence:

3 Does this person show flexibility in selecting problem-solving strategies? Through interviews or paper-and-pencil tests, determine rigidity in choosing to alter self, others, or the situation in solving problems.

    a. Interview evidence:

    b. Reference evidence:

    c. Test evidence (*Tacit Knowledge Inventory, Hersey-Blanchard Situational Leadership Inventory,* or other measures of flexibility or rigidity found in multidimensional instruments):

4 Does this person have the ability to plan a sequence of events in a logical, effective manner?

    a. Interview evidence (ask about time management practices, use of tickle files, and use of various planning techniques; look at the individual's "calendars," such as daily agendas):

    b. Reference evidence:

    c. In-basket exercise (this shows the ability to prioritize a diverse set of documents):

5   Does this person have the ability to be appropriately creative?

      a. Interview evidence:

      b. Reference evidence:

      c. Test evidence (using multidimensional or single-dimension tests):

6   Does this person have the ability to execute through fluent use of words, numbers,
and other materials?

      a. Test evidence (from the *Wunderlich Personnel Test* or some other similar test):

      b. Artifactual evidence (sample reports, drawings, etc.):

      c. Interview evidence (ability to grasp complex patterns and concepts presented
in organizational reports, charts, spreadsheets, etc.):

Appendix F

Personal checklist for intelligent behaviors

This self-evaluation is based on Robert Sternberg's theory of intelligence presented in Chapter Twelve. More intelligent persons will answer affirmatively to many of the items in all of the sections. Consider increasing your "intelligent behavior" repertoire in any section in which you check few or no items.

1 *Administrative behaviors*

_____ a. Do I keep a prioritized To-Do list?

_____ b. Do I use a tickler file?

_____ c. Do I take time to evaluate my progress toward goals?

_____ d. Do I regularly solicit feedback from others on how I'm doing?

_____ e. Am I aware of my weaknesses, and do I delegate to compensate for them?

_____ f. Do I consciously devote resources to developing in areas that need improvement?

_____ g. Do I keep myself in good condition and full of energy?

2 *Research behaviors*

_____ a. Do I regularly read periodicals that are relevant to my goals?

_____ b. Do I regularly read sections of the newspaper that are relevant to my goals?

_____ c. Do I scan the television schedules (especially public, educational stations) for programs of value to my goals, and then either view them or tape them for future viewing?

_____ d. Do I visit and use one or more libraries regularly?

_____ e. Do I call reference librarians with my questions?

_____ f. Do I practice the art of asking open-ended questions of all the significant people in my life?

_____ g. Do I attend seminars and courses to update my knowledge and skills?

3   *Problem-solving behaviors*

Altering self

_____ a. Do I learn new skills or bodies of knowledge?

_____ b. Do I consciously try to improve old skills or bodies of knowledge?

_____ c. Do I discontinue ineffective habits?

_____ d. Do I consult a therapist or counselor when the need arises?

_____ e. Do I ask for feedback from the significant people in my life, then act on it by changing my behavior or habits when appropriate?

Altering others

_____ a. Am I a consistently good listener?

_____ b. Do I take time to train others when they need training?

_____ c. Do I consciously make the effort to be a helper when others have problems?

_____ d. Do I offer sufficient praise and encouragement to others?

_____ e. Do I take the time to give nonblameful, constructive criticism when it is needed? Do I allow time to discuss corrective measures?

_____ f. When conflict arises, do I take time to discuss its causes and to explore possible solutions?

Altering the situation

_____ a. Do I know when to call it quits?

_____ b. Can I let go of existing ways of doing things and explore new, improved designs or processes?

_____ c. Do I regularly observe others' ways of accomplishing tasks similar to mine with an eye out for how I might change my situation for the better?

4   *Planning behaviors*

_____ a. Do I take time to map out complex projects using timelines, PERT charts, Gantt charts, outlines, etc?

_____ b. Do I take time to test my project design or outline before actually implementing it by using potential problem analysis (Kepner & Tregoe, 1981), visualization techniques, simulations, modeling, etc.?

_____ c. Do I start a project with the end in mind and then determine the best way to get there?

5 *Creativity behaviors*

_____ a. Do I practice the habit of seeing old patterns in new ways (e.g., seeing the half-empty
_____ glass as half-full, or letting go of old perceptual sets)?

_____ b. Do I occasionally let go of old skills or ways of doing things and explore new, different,
and possibly improved ways?

_____ c. Do I ask W. Edwards Deming's question: "What can I do to improve, today?"

_____ d. Do I tolerate ambiguity long enough to explore effective resolutions?
(Or do I jump to find answers?)

_____ e. Do I enjoy trying to understand complex situations?

_____ f. Can I keep my options open long enough to find the best one?

_____ g. Can I suspend judgment while exploring ideas?

_____ h. Do I resist peer and social pressures to conform?

6 *Execution behaviors*

_____ a. Do I look up words when I don't know them?

_____ b. Do I work puzzles such as crossword puzzles and math riddles?

_____ c. Do I take pride in having my presentations show careful crafting?

_____ d. Do I regularly edit my work for accuracy, completeness, and effectiveness?

_____ e. Do I watch for feedback during my presentations and alter my behavior according
to the feedback?

_____ f. Do I ask for feedback after my presentations and incorporate suggestions
into future presentations?

_____ g. In general, am I genuinely interested in improving myself in most facets of my being?

Appendix G

Checklist for the self-evaluation of learning practices

1 _____ Do I design activities aimed at helping students remember what they are learning?

2 _____ Do I periodically check with learners to see if they remember what they've learned in an earlier session?

3 _____ Do I consciously assess my learning environment for stressors and attempt to keep it as stress-free as possible?

4 _____ Do I provide learners with an opportunity to organize new learning into a form that is meaningful to them?

5 _____ Do I provide learners with opportunities to rehearse or practice their newly acquired information as an aid in converting it to long-term memory?

6 _____ Do I administer tests as a means to encourage learning?

7 _____ Do I help learners identify preexisting schemas that could help or hinder new learning?

8 _____ Do I provide opportunities for learners to apply new learnings to situations that are meaningful to them?

9 _____ Do I ensure that distractions are eliminated so learners can focus on the subject at hand?

10 _____ Do I maintain appropriately high expectations for all my learners?

11 _____ Do I expect and measure mastery on the part of all my learners?

12 _____ Do I use a variety of methods and materials, resisting the temptation to use printed material alone?

13 _____ Do I communicate with learners ahead of time to prepare them for what they are about to learn?

14	_____	Do I avoid trying to cover too many different lessons at one sitting by spacing lessons for maximum retention?
15	_____	Do I allow and encourage both scheduled and spontaneous breaks?
16	_____	Do I build into my lesson plans follow-up for previous sessions as well as pointing to follow-up for the current session?
17	_____	Do I solicit learner feedback and respond appropriately?
18	_____	Do I practice effective listening skills with learners?
19	_____	Do I consciously do things to establish better rapport with learners?
20	_____	Do I engage in specific activities at the beginning of each session that help learners feel at ease?
21	_____	Do I vary my voice, posture, gestures, and location enough to prevent learners from
	_____	habituating to me?
22	_____	Do I consciously do things to enhance my prestige and respect vis-à-vis the learners?
23	_____	Do I ensure that the learning environment has sufficient visual, tactile, and auditory stimulation to keep learners alert?
24	_____	Do I provide opportunities for learners to get feedback from their peers?

Appendix H

Brainstorming

Goals

1 To generate an extensive number of ideas or solutions to a problem by suspending criticism and evaluation.

2 To develop skills in creative problem solving.

Group size

Any number of small groups composed of approximately six participants each.

Materials

Newsprint and felt-tipped marker for each group.

Procedure

1 The facilitator forms small groups of approximately six participants each. Each group selects a secretary.

2 The facilitator instructs each group to form a circle. He or she provides newsprint and a felt-tipped marker for each secretary and asks the secretary to record every idea generated by the group.

3 The facilitator states the following rules:

a. There will be no criticism during the brainstorming phase.

b. Farfetched ideas are encouraged because they may trigger more practical ideas.

c. Many ideas are desirable. Go for quantity, not quality.

d. Let others' ideas suggest new ideas to you; "piggyback" on their ideas.

4 The facilitator announces the topic, for example, "How could we reduce costs?" She or he tells the groups that they have five or ten minutes to generate ideas.

5 At the end of the generating phase, the facilitator tells the groups that the ban on criticism is over, then directs them to evaluate their ideas and to select the best ones.

Appendix I

Brainwriting

A procedure for generating ideas, brainwriting is a form of brainstorming. It is particularly useful in more introverted groups with less outward verbal energy.

Procedure

1 Each member of the group makes a list of ideas to address the issue at hand. The groups are directed to go for quantity, not quality, and to refrain from talking.

2 After five to ten minutes, the members pass their papers to the member on their left. Then each member reads the items on his or her new list and allows these items to "suggest" new items, which are added to the list.

3 This continues until each member has had an opportunity to read and add ideas to each of the other lists.

4 The lists are circulated and some voting system is used to evaluate the ideas, for example, one to five stars. The scores are tallied and the top ten or so ideas are written on the board for everyone to see. The group continues to evaluate the ideas, either by consensus or by a rational decision analysis process, such as the Five-Step Rational Decision Analysis (Plunkett & Hale, 1982; Kepner & Tregoe, 1981) or the Precedence Chart (Saaty, 1982).

Appendix J

Universities offering interdisciplinary cognitive science degree programs

Boston University, Boston, Massachusetts: M.A. and Ph.D.

Brigham Young University, Provo, Utah: B.S., M.S., and Ph.D.

Brown University, Providence, Rhode Island: B.A., B.S., and Ph.D.

California Institute of Technology, Pasadena: Ph.D.

Carnegie Mellon University, Pittsburgh, Pennsylvania: B.S. and Ph.D.

      (joint program with the University of Pittsburgh)

Georgia Institute of Technology, Atlanta: Certificate

Indiana University, Bloomington: Ph.D.

Massachusetts Institute of Technology, Cambridge: Ph.D.

Stanford University, Stanford, California: B.S. and minor as part of related Ph.D.

University of California, San Diego: Ph.D.

University of Colorado, Boulder: Certificate

University of North Carolina at Chapel Hill: Ph.D.

University of Pittsburgh, Pittsburgh, Pennsylvania: B.S. and Ph.D.

      (joint program with Carnegie Mellon University)

Glossary

Acetylcholine. A neurotransmitter released in the neuron that is essential to the health of the neuronal membrane itself and to learning and memory; it is derived from fat in the diet.

Action potential. An electrical charge in response to a stimulus that, if sufficiently strong, results in the release of neurotransmitters at the synapse; a basic measure of neural activity. See also Latency; Amplitude.

Adrenaline. See Epinephrine.

Agonist. Said of a drug that mimics (i.e., can occupy the same receptor sites as and send the same signals as) a particular neurotransmitter (e.g., sumitriptan is an agonist for seratonin); the opposite of an antagonist.

Amplitude. The height of the wave resulting from measuring action potential; a measure of the amount of neural resources brought to bear on a particular stimulus. See also Latency.

Androgens. The family of male sex hormones (and drugs), the most familiar of which is testosterone; their level in the body is associated with degree of male gender characteristics, from body hair to aggression. It is present in both males and females, but is usually higher in males.

Antagonist. A drug that blocks the receptor site for a particular neurotransmitter. The opposite of an agonist.

Arousal. The level of activity of a bodily system: high limbic arousal indicates rapid pulse, for example, and low limbic arousal suggests a far slower pulse. The absence of arousal is associated with sleep.

Attention. The capacity to focus the senses on a specific stimulus source; it is possible to focus on only one stimulus source at a time. When we appear to be focusing on two sources simultaneously (e.g., using a car phone and driving), we are actually alternating attention. Attempting to focus on more than one stimulus source increases error proneness, unless one of the perceptual activities is completely routinized (we can suck a mint and drive at the same time).

Attributional style. The manner in which an individual attributes the causes of success or failure; it is usually described as either external (the causes are outside the individual, such as luck or sour grapes) or internal (the causes are inside the individual, such as hard work or talent). Also called explanatory style and locus of control.

Automatic behavior. See Automation.

Automation. The process by which a new learning becomes automatic or routine; refers to a skill or behavior that, when first learned, requires intense attentional focus, but that eventually demands little or no attentional focus, as in learning to tie one's shoes. Also called automization and automatization.

Automatization. See Automation.

Automatizer. See Automizer.

Automization. See Automation.

Automizer. Said of a person who can perform routine and repetitive activities for long periods with relatively little fatigue; associated with higher levels of testosterone. Also called automatizer.

Average evoked potential (AEP). The printed wave that represents the average on many actual waves; it is described in terms of its amplitude and latency.

Axon. The connective branch of a neuron that conveys messages through the synapse to other neurons.

Behaviorism. A school of psychology popular through the 1960s that maintained a monistic view of the mind-brain, saying that humans display no mental activity between stimulus and response. Behaviorism is associated with B. F. Skinner and J. B. Watson; it is also called stimulus-response psychology. It has generally been replaced today by cognitive psychology.

Biofeedback. Information about a bodily function; used in biofeedback training to gain personal control over that function.

Blocker. Generally speaking, any chemical that prevents passage of a neurotransmitter at the synapse.

Calpain. A neurotransmitter associated with efficiency of synaptic transmission. It is a calcium-activated intracellular proteinase.

Catecholamine. A family of neurotransmitters including dopamine, norepinephrine, and epinephrine.

Cerebral cortex. The part of the brain associated with rational thought; the most recent to appear, evolution-wise. Also called the cerebrum.

Cholecystokinin (CCK). A neurotransmitter influential in controlling appetite. It is found at lower levels in bulimia cases.

Chunk. A single element of learning or memory; chunks are pieced together to create memories.

Classical conditioning. The learning procedure in which a neutral stimulus (a stimulus that does not elicit any particular response, such as a ringing bell) precedes an unconditioned stimulus (a stimulus that elicits a predictable response, as when red meat causes a dog to salivate) and thereby becomes a conditioned response (e.g., the dog starts salivating after hearing the bell and before seeing meat); the meat is said to have been associated to the bell).

Cognitive dissonance. The situation that occurs when a person's behavior (e.g., eating snails and enjoying them) conflicts with his or her attitude toward that behavior (the person believes that snails are disgusting).

Cognitive therapy. The practice of changing the way a person thinks about the world for the purpose of improving his or her mental health.

Commissurotomy. A surgical procedure in which the corpus callosum is severed.

Corpus callosum. A bundle of neurons that connects and permits communication between the two hemispheres of the brain.

Cortex. The outer layer of a bodily organ. From the Latin *cortex,* or bark (of a tree). See also Cerebral cortex.

Cortisol. A hormone produced by the adrenal gland that contributes to sympathetic arousal and the general adaptation syndrome. See also Hydrocortisol.

Dementia. A general loss of mental ability (memory, quickness, accuracy, etc.) that is often associated—wrongly—with aging. It is more likely to be due to the prolonged effects of brain toxins such as medication, malnutrition, illness, or disuse.

Dendrite. The connective branching of the neuron that receives messages across the synapse from other neurons.

Deoxyribonucleic acid. See DNA.

DNA (deoxyribonucleic acid). The molecular basis of heredity found in cell nuclei.

Dopamine. One of the neurotransmitters associated with mood and movement.

Dualism. The view that the mind and brain are two separate entities that act independently of one another.

Dvorak keyboard. A redesigned keyboard in which the most frequently used keys are assigned to the strongest fingers, to increase speed and accuracy and reduce fatigue. See also Qwerty keyboard.

Endorphins. Literally "morphine within," these neurotransmitters are triggered by aerobic exercise, pain, and laughter and result in a noticeably pleasurable sensation, as in "runner's high."

Epinephrine. A hormone and neurotransmitter produced by the adrenal gland that is associated with sympathetic arousal. Also called Adrenaline.

Epistemology. The branch of philosophy that studies the structure of knowledge.

Estrogens. The family of female sex hormones that is responsible for the development of female gender characteristics, from reproduction to calmness.

Evoked potential. An electroencephalographic measurement of a neural impulse in response to a controlled stimulus, which may take the form of a light flash or an audible beep.

Explanatory style. See Attributional style.

Extrinsic motivation. The condition in which an activity is performed in expectation of rewards that are controlled by someone other than oneself (e.g., teacher, boss, or parent). See also Intrinsic motivation.

Fight-or-flight syndrome. See General adaptation syndrome.

General adaptation syndrome (GAS). The condition in which the body reacts to stress through activation of the sympathetic nervous system in preparation for having to fight, flee, or freeze. Also called the fight or flight syndrome.

Glial cells. Cells that support the networked structure of neurons; a kind of skeleton for the nervous system.

Habituation. A loss of sensitivity resulting from a prolonged pattern of stimulation; for example, the steady blinking of a neon sign will soon become unnoticeable (i.e., we habituate to it), but a random blinking will keep our attention.

Hard-wired. In computerese, a program that is built into the computer and can't be changed without major surgery. In brain lingo, the term refers to behaviors, traits, and instincts that we are born with.

Hydrocortisol. Pharmaceutical version of cortisol.

Hypothalamus. A part of the limbic system that is regarded as the body's main thermostat; it coordinates basic metabolism and related functions and the alternation between sympathetic and parasympathetic arousal.

Intrinsic motivation. The condition in which an activity is performed for its own enjoyment, with no expectation of rewards from other persons. See also Extrinsic motivation.

Latency. the width of the wave that measures action potential; a measure of the speed of response.

Limbic system. The portion of the midbrain (including the hippocampus, amygdala, hypothalamus, and olfactory area) that is associated with activating the general adaptation syndrome, or preparing the body for fight or flight; the main housing of emotional functions.

Locus of control. See Attributional style.

Massed learning. An approach to learning in which a single topic of instruction is executed without significant interruptions (or "spaces") between modules; it is the opposite of spaced learning.

Melatonin. A neurotransmitter originating in the pineal gland (a catabolite of serotonin), whose production is suppressed by natural light. It plays a key role in setting the body clock and in sleep onset and is available in some countries in pill form.

Mentation. A shorter expression than (but meaning the same thing as) mental activity.

Meta-analysis. A statistical technique by which a large number of separate studies on the same subject are analyzed for patterns.

Modular perspective. See Molar perspective.

Molar perspective. A big-picture, or top-down, look at a subject, as in studying the behaviors associated with a personality trait; the opposite of molecular perspective. Also called modular perspective.

Molecular perspective. A microscopic, or bottom-up, look at a subject, as in studying the body chemistry associated with personality traits; the opposite of molar perspective.

Monism. The view that brain and mind are one and the same, or that spirit cannot exist without matter.

Monozygotic twins. Twins that develop from one single fertilized egg and possess identical genetic structure.

Myelin sheath. The coating of the neural fiber; the thicker it is, the more efficient the neural transmission. Poor nutrition prevents normal myelin development.

Negative feedback. In neurophysiology, the tendency of a system that has changed to return to a normal state, as when a fire is doused; this happens with the general adaptation syndrome. See also Positive feedback.

Nerve growth factor (NGF). One of many trophic agents; it is released as a result of neural transmission and supports the growth of neural processes.

Neurolinguistic programming (NLP). The theory that asserts that people are programmed to communicate through one or more of three channels—visual, auditory, or kinesthetic—and can communicate more effectively by matching another person's preferred channel.

Neuron. A nerve cell; its major parts are the nucleus, axon, and dendrite.

Neuropeptide. A large group of peptides that act as neurotransmitters; they are involved particularly in emotions, hunger (e.g., cholecystokinin), pain (e.g., endorphins), and sleep (e.g., melatonin).

Neuropharmacology. The study of the effect of pharmaceuticals on the nervous system.

Neurotransmitters. A general term for chemicals that pass through the nervous system, transmitting nerve impulses across synapses. Different combinations of neurotransmitters, each of which can exhibit different states (e.g., weak vs. strong), result in different behaviors, thoughts, and emotions. Neurotransmitters, along with genes and ionic concentrations, make up the basic communication elements of the nervous system.

Nootropics. A family of drugs that purportedly enhance brain structure and function.

Noradrenaline. See Norepinephrine.

Norepinephrine. Like epinephrine, a hormone and neurotransmitter from the adrenal gland that is associated with sympathetic arousal. Also called noradrenaline.

Ontogeny recapitulates phylogeny. This terse phrase states that the development of each individual organism (ontogeny) reproduces the development of its species (phylogeny) from its origins to the present. In other words, during a human embryo's time in the womb, one can trace the stages of development from lizard through ape to human: the reptilian brain is the first to be identified (hindbrain), followed by the mammalian brain (midbrain) and culminating with the human brain (forebrain).

Paradigm. A set of assumptions in a defined area of knowledge that guides both research and applications in that area of knowledge, such as the assumption in pre-Copernican cosmology that the earth was at the center of the universe.

Paradigmatic shift. A fundamental change in one or more assumptions in a defined area of knowledge, such as Copernicus' assertion that the sun, not the earth, occupied the center of our solar system.

Parasympathetic arousal. See Sympathetic arousal.

Peptide. A compound formed by so-called head-to-tail linkups of two or more amino acids.

Phylogeny. See Ontogeny recapitulates phylogeny.

PNI. See Psychoneuroimmunology.

Positive feedback. In neurophysiology, the tendency of a change in a system to continue increasing in intensity, as in fanning a fire. See also Negative feedback.

Progesterone. A female sex hormone that is associated with preparation of the woman's body to care for a fertilized egg; levels increase at ovulation and decrease at menses.

Proto-oncogenes. About 100 genes that, when activated in certain combinations, cause cancer.

Psychoneuroimmunology (PNI). The study of how the body's immune system is affected by changes in mental and physical states. Its premise is that negative emotions lower resistance and positive emotions increase resistance.

Qwerty keyboard. The traditional keyboard in which the second row from the top begins, from the left side, "q...w...e...r...t...y." See also Dvorak keyboard.

Rapid eye movement (REM). The phase of the sleep cycle that consists of dreaming and motor neuron activity (but without physical movement other than eye movement); it is also called paradoxical sleep, since the motor neuron activity makes it appear on a brain scan that the sleeper is awake.

Receptor. A point on a dendritic terminal that receives a neurotransmitter from the axon connected at its synaptic gap.

Relaxation response. The body's response to an activity, such as meditation or aerobic exercise, that helps to return a stressed or sympathetically aroused person to a more relaxed state (parasympathetic arousal). See also Sympathetic arousal.

Reticular activating system (RAS). An area of the brain that acts like a kind of toggle switch so that, when the cerebral cortex is fully functional (e.g., relaxing, problem solving, planning, or creating), the limbic system (stress response) is not, and vice versa. Under stress, the RAS shuts the cerebral cortex down, and in the absence of stress it allows the cerebral cortex to fully function.

Reuptake inhibitor. Any chemical agent that prevents a neurotransmitter that has not reached the postsynaptic region from returning to the presynaptic region and hence prevents it from being retained for later use.

Routinize. To practice a skill to the point of being able to do it without consciously thinking about it.

SD. See Standard deviation.

Serotonin. A neurotransmitter involved in depression (too little), relaxation and sleep (just right), and aggression (too much); it is associated with vasoconstriction and headache relief.

Somatosensory. The part of the brain and nervous system that conveys messages that deal with bodily sensations of touch and movement.

Spaced learning. An approach to learning in which a single topic of instruction is broken up into modules and scheduled over time with breaks (or "spaces") between modules; it is the opposite of massed learning.

Standard deviation (SD). A measure of how closely members of a group score to the mean; roughly one-third of a group score within 1 SD above the mean, another one-third score within 1 SD below the mean, and the rest score higher or lower.

Stimulus-response psychology. See Behaviorism.

Sympathetic arousal. Mobilization by the body of its vast energy resources to fight off threat; parasympathetic arousal is the body's return to a more normal, relaxed state. See also General adaptation syndrome; Relaxation response.

Synapse. The synapse is the point of connection between two neurons, the area where a branch of an axon of one neuron has established a connection (they don't actually touch!) with the branch of a dendrite of another neuron. The synapse is the basic unit of learning. Knowledge can be measured by the number of existing synapses; effective use of knowledge is a reflection of their physical condition. The actual space through which neurotransmitters pass from one neuron to another is called the synaptic gap. As with the gap in a spark plug, the adjacent membranes of the axon and dendrite that form the synapse must be clean and healthy.

Synaptic gap. See Synapse.

Talking therapy. The practice of talking with a therapist for relief of psychological distress; it may be used instead of, or in addition to, drug therapy.

Testosterone. See Androgens.

Trophic. Contributing to growth; nutritional.

Type I, II error. Terms used in research to describe two related cases: when a difference in means is claimed although in fact no difference exists (Type I error) and when an equality of means is claimed although in fact the means are different (Type II error); that is, in Type I, an effect is claimed and none is present, and in Type II, no effect is claimed when one is in fact present.

Vasoconstriction. Shrinkage of the walls of a blood vessel; it is thought to be associated with headache relief. See also Vasodilation.

Vasodilation. Stretching, dilation, or relaxation of the walls of a blood vessel; vasodilation of blood vessels in the brain is associated with the onset of headaches. See also Vasoconstriction.

Visualization. Using the mind to review a series of bodily movements such as a downhill ski run or to prepare for a speech by giving it without actually going through the bodily movements. Visualization may be accompanied by either a running verbal commentary, some limited physical movement (such as so-called body English), or both. It is usually performed with the eyes closed.

Bibliography

Ackerman, D. (1990). *A Natural History of the Senses*. New York: Random House.

Adams, J. L. (1980). *Conceptual Blockbusting: A Guide to Better Ideas*. (2nd ed.). New York: W. W. Norton.

Adams, J. L. (1986). *The Care and Feeding of Ideas: A Guide to Encouraging Creativity*. Reading, MA: Addison-Wesley.

Albrecht, K. (no date). *Mind Mapping: A Tool for Clear Thinking*. [Videotape]. (10 minutes). San Diego, CA: Shamrock.

Allison, M. (1991, October). "Stopping the Brain Drain." *Harvard Health Letter, 16*, 6 ff.

Amabile, T. M. (1983). *The Social Psychology of Creativity*. New York: Springer-Verlag.

Anderson, J. R. (1993, January). "Problem Solving and Learning." *American Psychologist, 48*(1), 35–44.

Arkin, A. M., Antrobus, J. S., & Ellman, S. J. (Eds.). (1978). *The Mind in Sleep*. Hillsdale, NJ: Lawrence Erlbaum.

Armstrong, T. (1993). *Seven Kinds of Smart: Identifying and Developing Your Many Intelligences*. New York: Plume.

Atkins, S. (1978). *LIFO Training: Discovery Workbook*. Beverly Hills, CA: Stuart Atkins.

Bailey, C. (1991). *The New Fit or Fat*. Boston: Houghton Mifflin.

Bales, J. (1991, November). "Work Stress Grows, But Services Decline." *APA Monitor*, p. 32.

Bandler, R., & Grinder, J. (1982). *ReFraming: Neuro-Linguistic Programming and the Transformation of Meaning*. Moab, UT: Real People Press.

Bartlett, F. C. (1932). *Remembering*. Cambridge, England: Cambridge University Press.

Behn, R. D., & Vaupel, J. W. (1982). *Quick Analysis for Busy Decision Makers*. New York: Basic Books.

Bennett, W. (1991, October). "Obesity Is Not an Eating Disorder." *Harvard Mental Health Letter, 8*(4).

Benson, H., with Klipper, M. Z. (1976). *The Relaxation Response*. New York: Avon.

Bertalanffy, L. von. (1967). *Robots, Men and Minds: Psychology in the Modern World*. New York: Braziller.

Birdwhistell, R. L. (1970). *Kinesics and Context: Essays on Body Motion Communication*. Philadelphia: University of Pennsylvania Press.

Birren, F. (1978a). *Color and Human Response*. New York: Van Nostrand Reinhold.

Birren, F. (1978b). *Color in Your World*. New York: Collier.

Black, I. B. (1991). *Information in the Brain: A Molecular Perspective*. Cambridge, MA: MIT Press.

Block, P. (1987). *The Empowered Manager: Positive Political Skills at Work*. San Francisco: Jossey-Bass.

Boden, M. A. (1990). *The Creative Mind: Myths and Mechanisms*. New York: Basic Books.

Bois, J. S. (1966). *The Art of Awareness: A Textbook on General Semantics*. Dubuque, IA: William. C. Brown.

Bok, S. (1979). *Lying: Moral Choice in Public and Private Life*. New York: Vintage.

Bolles, E. B. (1988). *Remembering and Forgetting: An Inquiry into the Nature of Memory.* New York: Walker.

Bransford, J. D., & Stein, B. S. (1984). *The Ideal Problem Solver.* New York: W. H. Freeman.

Brody, N. (1992). *Intelligence.* (2nd ed.). San Diego: Academic Press.

Buss, A. H. (1989). "Personality as Traits." *American Psychologist, 44*(11), 1378–1388.

Buss, D. M. (Ed.). (1990, March). "Biological Foundations of Personality: Evolution, Behavioral Genetics, and Psychophysiology." *Journal of Personality* [Special Issue], *58*(1).

Buzan, T. (1991). *Use Your Perfect Memory.* (3rd ed.). New York: Penguin.

Cacioppo, J. T., & Berntson, G. G. (1992, August). "Social Psychological Contributions to the Decade of the Brain: Doctrine of Multilevel Analysis." *American Psychologist, 47*(8), 1019–1028.

Cacioppo, J. T., & Tassinary, L. G. (Eds.). (1990). *Principles of Psychophysiology: Physical, Social, and Inferential Elements.* Cambridge, England: Cambridge University Press.

Caine, R. N., & Caine, G. (1991). *Making Connections: Teaching and the Human Brain.* Alexandria, VA: Association for Supervision and Curriculum Development.

Campbell, R. J. (1989). *Psychiatric Dictionary.* (6th ed.). New York: Oxford University Press.

Capra, F. (1984). *The Tao of Physics.* (2nd ed.). Toronto: Bantam.

Cavett, D. (1992, August 3). "Goodbye, Darkness." *People Weekly, 38,* 88 ff.

Clark, W. V. (1956). "The Construction of an Industrial Selection Personality Test." *Journal of Psychology, 41,* 379–394.

Collin, F. (1992, May). "Sarah Leibowitz (Interview)." *OMNI, 14*(8), 73 ff.

"Combatting Stress at Work." (1993, January). *Conditions of Work Digest* [Special Issue], *12*(1).

Coren, S. (1992). *The Left-Hander Syndrome: The Causes and Consequences of Left-Handedness.* New York: Free Press.

Costa, P. T., Jr., & McCrae, R. R. (1992). *NEO Personality Inventory: Revised Professional Manual.* Odessa, FL: Psychological Assessment Resources.

Cousins, N. (1979). *Anatomy of an Illness.* New York: W. W. Norton.

Cousins, N. (1989). *Head First: The Biology of Hope.* New York: Dutton.

Covey, S. R. (1990). *The Seven Habits of Highly Effective People.* New York: Simon & Schuster

Crawford, M., & Gentry, M. (Eds.). (1989). *Gender and Thought.* New York: Springer-Verlag.

Crichton, M. (1990). *Jurassic Park: A Novel.* New York: Knopf.

Csikszentmihalyi, M. (1990). *Flow: The Psychology of Optimal Experience.* New York: HarperCollins.

Dahlitz, M., Alvarez, D., Vignau, J., English, J., Arendt, J., & Parkes, J. D. (1991, May 11). "Delayed Sleep Phase Syndrome Response to Melatonin." *The Lancet, 337,* 1121 ff.

Dalton, K. (1987). *Once a Month.* (4th ed.). Glasgow: Fontana Original.

Dawkins, R. (1989). *The Selfish Gene.* (2nd ed.). Oxford: Oxford University Press.

Dean, W., & Morgenthaler, J. (1990). *Smart Drugs & Nutrients.* Santa Cruz, CA: B & J Publications.

DeAngelis, T. (1992, February). "Cutting Cholesterol: Feeling Feisty?" *The APA Monitor,* 8–9.

de Bono, E. (1967). *New Think.* New York: Basic Books.

Deming, W. E. (1986). *Out of the Crisis.* Cambridge, MA: MIT Center for Advanced Engineering Study.

Diamond, M. (1988). *Enriching Heredity: The Impact of the Environment on the Anatomy of the Brain.* New York: Free Press.

Digman, J. M., & Inouye, J. (1986). "Further Specification of the Five Robust Factors of Personality." *Journal of Personality and Social Psychology, 50,* 116–123.

Dinges, D. F., & Broughton, R. J. (1989). *Sleep and Alertness: Chronobiological, Behavioral, and Medical Aspects of Napping.* New York: Raven Press.

Dreikurs, R., & Cassel, P. (1972). *Discipline Without Tears.* (rev. ed.). New York: Hawthorne Books.

Druckman, D., & Bjork, R. A. (Eds.). (1991). *In the Mind's Eye: Understanding Human Performance.* Washington, DC: National Academy Press.

Druckman, D., & Swets, J. A. (Eds.). (1988). *Enhancing Human Performance: Issues, Theories, and Techniques.* Washington, DC: National Academy Press.

Eaves, L. J., Eysenck, H. J., & Martin, N. G. (1989). *Genes, Culture and Personality.* London: Academic Press.

Eckles, R. W., Carmichael, R. L., & Sarchet, B. R. (1981). *Supervisory Management.* New York: Wiley.

Edelman, G. M. (1987). *Neural Darwinism: The Theory of Neuronal Group Selection.* New York: Basic Books.

Edelman, G. M. (1992). *Bright Air, Brilliant Fire: On the Matter of the Mind.* New York: Basic Books.

Education Research. (1987). *Problem Solving.* Education Research, 370 Lexington Ave., New York, NY 10017.

Education Research. (1988). *Decision Making.* Education Research, 370 Lexington Ave., New York, NY 10017.

Edwards, B. (1989). *Drawing on the Right Side of the Brain.* (rev. ed.). Los Angeles: Tarcher.

Ekman, P. (1985). *Telling Lies.* New York: W. W. Norton.

Epstein, S., & Meier, P. (1989). "Constructive Thinking: A Broad Coping Variable with Specific Components." *Journal of Personality and Social Psychology, 57*(2), 332–350.

Escher, M. C. (1983). *M. C. Escher: Twenty-Nine Master Prints.* New York: Abrams.

Eysenck, H. J. (1967). *The Biological Basis of Personality.* Springfield, IL: Charles C Thomas.

Eysenck, H. J. (1970). *The Structure of Human Personality.* (rev. ed.). London: Methuen.

Eysenck, H. J. (Ed.). (1981). *A Model for Personality.* Berlin: Springer-Verlag.

Eysenck, H. J., & Eysenck, M. W. (1985). *Personality and Individual Differences: A Natural Science Approach.* New York: Plenum.

Eysenck, H. J., & Kamin, L. (1981). *The Intelligence Controversy.* New York: Wiley.

Falletta, N. (1983). *The Paradoxicon.* Garden City, NY: Doubleday.

Fisher, M. (1981). *Intuition: How to Use It for Success and Happiness.* New York: Dutton.

Flanders, N. A. (1970). *Analyzing Teacher Behavior.* Reading, MA: Addison-Wesley.

Fluegelman, A. (Ed.). (1976). *The New Games Book.* Garden City, NY: Dolphin/Doubleday.

Folkins, C. H., & Sime, W. E. (1981, April). "Physical Fitness Training and Mental Health." *American Psychologist, 36*(4), 373–389.

Fowler, J. W. (1982). *Stages of Faith: The Psychology of Human Development and the Quest for Meaning.* New York: HarperCollins.

Fox, N. A. (1991). "If It's Not Left, It's Right: Electroencephalograph Asymmetry and the Development of Emotion." *American Psychologist, 46,* 863–872.

Gallagher, R. M. (Ed.). (1990). *Drug Therapy for Headache.* New York: Marcel Dekker.

Gardner, H. (1983). *Frames of Mind: The Theory of Multiple Intelligences.* New York: Basic Books.

Gardner, H. (1985). *The Mind's New Science: A History of the Cognitive Revolution.* New York: Basic Books.

Gardner, H. (1991). *The Unschooled Mind: How Schools Should Teach*. New York: Basic Books.

Gardner, M. (1979). *The Ambidextrous Universe: Mirror Asymmetry and Time-Reversed Worlds*. (2nd ed.). New York: Scribner's.

Gawain, S. (1978). *Creative Visualization*. Berkeley, CA: New World Library.

Gazzaniga, M. S. (1985). *The Social Brain*. New York: Basic Books.

Gazzaniga, M. S. (1988). *Mind Matters: How Mind and Brain Interact to Create Our Conscious Lives*. Boston: Houghton Mifflin.

Geen, R. G., Beatty, W. W., and Arkin, R. M. (1984). *Human Motivation: Physiological, Behavioral, and Social Approaches*. Boston: Allyn & Bacon.

Gitlow, H., Gitlow, S., Oppenheim, A., & Oppenheim, R. (1989). *Tools and Methods for the Improvement of Quality*. Homewood, IL: Irwin.

Glasser, W. (1990). *The Quality School: Managing Students Without Coercion*. New York: Harper Perennial Library.

Gleick, J. (1987). *Chaos: Making a New Science*. New York: Viking.

Goldberg, L. R. (1993, January). "The Structure of Phenotypic Personality Traits." *American Psychologist, 48*(1), 26–34.

Goldberg, P. (1983). *The Intuitive Edge*. Los Angeles: Tarcher.

Goleman, D., Kaufman, P., & Ray, M. (1992). *The Creative Spirit*. New York: Dutton.

Golembiewski, R. T. (1988). *Phases of Burnout*. New York: Praeger.

Gray, J. A. (1971). *The Psychology of Fear and Stress*. New York: McGraw-Hill.

Gregory, R. L. (Ed.). (1987). *The Oxford Companion to the Mind*. New York: Oxford University Press.

Hart, L. A. (1983). *Human Brain and Human Learning*. New York: Longman.

Hayes, J. R. (1989). *The Complete Problem Solver*. (2nd ed.). Hillsdale, NJ: Lawrence Erlbaum.

Healy, J. (1990). *Endangered Minds: Why Our Children Don't Think*. New York: Simon & Schuster.

Heisenberg, W. (1962). *Physics and Philosophy: The Revolution in Modern Science*. New York: HarperCollins.

Herber, H. (1978). *Teaching Reading in Content Areas*. (2nd ed.). Englewood Cliffs, NJ: Prentice-Hall.

Herrmann, D. J. (1991). *Super Memory: A Quick-Action Program for Memory Improvement*. Emmaus, PA: Rodale.

Herrmann, N. (1989). *The Creative Brain*. Lake Lure, NC: Brain Books.

Hersey, P., & Blanchard, K. H. (1976). *Management of Organization Behavior: Utilizing Human Resources*. (3rd ed.). Englewood Cliffs, NJ: Prentice-Hall.

Hobson, J. A. (1988). *The Dreaming Brain*. New York: Basic Books.

Hofstadter, D. R. (1979). *Gödel, Escher, Bach: An Eternal Golden Braid*. New York: Basic Books.

Holland, J. L. (1985). *Making Vocational Choices: A Theory of Vocational Personalities and Work Environments*. Englewood Cliffs, NJ: Prentice-Hall.

Hooper, J., & Teresi, D. (1986). *The Three-Pound Universe*. New York: Macmillan.

Horney, K. (1945). *Our Inner Conflicts*. New York: W. W. Norton.

Huff, D. (1954). *How to Lie with Statistics*. New York: W. W. Norton.

Hunt, M. (1982). *The Universe Within: A New Science Explores the Human Mind*. New York: Simon & Schuster.

"Hypnosis." (1991). *Harvard Mental Health Letter, 7*(10), 1–4.

Ingelfinger, F. (1980). "Arrogance." *New England Journal of Medicine, 303*, 1506–1511.

Ironson, G., et al. (1992, August). "Effects of Anger on Left Ventricular Ejection Fraction in Coronary Artery Disease." *American Journal of Cardiology, 70,* 281–285.

Izard, C. E., Kagan, J., & Zajonc, R. B. (Eds.). (1984). *Emotions, Cognition, and Behavior.* Cambridge, England: Cambridge University Press.

Jaffe, C. L., Jr. (1991). *Using "Practical Knowledge" Versus Cognitive Ability to Predict Job Performance for Personnel in Customer Oriented Jobs.* Unpublished doctoral dissertation, University of South Florida, Tampa.

John, O. P., Angleitner, A., & Ostendorf, F. (1988). "The Lexical Approach to Personality: A Historical Review of Trait Taxonomic Research." *European Journal of Personality, 2,* 171–203.

Johnson-Laird, P. (1988). *The Computer and the Mind: An Introduction to Cognitive Science.* Cambridge, MA: Harvard University Press.

Jung, C. G. (1971). *Psychological Types.* Princeton, NJ: Princeton University Press.

Kallan, C. (1991, October). "Probing the Power of Common Scents." *Prevention, 43*(10), 39–43.

Katahn, M. (1991). *One Meal at a Time.* New York: W. W. Norton.

Keeton, K. (1992). *Longevity: The Science of Staying Young.* New York: Viking.

Keirsey, D., & Bates, M. (1978). *Please Understand Me.* Del Mar, CA: Prometheus Nemesis.

Kepner, C. H., & Tregoe, B. B. (1981). *The New Rational Manager.* Princeton, NJ: Princeton Research Press.

Kiecolt-Glaser, J. K., & Glaser, R. (1992). "Psychoneuroimmunology: Can Psychological Interventions Modulate Immunity?" *Journal of Consulting and Clinical Psychology, 60*(4), 569–575.

Kimura, D., & Hampson, E. (1990, April). "Neural and Hormonal Mechanisms Mediating Sex Differences in Cognition." *Research Bulletin No. 689.* London, Ontario: Department of Psychology, University of Western Ontario.

Kinlaw, D. C. (1990). *Developing Superior Work Teams.* New York: Free Press.

Kline, M. (1953). *Mathematics in Western Culture.* New York: Oxford University Press.

Koestler, A. (1964). *The Act of Creation.* New York: Macmillan.

Kogan, Z. (1956). *Essentials in Problem Solving.* New York: Arco.

Kohlberg, L. (1984). *The Psychology of Moral Development: The Nature and Validity of Moral Stages.* New York: HarperCollins.

Kolata, G. B. (1976). "Brain Biochemistry: Effects of Diet." *Science, 192,* 41–42.

Kolata, G. B. (1979). "Mental Disorders: A New Approach to Treatment?" *Science, 203,* 36–38.

Kolbe, K. (1990). *The Conative Connection.* Reading, MA: Addison-Wesley.

Korzybski, A. (1948). *Science and Sanity: An Introduction to Non-Aristotelian Systems and General Semantics.* (3rd ed.). Lakeville, CT: International Non-Aristotelian Library.

Kuhn, T. S. (1970). *The Structure of Scientific Revolutions.* (2nd ed.). Chicago: University of Chicago Press.

Laborde, G. Z. (1983). *Influencing with Integrity.* Palo Alto, CA: Syntony.

Laborde, G. Z. (1988). *Fine Tune Your Brain.* Palo Alto, CA: Syntony.

Latané, B., & Darley, J. (1970). *The Unresponsive Bystander: Why Doesn't He Help?* New York: Appleton-Century-Crofts.

Lazarus, R. S. (1991a). *Emotion and Adaptation.* New York: Oxford University Press.

Lazarus, R. S. (1991b, August). "Progress on a Cognitive-Motivational-Relational Theory of Emotion." *American Psychologist, 46,* 819–834.

Lee, C. (1987, September). "Mindmapping: Brainstorming on Paper." *Training, 24*(9), 71–76.

Lefton, R. E., Buzzotta, V., & Sherberg, M. (1985). *Improving Productivity Through People Skills.* Boston: Ballinger.

Lenneberg, E. H. (1967). *Biological Foundations of Language.* New York: Wiley.

LeShan, L. (1989). *Cancer as a Turning Point.* New York: Dutton.

Long, M. E. (1987, December). "What Is This Thing Called Sleep?" *National Geographic, 172*(6), 787–821.

Lorayne, H., & Lucas, J. (1974). *The Memory Book.* New York: Stein & Day.

MacLean, P. D. (1990). *The Triune Brain in Evolution.* New York: Plenum.

Marston, W. M. (1987). *The Emotions of Normal People.* Minneapolis, MN: Carlson Learning.

Maslow, A. H. (1943). "A Theory of Human Motivation." *Psychological Review, 50,* 370–396.

McClelland, D. C. (1986). "Some Reflections on the Two Psychologies of Love." *Journal of Personality, 54,* 334–353.

McClelland, D. C., & Kirshnit, C. (1988). "The Effect of Motivational Arousal Through Films on Immunoglobulin A." *Psychology and Health, 2,* 31–52.

McCrae, R. M., & Costa, P. T. (1989). "Reinterpreting the Myers-Briggs Type Indicator from the Perspective of the Five-Factor Model of Personality." *Journal of Personality, 57*(1), 17–40.

McCrae, R. M., & Costa, P. T. (1990). *Personality in Adulthood.* New York: Guilford Press.

McGuire, C. B., & Radner, R. (Eds.). (1972). *Decision and Organization.* Amsterdam: North-Holland.

McNamee, P., & Celona, J. (1987). *Decision Analysis for the Professional with Supertree.* Redwood City, CA: Scientific Press.

Mehrabian, A. (1971). *Silent Messages.* Belmont, CA: Wadsworth.

Merrill, D. W., & Reid, H. H. (1981). *Personal Style and Effective Performance.* Radnor, PA: Chilton.

Merzbacher, C. F. (1979, April). "A Diet and Exercise Regimen: Its Effect upon Mental Acuity and Personality. A Pilot Study." *Perceptual and Motor Skills, 48*(2), 367–371.

Miller, G. A. (1956). "The Magical Number Seven, Plus or Minus Two: Some Limits on Our Capacity for Processing Information." *Psychological Review, 63,* 81–97.

Minninger, J. (1984). *Total Recall: How to Boost Your Memory Power.* Emmaus, PA: Rodale.

Mischel, W. (1968). *Personality and Assessment.* New York: Wiley.

Moir, A., & Jessel, D. (1991). *Brain Sex: The Real Difference Between Men and Women.* New York: Carol.

Moody, P. E. (1983). *Decision Making: Proven Methods for Better Decisions.* New York: McGraw-Hill.

Murray, H. A. (1938). *Explorations in Personality.* New York: Oxford University Press.

Myers, I. B., & McCauley, M. H. (1985). *Manual: A Guide to the Development and Use of the Myers-Briggs Type Indicator.* Palo Alto, CA: Consulting Psychologists Press.

Nadler, G., & Hibino, S. (1990). *Breakthrough Thinking.* Rocklin, CA: Prima.

National Research Council, Committee on Diet and Health. (1989). *Diet and Health: Implications for Reducing Chronic Disease Risk.* Washington, DC: National Academy Press.

Neubauer, P. B., & Neubauer, A. (1990). *Nature's Thumbprint: The New Genetics of Personality.* Reading, MA.: Addison-Wesley.

Nierenberg, G. I. (1985). *The Idea Generator.* Berkeley, CA: Experience in Software.

Norman, W. T. (1963). "Toward an Adequate Taxonomy of Personality Attributes: Replicated Factor Structure in Peer Nomination Personality Ratings." *Journal of Abnormal and Social Psychology, 66,* 574–583.

Northrop, F.S.C. (1946). *The Meeting of East and West: An Inquiry Concerning World Understanding.* New York: Macmillan.

Northrop, F.S.C. (1947). *The Logic of the Sciences and the Humanities.* Cleveland, OH: World.

Okogbaa, O. G., & Shell, R. L. (1986, December). "The Measurement of Knowledge Worker Fatigue." *IEEE Transactions, 18*(4), 335–342.

Ornstein, R., and Sobel, D. (1987) *The Healing Brain.* New York: Simon & Schuster.

Peck, M. S. (1987). *The Different Drum: Community-Making and Peace.* New York: Simon & Schuster.

Pemberton, W. H. (1989). *Sanity for Survival: A Semantic Approach to Conflict Resolution.* San Francisco: Graphic Guides.

Petri, H. L. (1991). *Motivation: Theory, Research, and Applications.* (3rd ed.). Belmont, CA: Wadsworth.

Piaget, J. (1977). *The Essential Piaget,* Ed. Guber, H. E., & Vaneche, J. J. New York: Basic Books.

Pirsig, R. M. (1974). *Zen and the Art of Motorcycle Maintenance: An Inquiry into Values.* New York: Morrow.

Plunkett, L. C., & Hale, G. A. (1982). *The Proactive Manager: The Complete Book of Problem Solving and Decision Making.* New York: Wiley.

Plutchik, R., & Kellerman, H. (Eds.). (1989). *The Measurement of Emotions.* (Vol. 4 in *Emotions: Theory, Research, and Experience,* Ed. Plutchik, R., & Kellerman, H.). San Diego, CA: Academic Press.

Pollitt, E., Leibel, R. L., & Greenfield, D. (1981). "Brief Fasting, Stress, and Cognition in Children." *American Journal of Clinical Nutrition, 34,* 1526–1533.

Polya, G. C. (1971). *How to Solve It: A New Aspect of Mathematical Method.* (2nd ed.). Princeton, NJ: Princeton University Press.

Poundstone, W. (1988). *Labyrinths of Reason: Paradox, Puzzles, and the Frailty of Knowledge.* New York: Doubleday/Anchor.

Prince, G. M. (1970). *The Practice of Creativity.* New York: Collier.

Raloff, J. (1991, October 5). "Searching Out How a Severe Diet Slows Aging." *Science News, 140*(14).

Reid, D. P. (1989). *The Tao of Health, Sex, and Longevity: A Modern Guide to the Ancient Way.* New York: Simon & Schuster.

Restak, R. M. (1984). *The Brain.* New York: Bantam.

Restak, R. M. (1988). *The Mind.* New York: Bantam.

Restak, R. M. (1991). *The Brain Has a Mind of Its Own.* New York: Harmony.

Rickards, T. (1974). *Problem-Solving Through Creative Analysis.* Epping, England: Gower.

Rogers, R. (Ed.). (1988). *Clinical Assessment of Malingering and Deception.* New York: Guilford Press.

Rosenfield, I. (1988). *The Invention of Memory: A New View of the Brain.* New York: Basic Books.

Rosenthal, R., & Jacobson, L. (1968). *Pygmalion in the Classroom.* New York: Holt, Rinehart & Winston.

Rossi, E. L., & Nimmons, D. (1991). *The 20-Minute Break: Using the New Science of Ultradian Rhythms.* Los Angeles: Tarcher.

Rowan, R. (1986). *The Intuitive Manager.* Boston: Little, Brown.

Saaty, T. L. (1982). *Decision Making for Leaders: The Analytical Hierarchy Process for Decisions in a Complex World.* Belmont, CA: Lifetime Learning.

Schachter, S., & Singer, J. E. (1962). "Cognitive, Social, and Physiological Determinants of Emotional States." *Psychological Review, 69,* 379–399.

Schlosberg, H. S. (1954). "Three Dimensions of Emotion." *Psychological Review, 61*, 81–88.

Schmidt, D. E., & Keating, J. P. (1979). Human Crowding and Personal Control: An Integration of the Research." *Psychological Bulletin, 86*, 680–700.

Seligman, M.E.P. (1984). *Seligman Attributional Style Questionnaire.* (Available by calling Martin Seligman or Peter Schulman at 215-898-2748.)

Seligman, M.E.P. (1991). *Learned Optimism.* New York: Knopf.

Selye, H. (1952). *The Story of the Adaptation Syndrome.* Montreal: Acta.

Senge, P. (1990). *The Fifth Discipline.* New York: Doubleday/Currency.

Siegel, B. (1987). *Love, Medicine and Miracles.* New York: HarperCollins.

Simon, H. (1969). *Sciences of the Artificial.* Cambridge, MA: MIT Press.

Simonton, O. C., Simonton, S., and Creighton, J. (1980). *Getting Well Again.* New York: Bantam.

Sternberg, R. J. (1988). *The Triarchic Mind: A New Theory of Human Intelligence.* New York: Viking.

Stevens, W. (1951). *The Necessary Angel.* New York: Knopf.

Stevens, W. (1967). *The Collected Poems of Wallace Stevens.* New York: Knopf.

Tellagen, A., Lykken, D. T., Bouchard, T. J., Wilcox, K. J., Segal, N. L., & Rich, S. (1988). "Personality Similarity in Twins Reared Apart and Together." *Journal of Personality and Social Psychology, 54*(6), 1031–1039.

Thagard, P. (1992). "Adversarial Problem Solving: Modeling an Opponent Using Explanatory Coherence." *Cognitive Science, 16*, 123–149.

Thayer, R. E. (1989). *Biopsychology of Mood and Arousal.* New York: Oxford University Press.

Thomas, M. C., & Thomas, T. S. (1990). *Getting Commitment at Work: A Guide for Managers and Employees.* Chapel Hill, NC: Commitment Press.

Thompson, C. (1992). *What a Great Idea! The Key Steps Creative People Take.* New York: HarperCollins.

Thompson, J. G. (1988). *The Psychobiology of Emotions.* New York: Plenum.

Toates, F. (1986). *The Biological Foundations of Behavior.* Philadelphia: Open University Press.

Torrance, E. P. (1974). *Torrance Tests of Creative Thinking.* Bensenville, IL: Scholastic Testing Service.

Toufexis, A. (1989, March 13). "The Latest Word on What to Eat." *Time, 133*(11), 51–52.

Vernon, P. A. (Ed.). (1987). *Speed of Information-Processing and Intelligence.* Norwood, NJ: Ablex.

von Oech, R. (1983). *A Whack on the Side of the Head: How to Unlock Your Mind for Innovation.* New York: Warner.

Wallas, G. (1926). *The Art of Thought.* London: J. Cape.

Walton, M. (1986). *The Deming Management Method.* New York: Dodd, Mead.

Watzlawick, P., Weakland, J. H., & Fisch, R. (1974). *Change: Principles of Problem Formation and Problem Resolution.* New York: W. W. Norton.

Weatherall, D. (1987, September). "New Light on Light." *Management Services, 31*(9), 38–39.

Webb, W. B. (Ed.). (1982). *Biological Rhythms, Sleep, and Performance.* Chichester, England: Wiley.

Webb, W. B. (1992). *Sleep: The Gentle Tyrant.* (2nd ed.). Bolton, MA: Anker.

Wiertelak, E., Maier, S. F., & Watkins, L. R. (1992, May 8). "Cholecystokinin Antianalgesia: Safety Cues Abolish Morphine Analgesia." *Science, 256*, 830 ff.

Williams, C. L., et al. (1985). *The Negotiable Environment: People, White Collar Work, and the Office.* Ann Arbor, MI: Miller, Herman.

Williams, R. (1989). *The Trusting Heart: Great News About Type A Behavior.* New York: Times Books.

Winter, A., & Winter, R. (1988). *Eat Right, Be Bright.* New York: St. Martin's Press.

Woteki, C. E., & Thomas, P. R. (Eds.). (1992). *Eat for Life: The Food and Nutrition Board's Guide to Reducing Your Risk of Chronic Disease.* Washington, DC: National Academy Press.

Yepsen, R. B., Jr. (1987). *How to Boost Your Brain Power: Achieving Peak Intelligence, Memory and Creativity.* Emmaus, PA: Rodale.

Zdenek, M. (1985). *The Right-Brain Experience.* New York: McGraw-Hill.

Zeskine, P. S., Marshall, T. R., & Goss, D. M. (1992). "Rhythmic Organization of Heart Rate in Breast Fed and Bottle Fed Newborn Infants." *Early Development and Parenting, 1*(2), 79–87.

Zuckerman, M. (1991). *The Psychobiology of Personality.* New York: Cambridge University Press.

Index

Page numbers in italics refer to figures.

C

C-kinase, 241, 274
Cacioppo, J. T., 26, 41
Caffeine: during breaks, 206;
    dependence on, 85;
    jet lag and, 98;
    learning and, 266;
    multivitamins and, 79;
    negative consequences of, 84–85;
    normal effective dose of, 84–85, 183;
    simple activities when overstimulated by, 183;
    sleep and, 38;
    and staying awake, 96, 99;
    suggestions on, 85–86, 183
Caine, G., 192, 193, 203, 239, 259, 263, 268
Caine, R. N., 192, 193, 203, 239, 259, 263, 268
Calcium, 37, 40, 53, 54, 245–246
Calcium supplements, 72
California Institute of Technology, 25, 352
Calorie allowance, daily, 73
Calpain, 37, 40, 53, 245, 274, 355
Campbell, R. J., 178
Canasil, 215
Cancer, 65, 111
Capra, F., 133, 323, 324
Carbamazepine, 115
Carbohydrates: during breaks, 206;
    chemistry of urge for, 76;
    creativity and, 275, 285;
    learning and, 265;
    recommended daily allowance for, 70–72, 77, 334, 335;
    role of, 77;
    sleep and, 97, 98;
    and staying awake in early-morning hours, 96;
    time-zone changes and, 207;
    timing of consumption of, 77
Card sorts, 232
Caregivers, 114
Carmichael, R. L., 234
Carnegie Mellon University, 25, 352
Casals, P., 60
Case studies, 236, 238
Cassel, P., 193
Castro, F., 312
Catecholamines, 77, 355
CAVE (content analysis of verbatim explanations), 172
Cavett, D., 115
CCK. See Cholecystokinin (CCK)
CEDAC, 294

Celona, J., 290
Center for Applied Cognitive Studies, 20
Center on the Psychobiology of Ethnicity, 88
Cerebral cortex: animal versus human, 28, 28;
    definition of, 355;
    evolution of, 35;
    memory and, 243–244;
    motivation and, 176, 177;
    structure of, 36
Challenger, in Big Five, 136, 137, 224, 225, 274–275, 285, 289
Changeux, J. P., 108
Charthouse International, 313
Chemicals. See Alcohol consumption; Caffeine; Drugs; Medication
Chi, 174
Children: adopted children, 128;
    babysitting for, 181;
    breakfast for, 77;
    communication with, 322;
    creativity of, 282;
    experiences of, as building blocks for adult accomplishments, 62;
    food additives and, 74;
    games for, 296;
    intelligence of, 163;
    and irreversible brain damage, 61–62;
    mineral production spurts in, 62;
    nicotine used around, 87;
    personality of, 126, 128;
    rewards and punishments for, 193;
    seat belts for, 61;
    television watching of, 305–306. See also Infants
Chili peppers, 40–41
Chocolate, 38
Cholecystokinin (CCK), 73–74, 355
Cholesterol, in diet, 71
Cholinesterase, 245–246
Christie, A., 97
Chromosomal mutations, 48
Chunks and chunking, 205, 230–231, 242–243, 246–247, 248, 355
Circadian rhythm, 94–97, 99, 152
Circumplex model of emotions, 147
Clark, W. V., 132
Classical conditioning, 355
Closed-ended questions, 285
Clozapine, 115
Cocaine, 86, 89

Codeine, 90

Coffee. *See* Caffeine

Cognition, as referring to both mind and brain, 27

Cognitive, as referring to both mind and brain, 27

Cognitive dissonance, 355

Cognitive science: brain structure and hormones, 34–41;
    connectivity principle in, 29, 328;
    control principle in, 29, 328;
    core principles of, 29, 328;
    definition of, 15;
    difference between humans and animals, 27–28;
    historical development of, 24–26;
    interconnectivity principle in, 29, 328;
    interdisciplinary nature of, 24, 25–26;
    latest developments in, 24–32;
    mind-brain dichotomy and, 26–28;
    nativism principle in, 29, 328;
    paradigm shifts in, 329;
    resources on, 19;
    scientific method and, 29–32;
    unity principle in, 29, 328;
    universities offering interdisciplinary degree programs in, 352

Cognitive style, and motivation, 272

Cognitive therapy, 171–172, 355

Cohen, D., 124

Cohen, N., 111, 244

Color, 215–216, 265, 267

Color and Human Response (Birren), 215–216, 265

Color discrimination: gender differences in, 51

Color Rendering Index (CRI), 214

Commissurotomy, 355

Communication: of expectations, 197–198;
    males and, 56;
    of positive expectations, 262;
    process of, 322;
    proxemics and, 223–224;
    resources on, 322;
    skills of, 320–322;
    story on, 318–320

Comparison of means, 30, 32

Componential domain of intelligence, 158

Concentration, 217–218, 265, 283

Conflict management, 321

Connectivity, as principle in cognitive science, 29, 328

Conscientiousness dimension, of Big Five, 133, 136–137

Conscientiousness facets, in Big Five, 138, 139–140

Constructive criticism, 321

Contextual domain of intelligence, 159–160

Control: aging and, 64–65;
    creativity and, 286;
    immune system functioning and, 113;
    as principle in cognitive science, 29, 328;
    as response to stressors, 179

Coping mechanisms, for emotions, 152–153

Coren, S., 107, 117

Corpus callosum, 45, 46–47, 274, 355

Correlation, 30

Cortex, 355

Cortisol, 76, 181, 183, 188–189, 190, 355

Costa, P. T., Jr., 133, 134, 138, 140, 141, 142, 160

Couch-potato syndrome, 108, 168

Cousins, N., 63, 64, 110, 112, 113, 117, 173–174, 180, 197

Covey, S., 25, 88, 315, 322, 324

Creativity: assessment of, 280–282;
    biology of creative personality, 274–276;
    creativity-relevant skills in, 272–273, *277*;
    definition of, 270–271;
    development of, 282–284;
    domain-relevant skills for, 272, *277*;
    evaluation stage of, 276;
    incubation stage of, 276;
    inspiration stage of, 276;
    madness and, 278;
    measurement of, 161;
    versus novelty, 271;
    obstacles to, 284–286;
    personality and, 274–275;
    preparation stage of, 276;
    psychobiology of, 270–278;
    psychology of creative personality, 272–274;
    rewards for, 274;
    stages of creative process, 276–278, *277*;
    and Sternberg's definition of intelligence, 158–159;
    task motivation for, 272, 273, *277*;
    work style and, 272;
    workplace environment for, 283. *See also* Problem solving

"Creativity pill," 276

Creighton, J., 113

CRI. *See* Color Rendering Index (CRI)

Crichton, M., 323

Criminals, 37, 53

Critical nature, as obstacle to creativity, 285

Criticism, constructive, 321

Csikszentmihalyi, M., 279, 286

Cultural differences, in proxemics, 223

Culture, in Big Five, 133

Cunningham, I., 60

Notes

Reader
participation card

The Center for Applied Cognitive Studies continually scans the research literature to find new topics with practical applications. We plan to publish an updated edition of *The Owner's Manual for the Brain* every several years. If you know of Topics you would like to see included in the next edition, or if you know of an Application idea for one of the Topics included in this edition, please list them below and mail or fax them to us for inclusion in the next edition. Of course, we will credit you as the contributor. Items that you send in may also be printed in our quarterly newsletter.

Topics I'd like to see included in the next edition:

_____

_____

_____

Application ideas for Topics in this edition:

Topic number _____ : _____

Topic number _____ : _____

Topic number _____ : _____

Topic number _____ : _____

Topic number _____ : _____

(Add continuation page for additional contributions.)

Other comments:

Fax to 704-331-9408, send to Internet E-mail address centacs@fx.net, or send by regular mail to *Cent*ACS, 719 Romany Road, Charlotte, NC 28203-4849.

Submitted by:

_____
Name

_____
Street address

City	State/Province		Country	Zip code

Phone: Work (____) ____ - _____ Fax (____) ____ - _____ Home (____) ____ - _____

_____
E-mail address

Brain Update:
A quarterly newsletter
for keeping current

The Center for Applied Cognitive Studies publishes *Brain Update*, a quarterly newsletter that uses a format similar to the one in this book. We include Topics that have emerged since this volume was submitted for publication as well as new Application ideas for Topics included in this volume. The contents of these newsletters will eventually be integrated into subsequent editions of this book.

You may subscribe to the *Brain Update* newsletter by mailing a check to CentACS, 719 Romany Road, Charlotte, NC 28203-4849. The annual subscription fee is $45.00.

Sign me up! My check for $45.00 is enclosed.

_____
Name

_____
Street address

_____
City   State/Province   Country   Zip code

Phone: Work (   ) _____ - _____ Fax (   ) _____ - _____ Home (   ) _____ - _____

E-mail address _____

About $Cent$ACS

The Center for Applied Cognitive Studies

The Center for Applied Cognitive Studies is a consulting firm, headquartered in Charlotte, North Carolina, that is dedicated to providing assistance to clients in developing their people and the teams with which they work.

$Cent$ACS continually scans the cognitive science literature—through active library research, computer data base searches, personal correspondence, and participation in professional associations—looking for applications that can be helpful in people development. The results of this research are converted into a variety of usable formats, including:

- Team building
- Retreats
- Executive briefings
- Skill-building workshops
- Informational seminars
- Problem-focused consulting
- Meeting facilitation
- Program design
- Organization development
- Individual coaching and counseling
- A consultant-referral network
- A quarterly newsletter

The quarterly newsletter—*Brain Update*—is designed to provide periodic reports on practical applications of cognitive science research. It serves as an interim communication between editions of *The Owner's Manual for the Brain*.

A special interest of the Center is the Five-Factor Model of personality traits, also called the Big Five model. An evolution of the *Myers-Briggs Type Indicator,* the Five-Factor Model represents the most advanced and comprehensive approach to assessment and discussion of individual differences in personality traits. CentACS predicts that over the next ten years, the Big Five will become the most widely used and accepted trait model for team and individual development. The Center offers a four-day certification program in this model for trainers and consultants. Contact the Center for complete information on Big Five training opportunities.

CentACS' services are available to all segments of the workplace—business, government, education, and not-for-profit organizations. They work with CEOs and entry-level employees, sales and production divisions, teams and individuals, boards and management teams, and entire organizations, both large and small.

From bankers in California to pharmaceutical developers in Connecticut, from auto workers in Michigan to accountants in Florida, from a foundry in Texas to a utility in North Carolina, CentACS goes where the need is.

Order form

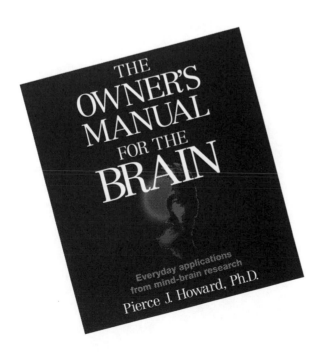